£40.99

Functional Anatomy of the Spine

SECOND EDITION

D1512637

For Elsevier:

Commissioning Editor: Heidi Harrison
Development Editor: Siobhan Campbell
Production Manager: David Fleming
Design: Judith Wright

Functional Anatomy of the Spine

SECOND EDITION

By

Alison Middleditch MCSP

Practice Principal, Surrey Physiotherapy Clinic, Coulsdon, Surrey

Jean Oliver MCSP

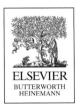

ELSEVIER
BUTTERWORTH
HEINEMANN

EDINBURGH LONDON NEW YORK OXFORD PHILADELPHIA ST LOUIS SYDNEY TORONTO 2005

ELSEVIER

BUTTERWORTH
HEINEMANN

An imprint of Elsevier Limited

© 2005, Elsevier Ltd
First published 1991
Reprinted 2002, (twice), 2004
Second edition 2005

ISBN 0 750 62717 4

British Library Cataloguing in Publication Data
A catalogue record for this book is available from the British Library.

Library of Congress Cataloging in Publication Data
A catalog record for this book is available from the Library of Congress.

Note
Knowledge and best practice in this field are constantly changing. As new research and experience broaden our knowledge, changes in practice, treatment and drug therapy may become necessary or appropriate. Readers are advised to check the most current information provided (i) on procedures featured or (ii) by the manufacturer of each product to be administered, to verify the recommended dose or formula, the method and duration of administration, and contraindications. It is the responsibility of the practitioner, relying on their own experience and knowledge of the patient, to make diagnoses, to determine dosages and the best treatment for each individual patient, and to take all appropriate safety precautions.

To the fullest extent of the law, neither the publisher nor the authors assumes any liability for any injury and/or damage.

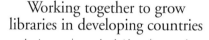
The
Publisher's
policy is to use
**paper manufactured
from sustainable forests**

Printed in China

Contents

Preface

During the last decade there has been much exciting research in the field of mechanical back and neck pain. In response to growing evidence there has been a change in emphasis in the management of patients with back pain so that active rehabilitation programmes are encouraged rather than passive therapeutic interventions. Self-care has become an integral part of the recovery process from back pain and the therapist must have a comprehensive understanding of functional anatomy and biomechanics of the region and the actions and interactions of muscles and fascia to effectively plan treatment strategies with the patient. Additionally, successful management of the patient requires knowledge of the pathophysiology of low back pain, and the effects of age related changes. Despite improvements in investigations and imaging techniques, the majority of patients with back pain do not require surgery or invasive intervention. We hope that this second edition provides necessary scientific information to assist the therapist in clinical decision making during rehabilitation of mechanical spinal pain.

Individuals with back pain often seek to identify the 'one' structure that is responsible for their problem. Mechanical back pain is never due to injury of a single structure because all the tissues of the back are interdependent; a normal healthy spine is reliant on normal function of these interdependent structures of the neuromuscular skeletal system. The different elements of the spine are represented by separate chapters and this has been done for ease of reference; we fully acknowledge that normal function and dysfunction of the spine is based on the integration of all these elements. Indeed, we also acknowledge the importance of psychosocial aspects such as fear and worry and recognise that these factors are significant in the development of chronic pain syndromes.

In this edition we have sought to identify new and relevant literature but at the same time have retained references to early research papers and original literature so that the student can consult papers from which knowledge has been based. We remain indebted to those who continue to research the expanding field of mechanical back and neck pain with such enthusiasm and dedication and have tried to report this research in a way that is relevant to the clinician. As clinicians ourselves, we continue to strive to provide the best possible treatment for our patients; in order to do this we need to be aware of good research and to be prepared to apply this thoughtfully and intelligently. We hope that this second edition will make therapists aware of new developments in the functional anatomy and biomechanics of the spine and go some way towards enabling the clinician to provide effective management of mechanical back and neck pain.

AJM
March, 2005

Preface to first edition

The need for a book on functional anatomy of the whole spine became obvious to us when we ourselves were studying for our diplomas in spinal manipulation. Up-to-date literature on the subject was only to be found by ploughing through books and journals which had to be specially ordered for us. More recently, while teaching spinal mobilization on postregistration physiotherapy courses, we found that the course participants were going through the same time-consuming process. Much excellent research on spinal function has been carried out over the last few decades but, for our purposes, it needed to be brought together in a book that would be directly relevant to therapists involved in assessing and treating spinal dysfunction. This we have attempted to do, and in the process our own approach to the management of spinal disorders has changed considerably.

As research continues, and much exciting and relevant work is still being carried out, for example in the field of adverse mechanical tension in the neuromeningeal structures, we hope to be able to keep this book up-to-date to enable therapists to expand on their knowledge of the anatomy, 'normal' biomechanics and the normal ageing process that occurs in the spine. Only then can we begin to comprehend spinal *dys*function. Inevitably as our understanding increases, the spinal assessments and treatments we carry out on patients will have deeper meaning; techniques can be used logically and can be adapted as necessary to suit the individual patient; advice can be given to the patient in a specific and appropriate way rather than at random. First and foremost, our attention should be directed to the field of prevention of back injuries, starting in schools, as we believe that much suffering and loss of working hours can be avoided.

The examination and treatment of any peripheral joint inevitably includes a consideration of the anatomy of that joint together with its pathological condition. As far as spinal lesions are concerned, however, this has not been general practice, and the tendency to treat solely signs and symptoms without due regard to the clinical diagnosis is fraught with danger. The spine is often regarded as being far too complex to attempt to form a specific diagnosis unless the lesion is overtly apparent, such as a prolapsed intervertebral disc with nerve root involvement. We hope that this text will go some way towards helping therapists form a clinical diagnosis before treating spinal lesions. This saves both patient and therapist time, as treatment is applied intelligently; signs and symptoms are not in any way disregarded but the interpretation of them is clearer. An accurate diagnosis will also prevent over-zealous manipulation of joints in the presence of, for example, instability or vertebral artery disease.

In concentrating on the functional anatomy of the spine, there is no suggestion that it should ever be considered as a separate entity from the remainder of the body. Our difficulty has been in deciding what to exclude from the text rather than what to include. The format of the book has been devised to help the reader use it for reference and study purposes; some repetition is, therefore, inevitable.

We are indebted to all those whose research has helped us to write this book, in particular M. A. Adams PhD; N. Bogduk DipAnat BSc(Hons) MBBS PhD; J. R. Taylor MD PhD and L. T. Twomey BApp Sc(Hons) PhD. Our grateful thanks are also due to P. Dolan PhD, J. P. G. Urban PhD and our colleagues listed below who painstakingly helped us with research or read various chapters and offered constructive advice:

Jack Balfour MCSP
Marilyn Berry MCSP
Sally Cassar MCSP Dip TP
Anna Edwards BSc MCSP Dip TP
Elizabeth Grieve MSc MCSP Dip TP
Anne-Marie Hassenkamp MSc MCSP
Ros Heron MCSP
Raymond Pinder CEng, MI Struct E
Sally Radmore MCSP
Ann Thompson MSc BA MCSP Dip TP

We also express gratitude for the use of the Library and Physiotherapy Department at the Royal National Orthopaedic Hospital, Bolsover Street, London and for the use of Cambridge University Medical Library.

We would also like to thank Jean Horn for her assistance in typing some of the manuscript and Richard Ledwidge, who with much patience and skill produced the fine illustrations which are an essential part of the book. Lastly, we would like to thank our husbands, Peter Oliver and John Middleditch, for their support and encouragement during the undertaking of this project.

July, 1991

Jean Oliver
Alison Middleditch

Chapter **1**

Structure of the vertebral column

CHAPTER CONTENTS

The vertebral column normally consists of 24 separate bony vertebrae (Fig. 1.1), together with 5 fused vertebrae that form the sacrum, and usually 4 fused vertebrae that form the coccyx. It is not unusual for variations to occur, particularly at the lumbosacral junction where the first sacral segment may exist as a separate vertebra. This is known as lumbarization of the first sacral vertebra. Sacralization of the fifth lumbar vertebra is another variant, in which there is complete or incomplete incorporation of the fifth lumbar vertebra into the sacrum. Hemivertebrae and fused vertebrae may also occur (see p. 299).

Figure 1.1 The vertebral column.

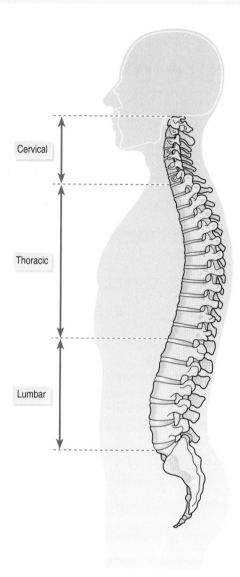

Cervical

Thoracic

Lumbar

The anterior pillar of the spine has weight-bearing and shock-absorbing functions. There is an intervertebral disc between adjacent vertebral bodies, with the exception of the first and second cervical vertebrae. The posterior pillar comprises the apophyseal joints that are formed by the articular facets on the articular processes.

The vertebral column has three principal functions:

- It supports the human in the upright posture
- It allows movement and locomotion
- It protects the spinal cord, cauda equina, meninges and vascular structures.

Humans are the only living creatures that have attained an upright posture in standing and walking. This bipedal posture has developed with certain anatomical changes. The fifth lumbar vertebra, lumbosacral disc and first sacral vertebra are all wedge-shaped with greater thickness anteriorly. Another factor that allows the upright position is the tilt of the sacrum, with its base at an acute angle of 41° to the horizontal (Rickenbacher et al, 1985). Other structural changes include an alteration in the angle of the hip joints as they have turned through 90°, inclination of the femur, torsion of the femur and tibia and development of the foot with its longitudinal arch.

When viewed from the side, the vertebral column displays five curves in the upright posture – two cervical and one each thoracic, lumbar and sacral.

The cervical curves. There are two normally occurring curves in the cervical spine: the upper cervical curve extending from the occiput to the axis, and the longer lordotic curve of the lower cervical spine extending from the axis to the second thoracic vertebra. The lower cervical curve is convex forwards and is the reverse of the upper cervical curve.

The thoracic curve is concave forwards, extending from T2 to T12. The concavity is due to greater depth of the posterior parts of the vertebral bodies in this region. In the upper part there is often a slight lateral curve with the convexity directed to either the right or left.

The lumbar curve is convex forwards and extends from T2 to the lumbosacral junction.

The sacral curve extends from the lumbosacral junction to the coccyx. Its anterior concavity faces downwards and forwards.

The shape of these curves varies in normal spines and it is frequently altered by pathological changes. Kendall et al (1993, pp. 71–103) describe ideal alignment in which, in the lateral view, the line of reference falls:

- Slightly anterior to the lateral malleolus
- Slightly anterior to the axis of the knee joint
- Slightly posterior to the axis of the hip joint
- Through the discs and bodies of the lumbar vertebrae
- Through the shoulder joint
- Through the bodies of the cervical vertebrae
- On the external auditory meatus
- Lightly posterior to the apex of the coronal suture.

Kendall et al (1993, pp. 416–417) also describe the neutral position of the pelvis as being when the anterior superior iliac spines are in the same horizontal plane and the anterior superior iliac spine and pubic symphysis are in the same vertical plane. The anterior superior iliac spines and the posterior superior iliac spines lie in approximately the same plane. However, structural variations of the pelvis make it impractical to use this as a standard postural test.

If the pelvis is in a neutral position the lumbar spine will have a slight anterior curve. When the pelvis is tilted anteriorly the lumbar lordosis is exaggerated, and when the pelvis is in posterior pelvic tilt the lower back is flattened.

In utero, the vertebral column is in total flexion. The upper cervical, thoracic and sacral curves, which are concave anteriorly during fetal life, retain the same curvature after birth and are therefore called *primary curves*.

The lower cervical curve begins to develop in the third month of intrauterine life and is accentuated as the child starts to hold its head upright at 3 months and as it sits upright at 6–9 months. Development of the lumbar curve occurs as the child learns to stand and walk. The lower cervical and lumbar curves are *secondary* or *compensatory curves*. The secondary spinal curves gradually develop during the first three months of life and become established by puberty (Rickenbacher et al, 1985).

The secondary spinal curves have an important function in helping to dissipate vertical compressive forces, thereby providing the spine with a shock-absorbing capacity. If the vertebral column were straight, vertical compressive forces would be transmitted through the vertebral bodies to the intervertebral discs alone. The curves of the spine thus ensure that the ligaments of the spine absorb some of the compressive forces.

Rickenbacher et al (1985) state that any major changes to the spinal curvature that occur are mechanically unsound. Muscle weakness or disease that affects the spinal curves will cause postural defects which lead to faulty biomechanics of the spinal joints and low back pain.

When the column is viewed from the back, a lateral curvature of the spine, termed a *scoliosis*, may be apparent in some individuals. Since lateral flexion of the spine occurs with rotation, scoliosis involves both lateral flexion and rotation. Two broad divisions of scoliosis are recognized: structural and non-structural.

Non-structural curves have no underlying structural abnormality and they can be corrected temporarily with a change of posture or traction. These curves are often reduced or absent in bending forward, or in lying, where the effect of gravity is eliminated. Postural curves are examples of non-structural scoliosis.

When a structural scoliosis is present, there are abnormalities of the vertebrae and ribs. The vertebral bodies are rotated towards the convexity of the curve, while the spinous processes deviate towards the concavity of the curvature. During forward flexion, rib and vertebral rotation occur towards the convexity of the structural curve. In some cases, the deformity may be three-dimensional, consisting of a flexion component in addition to a lateral flexion and rotational abnormality.

Scoliosis is more common in the white than the black population and is found more frequently in females than males with a ratio of 5:1 (Palastanga et al, 1989).

The aetiology of scoliosis is known in some instances but there are also many cases of scoliosis for which there is no known cause. In terms of aetiology and pathology, three classes of curves are recognized:

1. *Congenital* – structural, congenital abnormalities which can be readily identified
2. *Neuromuscular* – following muscular or neurological impairment, e.g. poliomyelitis

3. *Idiopathic* – the term given when the aetiology is unclear. There are four subgroups within this class: primary skeletal, neuromuscular, metabolic and hereditary.

Trabecular systems within the vertebral bodies

During childhood and early adult life the vertebral body has a thin, dense outer shell of cortical bone. This would tend to fail in compression by buckling, and is prevented from doing so by its filling of cancellous bone, the trabeculae of which act as struts, without being excessively heavy.

Approximately 66% of all vertebral bone is cancellous bone and it is arranged in irregular trabeculae 0.12–0.24 mm thick. The orientation of the trabeculae plates is parallel to the lines of stress and there are three main systems of trabeculae: a primary vertical, a secondary oblique and horizontal.

1. *Vertical system.* The vertical trabecular system is present throughout the entire vertebral column. The vertical trabeculae predominate in the anterior two thirds of the vertebral body (Singh, 1978). Within the vertebral body three zones of trabeculae run in a superoinferior direction. In the centre of the body, the trabeculae are vertically arranged, large-diameter cylinders whose walls are formed by thin, solid plates of lamellar bone. Trabeculae are also arranged in a circular pattern around the basivertebral veins. The zones above and below this central zone are directly adjacent to the vertebral end plates. In these areas, the trabeculae are regularly spaced longitudinally and transversely.

The vertical system sustains body weight and principally resists perpendicular compressive forces.

2. *Oblique system.* Four tracts of trabeculae form the oblique system: a superior and inferior tract on each side. The superior system extends from the superior articular process on one side, down through the pedicle to the lower surface of the vertebral body on the opposite side. Likewise, the inferior oblique system runs from the inferior articular processes on one side, up through the pedicle to the upper surface of the vertebral body on the opposite side. Posterior to the articular processes, the oblique systems are continuous with the trabeculae within the spinous process. The oblique systems do not reach the anterior margins on the vertebral body. They resist tension and, together with the vertical system, resist bending and shear.

3. *Horizontal systems.* The trabeculae are arranged horizontally within the transverse processes and pedicles. The trabeculae project into the vertebral body where they intersect in the midline.

There are fewer trabeculae in the anterior, superior and inferior regions of the vertebral bodies and these are, therefore, areas of mechanical weakness, collapse of which is evident in wedge-shaped compression fractures of the vertebral body.

Trabecular loss

Normally, bone mass increases gradually and reaches a peak in the fourth decade. Bone formation and resorption is an ongoing process and initially the formation of new bone occurs at a faster rate than old bone is lost. The peak bone density is significant in determining bone mass in an individual in later years. There is slow, progressive loss in both sexes from the fourth decade at a rate of approximately 0.3% of total bone mass per year. In women the rate of bone loss increases at the time of the menopause to 2–3% per year. The rate of bone loss in women declines 5–8 years after the menopause (Riggs et al, 1986).

Osteoporosis is the name given to bone loss with fracture; this is often confused with the term *osteopenia*, which is used to describe bone loss without fracture. In many texts the term osteoporosis is used to include both definitions (Twomey and Taylor, 1994).

At the age of 65, x-ray evaluation demonstrates that 66.8% of females and 21.5% of males have osteopenia. This increases by 8% for each additional decade in women, although in men the rate does not increase until after the age of 76 (Gitman and Kamholtz, 1965).

Both vertical and horizontal trabeculae are lost with age but it is the reduction in horizontal trabeculae that is particularly significant (Twomey et al, 1983). Atrophy of the trabecular system is resisted principally by the vertical system. In osteoporosis, the secondary systems atrophy first and their disappearance makes the lines of the vertical system stand out more clearly on x-rays. The horizontal trabeculae support the vertical trabeculae by forming 'cross braces' between them. Vertical force on a vertebral body is partly resolved along the cross braces. The loss of horizontal trabeculae will allow buckling of the vertical trabeculae.

Factors that affect bone density include diet, hormonal status, smoking and exercise.

CERVICAL SPINE

The cervical spine is designed for mobility and, under normal circumstances, this is not at the expense of stability. Movements of the head and neck are principally concerned with positioning of the eyes and hence the line of vision; therefore, the upper cervical muscles are highly innervated and enable movements to be made with a high degree of precision (see pp. 110–113).

The neck allows vision through a range of almost 180° in the horizontal plane and up to 120° in the vertical plane (Huelke and Nusholz, 1986). The cervical spine is designed to bear the weight of the head, which is approximately 3 kg. The cervical column also protects the spinal cord and blood vessels that supply the brain.

The cervical spine can be divided morphologically and physiologically into upper and lower segments at the second cervical vertebra. The craniovertebral region consists of the occiput, atlas and axis and forms the primary upper cervical curve. This region controls the head in a neutral position in an upright posture.

If the neck is viewed from the side in the neutral position, it can be seen that the lower cervical curve is longer, but the degree of curvature is greater in the upper cervical spine. In the lower cervical spine the cervical curve is a secondary curve imposed between the primary upper cervical and thoracic curves.

When the neck sustains an acute injury, for example a whiplash injury, the cervical spine loses its normal curvature and characteristically the x-ray view is of a loss or flattening of the normal cervical lordosis. Forces are dissipated less easily in a straight spine and the cervical spine will be subjected to even greater weight-bearing stresses.

Movements of the neck are influenced by the anatomical differences between the upper and lower cervical spine. It is important to note that in the sagittal plane independent movement is possible in the upper or lower cervical spine, and this must be considered when examining or treating the neck. For example, it is possible to extend the upper cervical spine and flex the lower cervical spine simultaneously. Regional and segmental movements of the neck are considered separately on page 186–192.

UPPER CERVICAL SPINE

The atlas

The first and second cervical vertebrae differ in structure from the lower cervical vertebrae.

The atlas (C1) is the first cervical vertebra (Fig. 1.2). It articulates superiorly with the occiput and inferiorly with the axis (C2), the second cervical vertebra.

The atlas differs from all the other vertebrae in that it does not have a body, but consists of two lateral masses that are joined together by an anterior arch and posterior arch.

The anterior arch is curved convexly forward. It becomes slightly thickened and roughened in the midline to form the anterior tubercle. The anterior longitudinal ligament and longus cervicis attach onto the anterior tubercle. On the dorsal surface of the anterior arch there is a facet which articulates with the dens of the axis.

The posterior arch is wider than the anterior arch. It is concave posteriorly and has a tubercle at the apex. The atlas does not have a spinous process, but this is represented by the posterior tubercle, which may be

Figure 1.2   The first cervical vertebra or atlas – superior aspect.

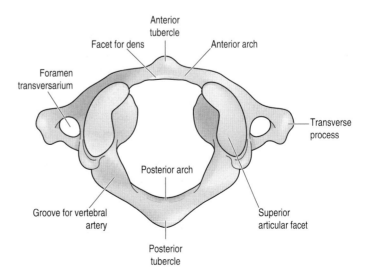

Anterior tubercle

Facet for dens

Anterior arch

Foramen transversarium

Transverse process

Posterior arch

Groove for vertebral artery

Superior articular facet

Posterior tubercle

palpated in some subjects (see p. 22). The nuchal ligament and rectus capitis posterior minor attach onto the posterior tubercle.

The lateral masses are directed forwards and medially. On the superior surface of each lateral mass is a concave facet that articulates with the corresponding occipital condyle. The facets are kidney-shaped and their lateral margins are higher than the medial margins. The orientation of these facets and their high margins ensure that movement at the atlanto-occipital joint is mainly flexion and extension. The orientation of the facets and depth of articular surface do not allow much rotation and lateral flexion to occur. The configuration of these facets means that if a large axial compressive force is applied the lateral masses are forced apart, fracturing the thinner anterior and posterior arches (Jefferson fracture). A prominent tubercle is attached to the medial side of the facets and provides attachment for the important transverse ligament of the atlas (see p. 13).

Posterior to each lateral mass is a groove in the posterior arch in which the vertebral artery and first cervical nerves are found. The vertebral artery is particularly susceptible to trauma at this point (see p. 162).

A study in which left–right asymmetries of the atlas were identified (Van Roy et al, 1997) demonstrated left–right asymmetries of the posterior arch of the atlas in 53 of 82 specimens. Variations observed included alteration in depth or width in the groove for the vertebral artery. In some vertebrae the groove was converted into a foramen by a thin plate of bone superiorly. The laminae also varied in shape and size and the posterior tubercle was observed to vary from a poorly developed spine to a large tubercle. In some vertebrae the posterior tubercle was absent.

Left–right asymmetries of the transverse processes were also observed and in many cases were due to differences in the size of the transverse foramen. The high number of asymmetries of the transverse foramina and grooves for the vertebral artery indicate the considerable variation in bony passage for the vertebral artery, surrounding veins and the C1 nerve.

Articular tropism of the superior zygapophyseal facets was also noted. Some of the superior zygapophyseal facets of the atlas were orientated mainly in a horizontal plane, showing poor curvature. Other facets had a more definitive curvature. Tropism of the joints was due to differences in shape, surface area and size. The inferior facets also demonstrated tropism with differences in size and surface area. Unlike the superior facets, tropism of the inferior facets was noted to be consistent in many instances with degenerative changes that had caused osteophytes and enlargement.

Van Roy et al (1997) comment that, apart from developmental failure and degenerative changes, there were no obvious explanations for the asymmetries observed. They hypothesize that many factors may influence the ultimate morphology of the vertebrae. These include genetic considerations, developmental aspects, left–right asymmetries of surrounding anatomical structures, asymmetrical loading of the cervical spine, postural positions and repetitive minor strains.

Furthermore, the authors raise the question as to whether asymmetrical facet joints lead to asymmetrical movement in the individual motion segment affected. Pearcy (1985) demonstrated that coupled motion in a specific intervertebral motion segment has to be differentiated from the global coupled motion in a specific region of the spine, which results from the cumulative motion in the constituent intervertebral motion segments. In vivo studies using 3D kinematic analysis and medical imaging techniques offer the possibility of linking abnormal motion to facet tropism.

The axis

The axis (Fig. 1.3) provides a pivot around which the atlas and head rotate. A vertical pillar of bone projects upwards from the superior surface of the body of the axis. This is the dens (odontoid process), approximately 1.5 cm long; its tip is pointed and provides attachment for the apical ligament. On either side of the apex, the dens is flattened where the alar ligaments attach.

The dens is narrower at its base, where it is grooved by the transverse ligament of the atlas. On the anterior surface of the dens is an oval

Figure 1.3   The second cervical vertebra or axis. A, Posterolateral aspect. B, Lateral aspect.

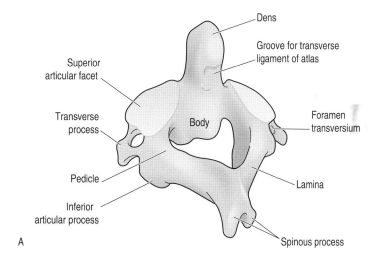

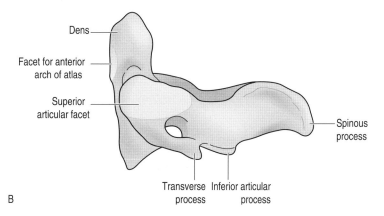

articular facet which articulates with a similar facet on the back of the anterior arch of the atlas. The bone of the dens is more compact than that of the body of the axis.

Large oval facets on either side at the base of the dens extend laterally over the body of the axis and the pedicles and articulate with the inferior facets of the atlas. As the superior facets of the axis are somewhat anterior to the inferior facets of the axis, they do not form part of the articular pillar in the cervical spine.

At the junction of the pedicles and laminae, the inferior facets of the axis face downwards and forwards as in a typical cervical vertebra. The pedicles of the axis are stout. The laminae are thicker than in any other vertebra and provide attachment for ligamenta flava.

The spinous process of the axis is large, usually bifid, and normally provides a prominent bony landmark for palpation. The suboccipital muscles attach onto the spinous process of the axis, which provides powerful leverage for the muscles' actions. Small transverse processes, which are much smaller than those of C1, have a single tubercle at their tip, and project laterally from the axis.

The foramina transversaria face superolaterally; this allows the vertebral arteries to pass upwards and laterally to the foramina of the atlas which are placed a little more laterally. The vertebral arteries are most prone to damage at the atlanto-axial joints (see p. 165).

Craniovertebral joints

Atlanto–occipital joints (Figs 1.4, 1.5).   These joints are formed by the articulation of the concave articular facets on the lateral masses of the atlas with the convex facets on the occipital condyles. The presence of articular tropism of the superior articular facets of the atlas will result in these being asymmetrical.

The lateral edges of the facets on the atlas are high and tend to restrict movements except those that occur in the sagittal plane.

Atlanto–axial joints (Figs 1.4, 1.5).   The atlanto-axial articulation comprises three synovial joints:

1. One central atlanto-odontoid joint
2. Two lateral atlanto-axial joints.

The atlanto-odontoid joint (median atlanto-axial joint). This is a pivot joint, comprising:

1. The articulation of the facet on the anterior surface of the odontoid with the reciprocally-shaped facet on the posterior arch of the atlas, and
2. A synovial cavity between the posterior arch of the odontoid and the cartilage-lined anterior surface of the transverse ligament of the axis.

As this joint consists of two articulations, it may be termed a 'double joint'. The stability of the atlanto-axial joint depends on the integrity of the transverse ligament, which holds the dens in place. The dens forms a pivot around which the atlas can rotate.

Figure 1.4   The atlanto-occipital and atlanto-axial joints. A, Posterior aspect. B, Anterior aspect. (Adapted from Williams P L, Warwick R 1980 *Gray's Anatomy*, 36th edn. Churchill Livingstone, Edinburgh, pp. 447, 448.)

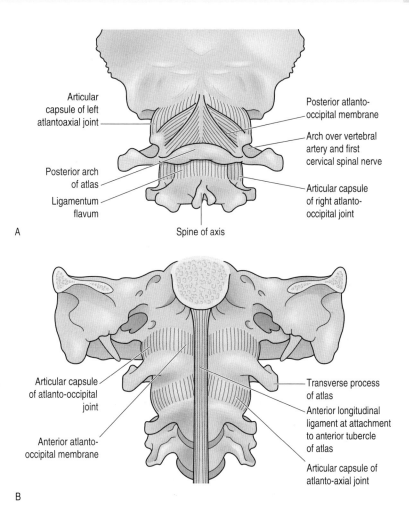

Figure 1.5   The atlanto-axial joints and atlanto-occipital joints. (Adapted from Williams PL, Warwick R 1980 *Gray's Anatomy*, 36th edn. Churchill Livingstone, Edinburgh, p. 449.)

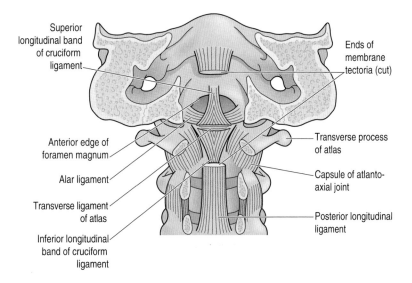

The lateral atlanto-axial joints. These bilateral joints have been described as plane joints as they are flat in the coronal plane. However, the articular surfaces are convex in the sagittal plane making the joints incongruous. The articular surfaces are covered with hyaline cartilage that is thicker centrally and thinner at the periphery. In elderly subjects, these surfaces are often well preserved (Twomey and Taylor, 1994). The facets lie at approximately 110° to the vertical.

The atlanto-axial joints have triangular-shaped meniscoid inclusions. The base of these meniscoids is attached to the inner surface of the fibrous capsule and their inner surfaces are lined with synovial membrane. The meniscoids are fat filled and have a good vascular supply in the young. Although they become fibrofatty in older subjects they normally maintain a good blood supply. During movements the meniscoids move and change shape in younger subjects but in older individuals they are stiffer and move less. These meniscoids are frequently injured during flexion/extension injuries.

Craniovertebral ligaments

Stability of the craniovertebral region is dependent upon the integrity of the ligaments of the upper cervical spine, and this is an important consideration when examining or treating the upper cervical spine.

From anterior to posterior, the ligaments of the region are:

1. The *anterior atlanto-occipital membrane* (see Fig. 1.4). This connects the foramen magnum above to the arch of the atlas below, and is continuous with the anterior longitudinal ligament. It overlies the capsules of the atlanto-occipital joints laterally.

2. The *apical ligament* (see Fig. 1.9, p.17). This is short and finer than the alar ligaments and attaches the tip of the dens to the anterior margin of the foramen magnum.

3. The two *alar ligaments* (Figs 1.5, 1.6). These are symmetrically placed, arising from the posterior part of the tip of the dens. The greater portion of the fibres insert onto the occipital condyles, while some fibres attach onto the lateral masses of the atlas. Rotation to the right is limited by the left alar ligament and vice versa, while the ipsilateral ligament is relaxed. During rotation, the inferior part of the ligament is stretched initially, but with increasing rotation, the load is transferred to the superior fibres.

During lateral flexion, the occipital part of the alar ligament on the same side is relaxed while the atlantal portion is stretched. The atlas moves in the same direction as the lateral flexion, but it does not rotate. As lateral flexion increases, the contralateral occipital portion of the ligament is stretched. The stretched occipital ligament on one side and the atlantal attachment on the opposite side induce rotation of the axis in the direction of the lateral flexion, so that the spinous process of the axis moves contralaterally (Dvorak and Panjabi, 1987).

If the suboccipital muscles are relaxed, flexion of the cervical spine is limited by the membrane tectoria, the longitudinal fibres of the cruciform ligament and the transverse ligament. The alar ligaments will resist flexion if these ligaments are ruptured.

Figure 1.6 Coronal aspect of alar ligaments.

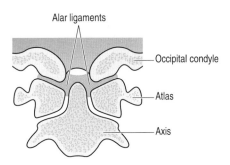

Alar ligaments

Occipital condyle

Atlas

Axis

Damage of the alar ligaments by impact trauma or inflammatory disease can result in increased axial rotation between the occiput and the atlas, and the atlas and axis. Excessive rotation may reduce blood flow in the vertebral artery (Fielding, 1957). There may also be increased lateral displacement between the atlas and axis during lateral flexion.

These ligaments are composed of collagen fibres, have a limited extensibility, and are most vulnerable when the head is rotated and additionally flexed, as in a rear collision whiplash injury. Following such injury, the transverse ligament of the atlas may remain intact even if one of the alar ligaments is ruptured.

4. The *transverse ligament of the atlas* (see Fig. 1.5). This is a thick band which holds the odontoid in place and passes between the tubercles on the medial side of the lateral masses of the atlas. The ligament is thicker centrally, where some fibres extend up to the occiput and others pass downwards to the body of the axis. The whole ligament is in the shape of a cross and is termed the *cruciform ligament of the atlas* (see Fig. 1.5). If the ligament is damaged by degenerative changes or traumatic tearing, the stability of the region is compromised, and the dens may impinge upon the spinal cord.

5. The *accessory atlanto-axial ligaments*. These pass upwards and laterally from the base of the dens to the inferomedial aspect of the lateral masses of the atlas.

6. The *membrane tectoria* (see Fig. 1.5). Connecting the posterior surface of the body of the axis to the basiocciput, the membrane tectoria is a prolongation of the posterior longitudinal ligament.

7. The *posterior atlanto-occipital membrane* (see Fig. 1.4). This connects the foramen magnum above with the posterior arch of the atlas below, and is continuous with the joint capsules laterally. It represents ligamentum flavum in this region of the spine, and forms a channel for the vertebral artery and first cervical nerve to run between itself and the groove on the posterior arch of the atlas.

8. The *lateral atlanto-occipital ligaments*. Reinforcing the capsules of the atlanto-occipital joints, the lateral atlanto-occipital ligaments pass

between the jugular processes of the occiput and lateral mass of the atlas on each side.

9. The *fibrous capsules* (see Fig. 1.4) of the craniovertebral joints. These are thin and baggy whereas those of the atlanto-axial joints are looser and permit relatively free movement to occur.

UPPER CERVICAL INSTABILITY

Instability of the upper cervical spine can be considered to be present when there is a loss of motion segment stiffness so that when a linear force is applied to the motion segment there is greater displacement than would be seen in a normal segment. This displacement may give rise to local or peripheral pain or other symptoms such as paraesthesiae and can put the neurological structures at risk.

The atlanto-dens interval (ADI) is the distance between the most anterior point of the dens and the posterior aspect of the arch of the atlas. The ADI is measured in flexion, extension and neutral position. In adults a normal ADI would be 2.5–3 mm and in children a normal ADI would be 4.5–5 mm. If the ADI is greater than these figures then a radiological diagnosis of instability may be made.

Instability in the upper cervical spine can result from trauma such as a whiplash accident (*ligamentous instability*), or it may be due to osteoarthrotic changes in the upper cervical spine (*arthrotic instability*). In the presence of a complete ligamentous tear there may be excessive movement and a soft, yielding end-feel. When the excessive motion has a hard, unyielding end-feel the intra-articular deterioration may be producing arthrotic instability (Pettman, 1994).

Other factors may also cause instability:

Congenital
- The body of the dens is too short to be restrained by the transverse ligament of the atlas
- Os odontoideum – the dens does not fuse with the body of the axis
- Congenital absence of the dens
- Underdeveloped dens

Pathological
- Osteoporosis of the dens
- Old undisplaced fracture of the dens

Inherited conditions
- Inherited collagen deficiency, e.g. Ehlers–Danlos syndrome where there is excessive laxity of collagenous tissues which may include the upper cervical ligaments
- Congenital laxity of the transverse ligament, e.g. Down's syndrome

> *Inflammatory conditions*
> - Inflammatory conditions such as rheumatoid arthritis or ankylosing spondylitis
> - Infections such as tonsillitis, dental caries, influenza and rheumatoid fever

Clinical instability can be difficult to identify. A number of clinical tests are used to test the integrity of the upper cervical spine but there is little evidence at present that clinical tests are sufficiently sensitive to detect minor instabilities that may be present in some individuals. Active movements of the head create angular motions in the cervical spine and create changes in the length of the vertebral artery. Linear tests do not normally affect the length of the vertebral artery but can cause transectory occlusion if excessive intersegmental linear motion is present (Pettman, 1994).

LOWER CERVICAL SPINE C3–7

The 3rd to 7th cervical vertebrae are similar in structure. Together with the craniovertebral region, this region allows movements and positioning of the head. Below the 2nd and subsequent cervical vertebrae are intervertebral discs between adjacent vertebrae. These discs contribute to more than one quarter of the length of the cervical column and are a factor in allowing considerable movement of the neck.

STRUCTURE OF A TYPICAL CERVICAL VERTEBRA
(Figs 1.7, 1.8)

Vertebral body

A typical cervical vertebra is composed of an anterior body and a posterior arch. The cervical vertebrae have the smallest bodies and the largest vertebral foramina of the vertebral column.

The vertebral body is roughly cylindrical; the superior surface is concave transversely and convex anteroposteriorly and on each side are prominent elevations known as the *uncinate (unciform) processes*. The inferior surface is reciprocally convex transversely and concave anteroposteriorly. Two articular facets on the inferior surface of the body articulate with the uncinate processes of the subjacent vertebra. These articulations are known as the *uncovertebral joints* or the *joints of Luschka*.

Considerable flexion and extension are possible in this region due to the convexity and concavity of the vertebral body, but lateral flexion is partially restricted by the uncinate processes.

The anterior surface of the vertebral body is convex transversely. At the superior and inferior margins it is marked by the fibres of the anterior longitudinal ligament. The posterior surface of the body is flattened and has foramina for two or more basivertebral veins.

Figure 1.7   A typical cervical vertebra – superior aspect.

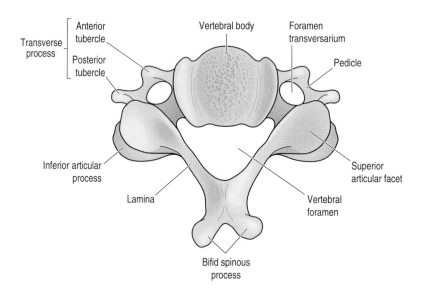

Figure 1.8   A typical cervical vertebra – anterior aspect.

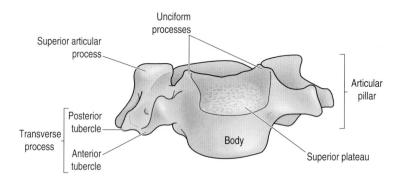

Posterior arch

The posterior arch is formed by the pedicles, articular processes, laminae and spinous processes.

The *pedicles* are short and thick, projecting backwards and slightly laterally from the vertebral body.

The *articular processes*. At the junction of the pedicles and laminae there are superior and inferior articular processes which form an *articular pillar*. The articular pillar is weight-bearing during axial loading. These articular processes contain the *articular facets*. The *superior* facets are oval, flat and face backwards and upwards, while the *inferior* facets correspondingly face forwards and downwards. The articular pillars of C3, 4 and 5 may be grooved anterolaterally by the dorsal rami of the cervical spinal nerves.

The *laminae* are long and thin, extending backwards and medially from the pedicles to meet in the midline, thereby completing the posterior arch.

The *spinous processes* project backwards from the junction of the laminae; they are short, bifid and often unequal in size (see Palpation, p. 22). The spinous process of C7 is long and thin and the C7 vertebra is called the *vertebra prominens*.

The *vertebral foramen* is bounded by the vertebral body anteriorly, the pedicles laterally and the laminae laterally and posteriorly. In the cervical spine, the foramen is comparatively large and triangular. It is occupied by the spinal cord, meninges and associated vessels.

The *transverse processes* arise from two roots. Anteriorly, they arise from the vertebral body and posteriorly from the articular processes. They project anterolaterally and are at an angle of 45° to the vertical. Laterally, the transverse processes are bifid, with anterior and posterior tubercles that give attachment to the scalene muscles. The *carotid tubercle* is the anterior tubercle of the 6th cervical vertebra. It is very large and is immediately posterior to the carotid artery, which can be compressed at this point. The transverse process contains the *foramen transversarium* in which lie the vertebral artery, venous and sympathetic plexuses. The medial section of the posterior root of the transverse process is homologous with a true transverse process, as in a thoracic vertebra. The rest of the transverse process constitutes the homologue of a rib.

LIGAMENTS OF THE LOWER CERVICAL SPINE

The *anterior longitudinal ligament* (Fig. 1.9) is a strong band which lies anterior to the vertebral body. It is attached to the basilar part of the occipital bone, from which it extends to the tubercle of the atlas and then attaches to the front of the vertebral bodies.

Figure 1.9   Additional ligaments of the cervical spine. Sectional lateral aspect of the upper three segments.

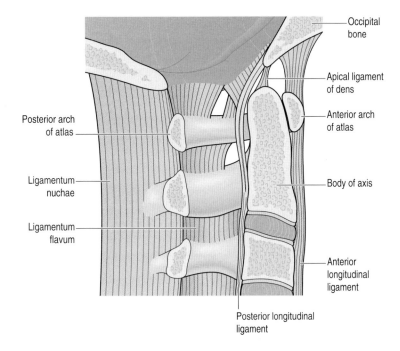

Occipital bone

Apical ligament of dens

Anterior arch of atlas

Posterior arch of atlas

Body of axis

Ligamentum nuchae

Ligamentum flavum

Anterior longitudinal ligament

Posterior longitudinal ligament

It consists of several layers of fibres fixed to the superior and inferior margins of the vertebral bodies and the intervertebral disc. The superficial fibres are long and extend over three or four vertebrae; the middle fibres extend over two or three vertebrae, while the deepest fibres are attached to the adjacent vertebrae.

The ligament is thicker and narrower opposite the vertebral bodies, and thinner opposite the intervertebral discs. It is relaxed in flexion and taut in extension.

The *posterior longitudinal ligament* is posterior to the vertebral body, lies inside the vertebral canal, and is attached to the body of the axis and then to the margins of the vertebral bodies and intervertebral discs. It consists of superficial fibres extending over three or four vertebrae and deep fibres which extend between adjacent vertebrae. This ligament is broad and uniform in width in the cervical spine. It is stretched during neck flexion and relaxed in extension.

The *articular capsules* of the apophyseal joints are attached to the margins of the articular facets. They are loose in the cervical spine and, therefore, allow considerable mobility.

The *ligamenta flava* are predominantly yellow elastic tissue and connect the laminae of the adjacent vertebrae. These ligaments, which are broad and long in the neck, allow flexion to occur, but prevent hyperflexion by braking the movement so that the end of range is not reached abruptly.

The *ligamentum nuchae* is a fibroelastic membrane which extends from the external occipital protuberance and external occipital crest to the spine of all the cervical vertebrae. It is homologous with the supraspinous and interspinous ligaments in the thoracic and lumbar spines, but is stronger than in other parts of the column. The ligament forms a septum for the attachment of the trapezius and splenius muscles, and it contributes to the stability of the head and neck with its strong fibres which are of particular importance in flexion/acceleration injuries. If an applied force is sufficient to tear the ligamentum nuchae, there is likely to be even greater damage to the intrinsic structures.

The *interspinous* ligaments are rudimentary in the cervical spine and connect adjoining spinous processes.

The *intertransverse ligaments* connect adjacent transverse processes. They are irregular in the cervical spine and are reinforced by the intertransverse muscles.

JOINTS BETWEEN TYPICAL CERVICAL VERTEBRAE

Three different types of joints link adjacent cervical vertebrae:

Interbody joints
(Fig. 1.10)

- Interbody joints
- Apophyseal joints
- Uncovertebral joints.

Below C2, adjacent cervical vertebrae are linked by an intervertebral disc at the interbody joint which is termed a *symphysis*. The discs allow and restrain movement and in the cervical region they allow considerable mobility. The joints between the vertebral bodies and discs are sad-

Figure 1.10   Apophyseal joint.
A, Posterolateral aspect of
typical cervical vertebra. B,
Anterolateral aspect of cervical
interbody joint and
uncovertable joints.

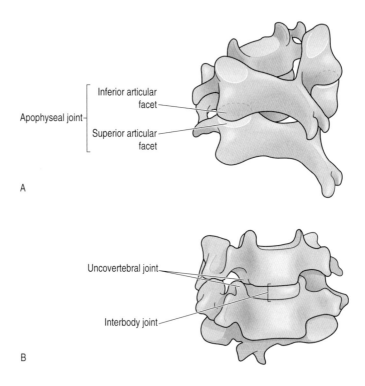

dle articulations; they are concave in the frontal and convex in the sagittal plane. They are reinforced anteriorly by the anterior longitudinal ligament and posteriorly by the posterior longitudinal ligament.

Apophyseal joints
(see Fig. 1.10)

The paired cervical apophyseal joints are plane joints formed by the articulation of the inferior facets of one cervical vertebra with the superior facets of the subjacent vertebra. Direction and range of movement at these joints is determined by the orientation of the articular facets. The inferior facets of a typical vertebra face forwards and downwards, articulating with the superior facets of the vertebra below, which face upwards and backwards. These joints allow flexion, extension, rotation and lateral flexion to occur (see pp. 188–192). The facet planes lie at approximately 45° to the vertical; the upper joints are more horizontally placed, lying at approximately 55° to the vertical, while the facet planes of the lower joints lie at approximately 25° to the vertical.

The joint surfaces are reciprocally concave and convex. Articular cartilage lines the apophyseal joints and is subjected to weight-bearing stresses as the apophyseal joints share the weight of the head with the vertebral bodies and discs. Degenerative changes at the cervical apophyseal joints are very common due to their weight-bearing function.

The lateral joint capsule is lax. It is fibrous and continuous with ligamentum flavum anteriorly but the posterior capsule is very thin, particularly where the fat pad at the inferior posterior joint margin is enclosed by the deep cervical muscles (Twomey and Taylor, 1994).

The loose capsules have a degree of elasticity, thereby allowing the large range of sagittal and axial rotation in this area. Apophyseal joint capsules are highly innervated and may, therefore, be a primary source of pain.

The uncovertebral joints (joints of Luschka)

In a child, the cervical intervertebral disc does not extend the transverse width of the vertebral body. Uncinate processes grow upwards from the superior, lateral borders of the vertebral bodies of C3–6. They project into the loose vascular fibrous tissue at the outer margins of the annulus (Kramer, 1981) and correspond with reciprocally-shaped cavities on the lower border of the vertebra above. The joints become apparent in the first or second decade of life, but can be seen microscopically much earlier (Hirsch et al, 1967).

By the age of 8, each uncus has grown to form a kind of adventitious joint called the uncovertebral joint. Opinion is divided as to whether these structures are joints or pseudoarthroses. They have been described as synovial articulations (von Luschka, 1858; Boreadis and Gershon Cohen, 1956), while others believe that they are a degenerative phenomenon (Hadley, 1957; Orofino et al, 1960; Hirsch et al, 1967).

The joints are lined by fibrocartilage that probably derives from the outer annulus. These clefts are bound medially by the intervertebral disc and posterolaterally by an extension of the annulus.

The clinical significance of these structures is in their tendency to develop marked degenerative changes and form bony exostoses which may impinge the vertebral artery, cervical nerve roots or the anterior part of the spinal cord (Clark, 1988).

During flexion and extension, gliding movements occur at these joints and this concentrates the plane of shear to a horizontal band within the annulus, between the uncovertebral joints. It is this shearing which is thought to cause the horizontal fissuring across the posterior annulus.

MENISCOID INCLUSIONS

Three types of intra-articular incisions have been identified in the cervical synovial joints. Each joint has at least one type of structure.

Intra-articular fat pads are formed of adipose tissue with some connective tissue and blood vessels. Fat pads are attached to the joint capsules and are at the periphery of the articular cartilage, remaining outside the joint space. They are most commonly found at the atlanto-occipital joints and rarely occur in the lower cervical apophyseal joints. They are considered to be mobile space fillers. In the neutral position the fat pads fill the non-articular parts of the joint and move during motion.

Fibroadipose meniscoids occur throughout the cervical apophyseal joints except at the atlanto-occipital joint. The base of each meniscoid is attached to the joint capsule, while the other end protrudes into the joint space for varying distances from 2 to 5 mm (Mercer, 1994). The free end of these meniscoids is mobile and moves over the articular surfaces. In the apophyseal joints the fibroadipose meniscoids occur at the ventrolateral and dorsomedial poles. They are covered with synovial membrane and lie along the axes of motion. Their function is to protect cartilage that is exposed during motion by maintaining a film of synovial fluid between themselves and the cartilage (Mercer, 1994).

Capsular rims are wedge-shaped structures at the margins of the articular surfaces. They do not enter the joint space, but occupy the space between the joint capsule and the facet margin. They occur most frequently at the atlanto-occipital joints. In the lower cervical apophyseal joints, when capsular rims and fibroadipose meniscoids are present they are often continuous at the anterior and posterior poles. They fill the space around the margins of the joint and assist in force dissipation.

Clinical implications

The role of the cervical intra-articular inclusions in cervical pathology is speculative. Imaging techniques are not yet sophisticated enough to show the structures in vivo.

It has been suggested that the inclusions may have a role in joint stiffness and the acute locked neck. When a knee is immobilized, the adipose tissue of the intra-articular fat poles proliferates. These changes could also occur in the cervical spine, where the fat pads may provide a source of proliferation of fatty tissue if the neck is immobilized.

The fibroadipose meniscoids may be the structure from which fibrous tissue develops to form adhesions. These could occur after trauma such as a whiplash injury when there is intra-articular hemorrhage and capsular tears.

The intra-articular inclusions have been implicated in the acute locked joint. During lateral flexion and rotation to one side the inferior articular facet of the apophyseal joint on the contralateral side glides superiorly and anteriorly, taking with it the fibroadipose meniscoid. The capsule becomes stretched because it is attached to the meniscoid. On the return movement, if the meniscoid becomes deflected on the articular margin it folds, increasing tension on the joint capsule and resulting in pain and muscle spasm (Bogduk and Jull, 1985).

CERVICAL INTERVERTEBRAL DISCS

The cervical discs differ in structure to the lumbar discs in that they are smaller and the nucleus pulposus is less distinct from the annulus fibrosus. Even in young children the cervical nucleus has higher fibrocartilage content and is tightly enclosed by fibrous and cartilaginous tissue. The proteoglycan content of the cervical discs is also lower and hence they have lower water content than the lumbar discs. In adolescence, cervical discs bear less axial loading than lumbar discs.

Horizontal fissuring occurs across the posterior annulus between the uncinate processes. In the adult, the horizontal fissures may extend through the posterior half of the disc so that the disc becomes bipartite with a 'gliding' joint between the upper and lower parts that allows several millimetres of forward or backward translation during flexion and extension. When the disc becomes bipartite the posterior longitudinal ligament, anterior annulus and anterior longitudinal ligament normally remain intact.

In the lumbar spine the discs tend to prolapse posterolaterally. Posterolateral disc herniations in the cervical disc are rare; degenerative changes produce a posterior bar-like bulge, which may compromise the central vertebral canal.

PALPATION OF THE CERVICAL SPINE (Figs 1.11, 1.12)

Palpation is an essential part of a patient assessment. Considerable differences may be felt between individuals. This may be due to congenital anomalies or occur as a result of degenerative changes. People with even minor degenerative changes may develop tightening of the overlying tissues, which makes palpation difficult.

When palpating the soft tissues, an alteration in skin temperature or sweating may be noted. In addition there may be thickening, tightness, nodules, swelling or muscle spasm that can be detected by careful palpation.

In the cervical spine the following bony points may be palpated:

- Posterior tubercle of the atlas
- Posterolateral arch of the atlas
- Transverse process of the atlas

Figure 1.11   Palpation points in the cervical spine – posterior aspect.

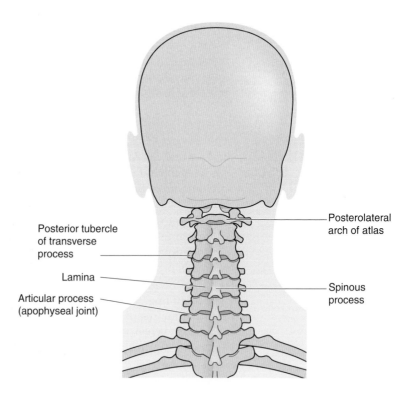

Posterior tubercle of transverse process

Lamina

Articular process (apophyseal joint)

Posterolateral arch of atlas

Spinous process

- Spinous processes C2–7
- Laminae C2–7
- Articular pillar/processes C2–7
- Transverse processes C1–7
- Superior and posterior border of the first rib

Most of the bony landmarks may be easily palpated with the subject in prone-lying with the forehead supported.

The surface mark of the *posterior tubercle* of the atlas (C1) is in the soft tissue sulcus between the base of the occiput and the large spinous process of C2. This is not palpable in everyone, but in many people the bony tubercle may be identified.

The *posterolateral arches* of the atlas can be palpated just below the base of the occiput on either side.

Between the angle of the jaw and the mastoid process, the lateral tip of the *transverse process* of the atlas can be palpated. The tip of the transverse process is frequently tender to even gentle palpation. In some individuals, it is easier to palpate the transverse process if the head is placed in slight extension. It may be best palpated with the person in side-lying.

The *spinous process* of C2 is large and is felt as the first prominent bony landmark below the base of the occiput. The spinous process of C3 is smaller and tucked under the larger process of C2, while those of C4 and 5 are slightly larger. Palpation of the spinous process of C3 is often difficult as it is tucked under the larger process of C2; it may be easier to feel

Figure 1.12   Palpation points in the cervical spine – anterolateral aspect.

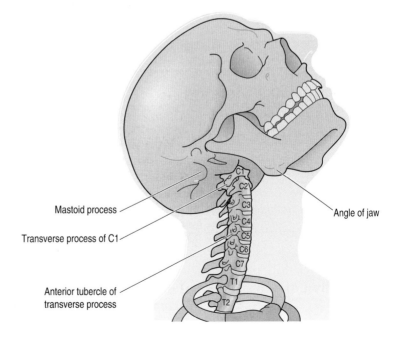

Mastoid process

Transverse process of C1

Anterior tubercle of transverse process

Angle of jaw

C1
C2
C3
C4
C5
C6
C7
T1
T2

if the direction of the palpating thumb is angled slightly cranially as well as anteriorly. The spinous processes of C3–5 are usually bifid and may feel asymmetrical on palpation.

The spinous processes of C6 and 7 are not usually bifid and that of C7 is particularly prominent, being known as *vertebra prominens*. In order to differentiate between C6 and 7, both spinous processes are palpated, the person is asked to extend the neck and the process of C7 remains palpable while that of C6 glides away. The tips of the spinous processes of C2–6 are at the level of the inferior articular facet. Hence, the spinous process of C5 is at the same level as the inferior margin of the C5/6 apophyseal joint.

Deeper and lateral to the spinous process, the *laminae* may be palpated on either side. Palpation of the laminae may give a good indication of symmetry of the vertebra if the spinous process is asymmetrically bifid.

The posterior surface of the inferior *articular processes* of C2–7 may be palpated bilaterally 2–3 cm from the midline. The processes of C2–4 are easier to find than those of the lower cervical spine. Because the lateral atlanto-axial joints lie anterior to the articular pillar, they are easier to palpate anteriorly.

In supine-lying, the anterior aspect of the *transverse processes* can be palpated and it may be necessary to lift the musculature gently to one side in order to make bony contact. This palpation must be performed with great care, as it is frequently uncomfortable and may produce neck and arm pain in a normal spine. In the long, slim-necked person, it has been reported (Grieve, 1986) that it is possible to palpate from C1 to T3.

The superior surface of the *first rib* may be palpated with the bulk of the upper fibres of trapezius gently lifted out of the way. The first rib curves anteriorly after its articulation at the costotransverse joint of T1 and it can therefore be palpated with greater ease close to the spine. The posterior border of the first rib can be palpated in prone-lying. The costotransverse joint of T1 is palpated, and the rib can be felt lateral to the articulation.

CERVICO-THORACIC JUNCTION

At the cervico-thoracic junction, where the relatively mobile lower cervical spine articulates with the stiff thoracic spine, the intervertebral discs and apophyseal joints are particularly subject to stress and strain. Degenerative changes commonly occur at C6/7 and C7/T1 segments. In cervical spondylosis, the spinous processes of C7 and T1 may become unduly prominent with an overlying fatty tissue pad. These spinous processes are often tender to palpation, and the characteristic stiffness that develops is frequently the source of pain in this area.

CERVICAL RIBS

Cervical ribs are the most common bony anomaly associated with the cervico-thoracic region. Although cervical ribs have been reported as high as C4, they most frequently originate from the body and transverse process of the seventh cervical vertebra (Brain et al., 1967). A true cervical rib has a head and neck, articulating with the transverse process and body of a cervical vertebra in a similar fashion to the articulation of a true rib with a thoracic vertebra. Cervical ribs may be long or short, unilateral or bilateral, symmetrical or asymmetrical. Soft tissue and nervous tissue anomalies are often associated with cervical ribs, e.g. supernumerary fascial bands, anomalies of the scalene muscles, or a pre- or post-fixed brachial plexus.

THORACIC OUTLET (OR INLET)

As the neurovascular bundle passes from the thorax into the upper extremity, it courses through the thoracic outlet. The thorax outlet can be likened to a series of tunnels made up of bones and muscles. The nerves and blood vessels may be compromised in their pathway through these tunnels (Edgelow, 1997). Narrowing or stenosis of the tunnels may be due to congenital factors or secondary to trauma.

Bones

The bony boundaries of the thoracic outlet consist of the clavicle anteriorly, the scapula posteriorly, the cervical vertebrae and discs medially and the glenohumeral joint laterally. The first to fifth ribs make up the floor of the thoracic outlet. In this area the brachial plexus is susceptible to compression or trauma from bony anomalies such as a large first rib, the presence of a cervical rib, the length of the clavicle, or a large transverse process of C7.

Hypertrophy or degenerative changes may also reduce the size of these tunnels and compromise the neural pathway. Examples include callus formation following a fracture of the clavicle or first rib. The neurovascular bundle passes under the coracoid process and may be stretched or compromised in an arthritic glenohumeral joint, particularly when the arm is taken into hyperabduction and lateral rotation.

Changes in the angulation of the clavicle or first rib may reduce the size of the costoclavicular interval through which the neurovascular bundle passes. Postural changes and dysfunctional breathing patterns are common causes of alteration of this space.

Muscles

There are two soft tissue tunnels. The first tunnel is formed by the middle and anterior scalene muscles which arise from the transverse processes of the cervical vertebrae and attach onto the first rib. The subclavian artery and lower portions of the brachial plexus pass through this triangle-shaped space. The pectoralis minor muscle, which arises from the third, fourth and fifth ribs, attaches onto the coracoid process of the scapula. This forms the second muscular tunnel.

The size of these tunnels can be reduced by anomalous insertions of the muscles, additional muscle fascicles, extra fascial strips or bands, and spasm or shortening of the muscles or fascia.

The cervical fascia is continuous with the axillary sheath that encases the neurovascular bundle. Post-traumatic scarring occurs in the deep cervical fascia and it is thought that scarring in one area of a tissue may reduce mobility throughout the rest of the structure.

Nerves   It is the lower portions of the brachial plexus that are particularly at risk in the thoracic outlet area. This includes the ventral rami of C8 and T1. The stellate ganglion, which gives autonomic fibres to the upper arm, lies on the neck of the first rib and may also be compromised.

Risk factors for the neural elements include anomalous pathway of the nerves. If a post-fixed plexus exists there may be an abnormally large contribution of T2 fibres to the T1 root; this lowers the T1 root so that it has a longer course to get over the first rib and into the arm. Scarring of the soft tissue structures through which the nerves pass may reduce the mobility of the plexus, giving rise to symptoms.

Blood vessels   Ninety per cent of thoracic outlet problems affect the neural structures while 10% affect the vascular structures. The subclavian artery is most susceptible to compromise in the scalene triangle area formed by the anterior and middle scalene muscles and the first rib. The subclavian vein passes in front of the anterior scalene muscle. The subclavian vessels become the axillary artery and vein distal to the first rib. The subclavian vein is vulnerable to compression in the tunnel formed by the first rib, the clavicle and the anterior scalene and subclavius muscle. Narrowing of this space would affect venous flow, altering fluid dynamics in the thoracic outlet and also in the carpal tunnel. Venous congestion immediately alters pressure within a tunnel and sets off a sequence of events that can lead to nerve damage.

THORACIC SPINE AND RIBS

Although the thoracic spine is an important source of pain, in comparison with the cervical and lumbar regions it has been less thoroughly researched. Present understanding of joint biomechanics is largely based on ex vivo studies (White 1969, Panjabi et al 1976).

> The thoracic vertebral column plays an important role in spinal dysfunction for the following reasons:
>
> - The thoracic spine is a source of local and referred pain.
> - Thoracic curvature affects the overall spinal posture.
> - Thoracic mobility affects motion in the cervical and lumbar spines and the shoulder girdle.

The thoracic region is the least mobile area of the spine. Individual components of the thorax are flexible, but the overall stability is due to:

1. Costotransverse, costovertebral and sternocostal joints
2. Rib cage and sternum
3. The thoracic intervertebral discs

4. The radiate ligament which attaches the head of the rib to adjacent vertebra and the intervening intervertebral disc
5. The strong intercostal fascia
6. Increased moment of inertia which stiffens the spine when rotatory forces are sustained.

An important function of the thoracic spine and rib cage is to prevent compression of the heart, lungs and major vessels. Protection of these structures is at the expense of mobility in this region. In addition to increasing stiffness, the rib cage has an energy-absorbing capacity, so that the load-bearing capacity of the thoracic spine is increased threefold (Andriacchi et al, 1974). Resection of the costovertebral joints increases the neutral zone and the range of movement in lateral flexion and rotation (Oda et al, 1996). In vitro studies of the thoracic vertebral column have shown that when the posterior elements or ligamentous structures are resected there is increased motion during bending loads (Panjabi et al, 1981; Shea et al, 1996).

Stability of the thoracic spine is also increased by rises in intrathoracic pressure which convert the thorax into a solid unit capable of transmitting large forces (Morris et al, 1961).

Thoracic curvature

In a standing position the line of gravity falls anterior to the vertebral bodies and therefore axial loading tends to increase the thoracic curvature. The thoracic vertebrae are wedge-shaped due to the shorter vertical height of the anterior vertebral body. The cumulative effect of thoracic vertebral body shape is to form the thoracic kyphosis. A radiological study comparing thoracic curvature measurements from vertebral columns at post mortem to curvature measurements from pre-morbid x-rays of the same individual showed that the degree of curvature in vivo and in vitro was strongly correlated. This suggests that the thoracic curvature is strongly influenced by the vertebral body shape and associated ligaments and that activity in the thoracic extensors has little effect on the thoracic kyphosis (Singer et al, 1994).

The thoracic discs also contribute to the thoracic kyphosis (Manns et al, 1996; Goh et al, 1999); like the thoracic vertebral bodies they are also wedge-shaped. This extends from T1–2 to T8–9 and is most evident in the mid-thoracic region (Giles and Singer, 2000).

Changes in thoracic vertebral shape occur due to changes in the material substance of the vertebra and in response to axial loading. Osteoporosis and osteochondrosis (Scheuermann's disease) cause increased wedging of the thoracic vertebrae, resulting in an increased thoracic kyphosis. An increase in thoracic curvature is associated with a reduction in thoracic mobility. This reduction in thoracic mobility may limit the ability to change thoracic posture. Edmondston and Singer (1997) suggests that posture correction is achieved primarily through compensatory changes in the relatively more mobile cervical and lumbar spines while the relatively stiff thoracic spine does not change.

The normal range of thoracic kyphosis is between 20° and 40°, but these values depend on age and gender. During the life span, thoracic kyphosis progresses faster in females. This has been attributed to biomechanical changes, weight alteration and soft tissue extensibility that are a feature of pregnancy, later perpetuated by the demands of nursing, feeding and carrying children (Grieve, 1989). Reduced physical activity, poor muscle tone and the effect of the breasts have also been implicated in the development of the female thoracic kyphosis (Milne and Lauder, 1974).

A slight lateral curve is often noticeable in the thoracic spine, and it has been suggested that this may be due to the dominance of either hand (e.g. in a right-handed individual there may be a slight curve convex to the right and vice versa) or the position of the aorta may influence this curve.

The structures that oppose forward bending are the interspinous ligaments, ligamentum flavum, the posterior longitudinal ligament, multifidus and the long thoracic extensors. In the transverse plane the intervertebral disc fibres resist translation (particularly anteriorly) and shear deformation. Anterior vertebral displacement is resisted by the planes of the apophyseal joints. Rotational stresses in the transverse plane are restricted by the intervertebral disc fibres and the articular facets.

The thoracic intervertebral discs form one seventh of the length of the thoracic spine. The nucleus is situated more centrally than in the cervical and lumbar regions, but it is smaller and has less capacity to swell (Koeller et al, 1984). The main functions of the thoracic discs are to sustain axial loading and allow and restrain thoracic motion.

Although the rib cage contributes to the stiffness of the thoracic spine, the most restricting element is the intervertebral disc. Thoracic discs behave in a more viscous manner than lumbar discs and this may be due to the difference in structure of the collagen network or their framework (Koeller et al, 1984).

Thoracic disc height is less than lumbar disc height. A larger disc height tends to decrease stiffness, whereas a larger cross-sectional area increases it. Flexibility of thoracic and lumbar discs is the same in flexion, extension and lateral flexion and this may be because the effect of the greater cross-sectional area of the lumbar disc is neutralized by the shorter height of the thoracic disc. The height of the upper thoracic discs is less than the rest of the thoracic spine and consequently may contribute to the relative increase in stiffness in the upper thoracic segments. The ratio of disc diameter to height results in fewer circumferential stresses in the thoracic discs, and is a reason why disc prolapses are less common in the thoracic than the lumbar spine.

The ribs which attach to the thoracic vertebrae and sternum present increased resistance to torsion whereas, in the lumbar spine, the apophyseal joints resist torsional stresses.

STRUCTURE OF A TYPICAL THORACIC VERTEBRA (Fig. 1.13)

Vertebral body

The vertebral body is more or less cylindrical and 'heart'-shaped, with its anteroposterior and transverse dimensions almost equal. The vertebral bodies diminish in size from T1 to T3 and then progressively increase in size to T12. The primary function of the thoracic vertebral body is to support the weight of the trunk, and the cancellous bone networks are aligned to withstand axial loading. On the vertebral body's upper and

Figure 1.13 A typical thoracic vertebra. A, Lateral aspect. B, Posterolateral aspect.

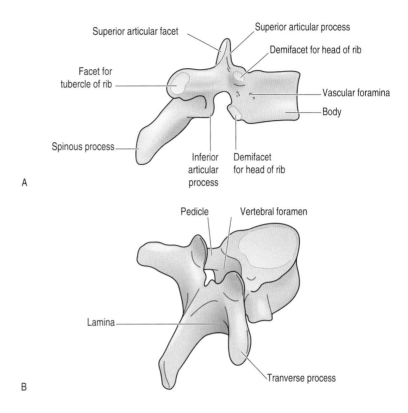

lower lateral borders are the demifacets for articulation with the heads of the ribs. The two superior facets are usually larger and near the root of the pedicle, while the two inferior facets lie anterior to the inferior vertebral notch.

Posterior arch

The *vertebral foramen* is circular in shape and relatively small. The canal is narrowest at T6, although a narrow zone extends from T4 to T9. In this region, the spinal cord is particularly vulnerable to any degenerative change or space-occupying lesion that further decreases the size of the vertebral foramen.

The *pedicles* are short, stout processes passing directly posteriorly from the posterolateral parts of the body. The two *superior articular processes* arise from the superior borders of the laminae near their respective pedicles. They are thin plates of bone projecting superiorly and bearing articular facets, which are almost flat and oval, and face posteriorly, slightly laterally and slightly superiorly. The *inferior articular facets* are fused to the lateral ends of the laminae. They have a facet on their anterior surfaces which faces anteriorly, slightly inferiorly and slightly medially. These facets on the articular processes form the *apophyseal joints*.

The *spinous process* is long. It arises from the junction of the laminae and is directed inferiorly and posteriorly. In the mid-thoracic region, the inferior angulation is particularly marked, the tip of the spinous process lying at the level of the subjacent vertebral body. In the upper and lower thoracic spine, however, the spinous processes face more posteriorly. This is relevant when performing mobilizing techniques on the spinous processes; 'posteroanterior' techniques usually need some modification and greater motion is likely to be achieved if the technique is applied in the plane of the facets. Transverse pressure on the spinous processes in the mid-thoracic region will probably have a different effect on the apophyseal joints than that exerted in the upper and lower thoracic spine due to differences in leverage from the length and angulation of the spinous processes.

The *two transverse processes* project laterally and slightly posteriorly from the junction of the pedicles and laminae. In the upper thoracic spine, they may extend laterally for 4–5 cm but they progressively decrease in size downwards.

The *costal facets*, which articulate with the tubercle of the rib, are found anteriorly on the transverse processes of T1–6 while the costal facets of T7–12 are placed more superiorly on the transverse processes.

PARTICULAR FEATURES OF THORACIC VERTEBRAE

T1

The superior costal facets lie on the sides of the body and are circular, as they alone articulate with the first rib. The lower facets are much smaller and semilunar in shape.

T10, T11 and T12

These usually articulate with the head of the rib of their numerically corresponding rib alone and so only bear one circular costal facet on each side. The transverse processes of T11 and T12 are small and do not bear articular facets.

THE RIBS

There are usually 12 ribs on each side except where a cervical (or lumbar) rib has developed. Cervical ribs have been found as high as C4. The nomenclature of R1–12 is as follows:

> R1–7: *true* ribs. These are connected via the costal cartilages to the sternum.
> R8–12: *false* ribs. The costal cartilages of R8–10 are joined to that of the rib above.
> R11–12: *floating* ribs, so called because they are not connected anteriorly to the sternum.

The direction of the ribs varies, the upper ones being more horizontal. They increase in obliquity down to R9 and then become more horizontal again, with the breadth of the ribs decreasing caudally. The spaces between the ribs are termed *intercostal spaces*.

Typical ribs (Fig. 1.14)

R3–9. Each rib consists of a shaft and an anterior and posterior end. The *shaft* is thin and flattened with a superior and inferior border and an internal concave and external convex surface. The internal surface is marked along its inferior border by the *costal groove*. It is gently curved and twisted in its long axis. The *rib angle*, where the rib is more bent, lies approximately 5–6 cm from the tubercle and provides useful leverage for performing mobilizing techniques aimed at the costovertebral and costotransverse joints.

At the *anterior end* there is a small, cup-shaped depression for connection with the costal cartilage. The *posterior end* has a head, neck and tubercle. The *head* of the rib bears an upper smaller and lower larger facet separated by a crest, which lies opposite the intervertebral disc. The upper facet articulates with the vertebra above and the lower larger facet articulates with the body of the numerically corresponding vertebra. The *neck* is flattened and lies between the head and tubercle of the rib. The *tubercle* is situated on the external surface of the posterior part of the rib at the junction of the neck with the shaft. It has a roughened lateral non-articular part for ligamentous attachment, and a medial articular part with a small, oval facet for articulation with the transverse process of the numerically corresponding vertebra.

Atypical ribs

R1. The first rib (Fig. 1.15) is usually the shortest, but has the largest curvature. Its flattened surfaces face superiorly and inferiorly, and its borders internally and externally. It is higher at its posterior end, sloping downwards towards its anterior end. The *head* has only one facet for articulation with the first thoracic vertebra. The *neck* is rounded and is directed superiorly, posteriorly and laterally. Angulation of the rib

Figure 1.14   A typical rib.

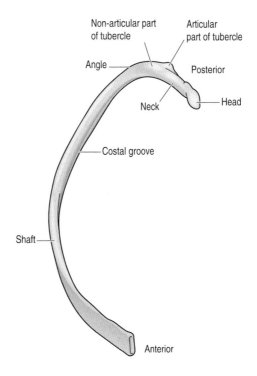

Figure 1.15 The first rib – superior aspect.

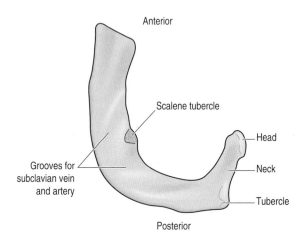

occurs at the *tubercle*, which has an oval facet for articulation with the transverse process of the first thoracic vertebra. Two shallow grooves for the subclavian artery and vein cross the upper surface of the shaft. Any change in obliquity of the rib may cause traction or entrapment of the inferior portions of the brachial plexus and subclavian vessels (see p. 25). A small ridge and scalene tubercle lie between the grooves on its internal border.

R2. The second rib is much longer than the first, its angle being near the tubercle. The shaft is not twisted and the rib has a convex external surface facing superiorly and slightly externally, and a concave internal surface facing inferiorly and slightly internally.

R10. The *head* has a single facet for articulation with the upper border of the 10th thoracic vertebra and also the T9/10 disc.

R11, 12. Each *head* bears a large articulating facet, but these ribs do not have necks or tubercles. R11 has a slight angle, but R12 does not and is much shorter, sometimes being almost insignificant. Their anterior ends are pointed and are covered with cartilage.

LIGAMENTS OF THE THORACIC SPINE

The thoracic portion of the *anterior longitudinal ligament* is thicker and narrower than the cervical and lumbar portions of the ligament. It is composed mainly of Type II collagen, which is virtually inextensible, and consists of several layers of longitudinally orientated fibres. The fibres attach directly to the cortical bone at the edges of the vertebrae and are closely interwoven with the anterior and lateral aspects of the vertebral bodies. Superficial fibres extend over three or four vertebrae and cross each other at an angle of about 20°; intermediate fibres extend over two or three vertebrae; the deep layers attach to adjacent intervertebral discs and cross each other at an angle of approximately 80°. These deep fibres are not well placed to control extension but help to limit rotation with the outer annular fibres.

The *posterior longitudinal ligament* is broad and almost uniform in width in the upper thoracic spine, but in the lower thoracic and lumbar regions it has a denticulate appearance, being narrower over the vertebral bodies and wider over the discs. It contains elastic and collagen fibres (Nakagawa et al, 1994) and is not as strong as the anterior longitudinal ligament. Fibres are attached to the vertebral bodies and intervertebral discs, and are arranged in superficial layers which extend over three or four vertebrae and blend with the deep layers opposite the intervertebral discs. The fibres of the deeper layers attach to the posterolateral aspect of the annulus fibrosus. This ligament helps to limit flexion and anterior translation at the limit of flexion.

Articular capsules of the thoracic apophyseal joints attach to the margins of adjacent vertebrae. They are reinforced anteriorly by ligamenta flava and posteriorly by multifidus.

The *ligamenta flava* connect adjacent laminae and are thicker in the thoracic spine than in any other region. Each ligament extends along the length of the lamina, forming the posterior boundary of the intervertebral foramen. It is composed mainly of elastic fibres embedded in a covering of collagen fibres (Yahia et al, 1990). This elastic property gives considerable static compression to the vertebral segment (Nachemson and Evans, 1968).

The thoracolumbar portion of this ligament can become heavily calcified (Hijioka et al, 1994) and extensive ossification has even been observed in young people. As this ligament helps to form a boundary of the intervertebral foramen these changes may compromise the spinal nerve as it passes through the foramen.

The ligamenta flava help to brake the movement of flexion and assist the paravertebral muscles in restoring the trunk to the upright posture. As the vertebral column moves from a flexed to an upright position, the elastic property of ligamenta flava prevents them from forming folds. If such folds were to occur, they could become trapped between adjacent laminae or press on the dura mater. Fibrosis of these ligaments occurs with increasing age and, as the elasticity decreases, the ligaments have a tendency to buckle, thereby decreasing the neural space of the intervertebral foramen (see p. 322).

Adjacent spinous processes are connected by the *supraspinous* and *interspinous* ligaments. The interspinous ligaments blend posteriorly with the supraspinous ligaments and anteriorly with the articular capsules. *Intertransverse* ligaments connect adjacent transverse processes.

JOINTS OF THE THORACIC SPINE

Thoracic apophyseal joints (Fig. 1.16)

A typical thoracic apophyseal joint is formed by the articulation of the inferior facets of one thoracic vertebra with the superior articular facets of the vertebra below. The superior articular facets are flat and face posteriorly, superiorly and slightly laterally, while the inferior articular facets face predominantly anteriorly, slightly medially and downwards. In the horizontal plane, the combined plane of these facets forms the arc of a circle. The position of the centre of this arc varies according to the individual level. In the first and second thoracic vertebrae, the centre of the arc lies in front of the vertebral body, in the mid-thoracic spine it lies in the vertebral body, whilst in the lower thoracic spine it once again lies

Figure 1.16 A typical thoracic apophyseal articulation – lateral aspect.

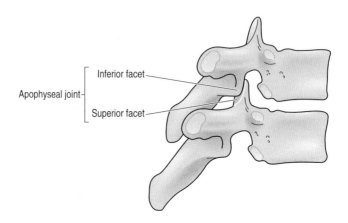

Apophyseal joint

Inferior facet

Superior facet

in front of the anterior border of the vertebral body. This difference is due to the change in medial orientation of the facets at various levels of the thoracic spine (Davis, 1959).

The planes of the apophyseal joints are orientated backward and upward. In the upper thoracic spine the angle between the planes of the joints and the horizontal is approximately 60°. In the mid-thoracic spine the angle becomes closer to the vertical, while the lower thoracic segments have characteristics of the lumbar spine and the joints lie more in the sagittal plane.

In the thoracic region, the vertebral bodies and intervertebral discs take most of the weight-bearing forces in the upright position. However, when the column is flexed and rotated, the apophyseal joints are stressed by compression forces and the upward-facing superior facets are subject to weight-bearing forces. If a thoracic spine deformity develops, e.g. kyphoscoliosis, the superior facets will be subject to greater axial loading and hence they may be more likely to undergo degenerative changes.

The backward-facing superior facets contribute to the stability of the motion segment by preventing forward translation of the superior vertebra on the inferior vertebra. In the horizontal plane the facets are orientated to allow axial rotation to occur.

The joint surfaces are covered with hyaline cartilage and they contain meniscoid structures (see p. 52).

Thoraco–lumbar junction

The thoraco-lumbar region is a transitional area between T10 and L1 where the apophyseal orientation changes from the nearly coronal plane in the thoracic spine to the sagittal plane in the lumbar spine. Many texts refer to an abrupt change of apophyseal orientation with individual vertebrae having superior facets with thoracic characteristics and inferior facets with lumbar characteristics (Hamilton, 1976; Williams and Warwick, 1980). However, a study using computed tomography archives and cadaveric histology demonstrated that in 70% of cases there is a progressive change of facet orientation from T10/11 to T12/L1. In only one third of cases is there an abrupt change of facet orientation (Singer, 1989). This gradual change in facet plane may help to minimize the stress at this transitional zone. An abrupt change of facet direction is considered to be a contributor to injury as forces tend to be localized specifically to that level.

Although the size of each vertebral body increases caudally, the mid-vertebral body area and vertebral trabecular density are similar for all vertebra in the region T10 to L1. This suggests that the thoracolumbar vertebrae sustain a similar amount of axial weight-bearing (Singer, 1997). The increased cross-sectional area of the pedicles at the thoracolumbar junction aids transmission between the anterior and posterior elements. The amount of weight-bearing sustained by the thoracolumbar apophyseal joints will vary depending on the distance between the joints and the line of gravity.

In *articular tropism* (see p. 55) there is a difference between the left and right apophyseal joint planes of an individual vertebra; this occurs commonly at the thoraco-lumbar junction. Tropism at one spinal level is often associated with spinal variants at other levels in the vertebral column.

The term 'mortice joint' was first used by Davis (1959) to describe interlocking apophyseal joints that occur commonly at T11/12 and T12/L1. When this level is fully extended, the upper vertebra forms a bony block with the subjacent vertebra, preventing any lateral flexion or rotation; only flexion is possible. The clinical significance of this is that, when the transitional level is in full extension, it is impossible to gain any movement other than flexion, and in treatment it is dangerous to attempt it. Malmivaara et al (1987) noted that the presence of unilateral mortise joints was associated with apophyseal joint tropism.

Mamillary processes are thickened bony elevations on the posterior border of the superior articular facets. They are found on the lumbar vertebrae and are also present at the thoraco-lumbar junction. These processes may develop due to activity in the multifidus muscle (Kaplan, 1945). Multifidus acts as an antagonist to rotation at the thoraco-lumbar junction, thereby reinforcing the role of the apophyseal joints and reducing torsion.

COSTOVERTEBRAL AND COSTOTRANSVERSE JOINTS (Fig. 1.17)

Each rib is connected to the thoracic vertebral column at two joints:

1. The costovertebral joint between the head of a rib, the bodies of two adjacent vertebrae and the intervening disc

2. The costotransverse joint between the tubercle of the rib and the transverse process of the numerically corresponding vertebra.

R1, 10, 11 and 12 articulate with their own numerically corresponding vertebral body, but the 11th and 12th ribs do not articulate with their transverse process.

Figure 1.17 Costovertebral and costotransverse joints. A, Superior aspect. B, Lateral aspect. (Adapted from Williams PL, Warwick R 1980 *Gray's Anatomy*, 36th edn. Churchill Livingstone, Edinburgh, pp. 450, 451.)

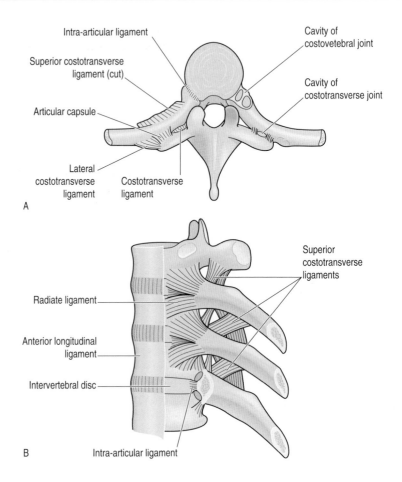

Costovertebral joints

The costovertebral joints are synovial, 'plane' joints. The two slightly convex facets on the head of a typical rib fit into the concavity formed by two costal facets on adjacent vertebrae and the intervertebral discs in between. The costal facets lie one on the inferior border of the vertebra above, and the other on the superior border of the subjacent vertebra to which the rib numerically corresponds. A single loose fibrous capsule surrounds the joint, the surfaces of which are covered with hyaline cartilage.

The joint cavity is divided into two by an *intra-articular ligament* which is attached laterally to the crest on the head of a typical rib and passes inside the joint to be attached medially to the intervertebral disc. The *radiate ligament* reinforces the joint anteriorly and is attached laterally to the anterior part of the head of the rib. It has three sets of fibres: the superior fibres are attached to the body of the vertebra above; the inferior fibres to the body below; and the horizontal fibres to the intervertebral disc. As the 1st, 10th, 11th and 12th ribs articulate with their own vertebral body only, they have a single joint cavity, no intra-articular ligament and a poorly developed radiate ligament.

Costotransverse joints

The costotransverse joints are also synovial joints and are formed by the articulation of the facet on the front of the transverse process with the oval facet on the posteromedial aspect of the tubercle of the rib. In the upper costotransverse joints, the facet on the rib is convex and that on the transverse process is reciprocally concave. In the lower costotransverse joints, the facets of the rib and transverse processes become flatter. This change in shape of the facets is one of the factors responsible for the different movements of the upper and lower ribs during respiration. The joint has a thin fibrous capsule lined with synovium.

The ligaments of the joint are strong, so that the movements are markedly limited to small gliding motions.

The *superior costotransverse ligament* has two layers: (1) the anterior fibres are attached below to the crest of the neck of the rib and pass upwards and laterally to the lower border of the transverse process above; (2) the posterior fibres are attached below to the posterior surface of the neck of the rib and pass upwards and medially behind the anterior fibres to the transverse process above. The two bands are separated by the external intercostal membrane, and fibres of the anterior band blend laterally with the internal intercostal membrane.

The *costotransverse ligament* attaches the posterior part of the neck of the rib to the anterior surface of the transverse process.

The *lateral costotransverse ligament* attaches the tip of the transverse process to the roughened articular portion of the tubercle of the rib. This ligament strengthens the posterolateral aspect of the joint capsule.

STERNOCOSTAL JOINTS

The sternocostal joints are formed by the articulation of the medial end of the costal cartilages of the 1st–7th ribs and sternum. The joint between the 1st costal cartilage and the sternum is a primary cartilaginous joint (synchondrosis) where the cartilage unites with the upper lateral border of the manubrium sterni. Movement does not occur at this joint; this is a relevant factor during respiration (see p. 199). The 2nd–7th joints are synovial and surrounded by a fibrous capsule.

An *intra-articular ligament* divides the joint cavity into two although, with increasing age, these joint cavities (except that of the 2nd costal cartilage) become obliterated. Movement at the sternocostal joints is restricted by the intra-articular ligament.

Anterior and posterior radiate ligaments pass from the medial end of the costal cartilage to the anterior and posterior aspects of the sternum. Anteriorly, from the costal cartilage, the superior fibres pass upwards and medially, the middle fibres horizontally and the lower fibres medially and downwards. The fibres interlace with those from the joints above and below. Tendinous fibres of pectoralis major fuse with the anterior radiate ligaments. The posterior radiate ligaments have a similar arrangement on the posterior aspect of the sternum.

INTERCHONDRAL JOINTS

The interchondral joints are formed by the tips of the costal cartilages of the 8th, 9th and 10th ribs with the lower border of the cartilage above.

The 8th and 9th interchondral joints are synovial, while the 10th is more fibrous. Small synovial joints also occur between the adjacent margins of the 5th–9th costal cartilages. A fibrous capsule surrounds these joints and they are strengthened anteriorly and posteriorly by the oblique interchondral ligaments.

The costochondral and interchondral joints may give rise to symptoms of local pain, tenderness, or localized swelling (Tietze, 1921), or they may simulate disease of the thoracic viscera or mimic the anterior referral of pain from vertebral joint problems. This condition may arise from torsion of the rib secondary to a segmental vertebral lesion of fixation (Patriquin, 1983).

PALPATION OF THE THORACIC SPINE AND RIB CAGE (Fig. 1.18)

The following bony points can be palpated:

Figure 1.18 Palpation points in the thoracic spine – posterior aspect.

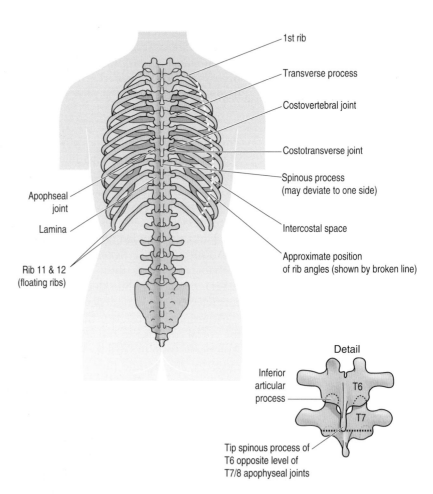

1st rib

Transverse process

Costovertebral joint

Costotransverse joint

Spinous process
(may deviate to one side)

Intercostal space

Approximate position
of rib angles (shown by broken line)

Apophseal
joint

Lamina

Rib 11 & 12
(floating ribs)

Detail

Inferior
articular
process

T6

T7

Tip spinous process of
T6 opposite level of
T7/8 apophyseal joints

Spinous processes

The tips of the spinous processes are slightly bulbous and sometimes deviate from the midline. Palpation of the levels of the *laminae* will clarify whether or not the vertebra is rotated. The tip of the spinous process of T1 is usually prominent (as is C7). The spinous processes project downwards more in the mid-thoracic spine and this should be taken into consideration when performing treatment techniques on them. The position of their tips relative to that of the apophyseal joints varies, so that in the upper and lower thoracic spine the tips are approximately on a level with the apophyseal joint formed from the inferior facets of the numerically corresponding vertebra and the superior facets of the vertebra below. In the mid-thoracic spine the spinous processes may project downwards as far as the subjacent apophyseal joints.

> *To clarify*: the tip of the spinous process of T6 lies at approximately the level of the T7/8 apophyseal joints.

Dorsal aspects of apophyseal joints (inferior articular processes)

These can be palpated in some subjects by gently probing through the paravertebral muscles until a bony ridge can be felt. The accuracy of palpating the apophyseal joints is improved by keeping the palpating thumb close to the spinous process laterally.

Transverse processes

The transverse processes (overlying the costotransverse joints) lie in a more posterior plane than the articular processes, approximately 3 cm from the midline, reducing to 2 cm in the lower thorax. Their tips lie more or less level with the tip of the spinous process of the vertebra above. Mobilization techniques can be used with great effect at these joints. The rib and vertebra can be mobilized together but also the thoracic vertebra can be fixed and the movement and position of the rib relative to transverse process can be established.

Ribs

Due to the obliquity of the direction of the ribs posteriorly, the *intercostal spaces* are narrower behind than in front. The *rib angles* are roughly level with their corresponding transverse process and with the tip of the spinous process of the vertebra above, and lie at a varying distance from the midline, the furthest away being that of R8. Caudally and cranially from this rib angle, they become progressively closer to the midline. They provide useful leverage for mobilizing the costotransverse and costovertebral joints. R12 is small and sometimes difficult to palpate. The flattened tendons of erector spinae arise and insert into the rib angles, and local soft tissue lesions here are not uncommon.

When the person is in prone-lying, R1 may be felt by lifting up the upper fibres of trapezius with the thumbs and palpating caudally; its upper surface faces superiorly and is often tender on palpation.

Anteriorly, R1 is covered mainly by the clavicle, its costal cartilage lying just under the sternal end. The narrow posterior border of R1 may also be palpated in prone-lying.

In supine-lying, the sternal notch and sternoclavicular joint can be palpated. The sternal angle is normally prominent and can be felt 3–4 cm inferiorly from the sternal notch. The first sternocostal joint on either side is at the upper lateral border of the manubrium sterni, just inferior to the sternoclavicular joint. The 2nd to 7th sternocostal joints can normally be palpated along the lateral border of the sternum in males, but accurate palpation in females may be difficult due to the breast tissue.

The costochondral junction of the ribs with the costal cartilage can be palpated by placing a thumb on an individual rib laterally and following its course anteriorly until a difference in resistance and resilience is felt, indicating a change from bony to cartilaginous tissue.

LUMBAR SPINE

The lumbar vertebral column comprises five vertebra and the intervening discs. When an upright normal lumbar spine is viewed from the side, it can be seen that the lumbar column has a curve that is concave posteriorly. This curve is known as the lumbar lordosis (Fig. 1.19).

In the standing position, the sacrum is tilted forwards so that its upper surface is inclined forwards and downwards forming an angle between the top of the sacrum and the horizontal which varies between 50° and 53° (Hellems and Keates, 1971). If the lumbar spine articulated in a straight line with the sacrum, the trunk would be inclined forwards. In order to compensate for the inclination of the sacrum and to allow the upright standing position to be achieved, the lumbar spine curves posteriorly.

Figure 1.19   The lumbar lordosis – lateral aspect.

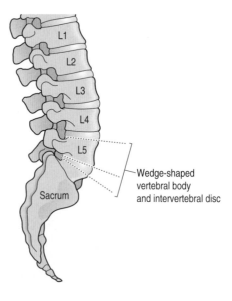

L1

L2

L3

L4

L5

Sacrum

Wedge-shaped
vertebral body
and intervertebral disc

Several factors contribute to the normal shape of the lumbar lordosis:

1. The L5 vertebral body is wedge-shaped: the anterior body wall is 3 mm higher than the posterior body wall (Gilad and Nissan, 1985). This brings the upper surface of the L5 body closer to the horizontal plane than the upper surface of the sacrum.

2. The L5/S1 disc is also wedge-shaped and its anterior vertical height is 6–7 mm greater than its posterior height. As a result of the wedge shape of the disc, the inferior surface of the L5 vertebral body is not parallel to the superior surface of the sacrum, so that the angle formed between the two surfaces may vary between 6° and 29° and has an average measurement of 16° (Schmorl and Junghanns, 1971).

3. Each vertebra above L5 is inclined slightly backwards in relation to the vertebra below.

4. In 75% of adults the centre of gravity lies anterior to the vertebral column. In these individuals there is constant slight activity in the erector spinae muscles, which work to prevent the trunk from falling forwards and hence assist in maintaining the lumbar lordosis.

In a normal spine in the upright posture, the body of L5 lies directly vertically above the sacrum (Bogduk and Twomey, 1987). Various attempts have been made to measure the lumbar lordosis, but as investigators have used different parameters the results differ substantially (Torgerson and Dotter, 1976; Ferdinand and Fox, 1985; Hansson et al, 1985a). In the standing position, measurements from radiographs of the angle between the top of L1 and the sacrum have been recorded as 67° (± 3° standard deviation) in children and 74° (± 7° standard deviation) in young males (Hansson et al, 1985a).

Development of the lumbar lordosis begins as an infant starts to stand, usually between 12 and 18 months of age, and it continues to develop until the completion of spinal growth, normally between 15 and 18 years in females and 17 and 21 years in males. In old age the lordosis often becomes flattened.

FACTORS AFFECTING THE LUMBAR LORDOSIS

Sex

The degree of curvature of the lumbar lordosis varies considerably between individuals, and in each individual it alters in different postures and positions. The following factors influence lumbar lordosis:

It has been shown that the L5/S1 angle of the lordosis is greater in women during childbearing years than in men (Twomey and Taylor, 1987), and it has been speculated that this difference may be, in part, due to hormones – and to one in particular known as relaxin. Relaxin is secreted by the ovary and has been shown to relax the spinal ligaments, symphysis pubis and the sacroiliac joints. During pregnancy, large amounts of this hormone are present in the blood, but it is also found in small amounts in the blood of non-pregnant women (Hytten and Leitch, 1971). The level of relaxin present between adolescence and middle age may be responsible for a relaxing of the spinal ligaments and an increase in lumbar lordosis in women. Before adolescence and after middle age, there is no difference in the lordosis of the two sexes.

Age

In most individuals the lumbar spine flattens with age (Schmorl and Junghanns, 1971) due in part, at least, to a flexed lifestyle. However, some individuals have an increase in lordosis which may become very pronounced in some instances. An increased lordosis is often accompanied by an increase in weight and size of the abdomen, together with a decrease in the strength of the abdominal muscles.

Position

In the standing position there is an increase in lumbar lordosis and consequent increase in anterior shear in the lumbar spine. The anterior shear is countered by the force of the abdominal wall as it holds the abdominal contents back against the anterior aspect of the spine. Those with an increase in lumbar lordosis have weak abdominal muscles, particularly transversus abdominis, and the force resisting lumbar anterior shear is greatly reduced. In the sitting position lumbar lordosis is decreased, hence anterior shear is also reduced in sitting.

If an individual stands in an upright position for a long period, the trunk muscles begin to fatigue and intervertebral disc height is reduced due to 'creep' (see p. 79), so that the natural tendency of the lumbar spine towards extension becomes exaggerated.

Pathology

Studies investigating the relationship between lumbar lordosis and the presence or absence of symptoms of back pain have failed to find any correlation between the two (Torgerson and Dotter, 1976: Hansson et al, 1985b). However, the causes of back pain are often multifactorial and the shape of the lumbar curve is but one factor. In clinical practice, it will be noted that in some individuals the presence of a mechanical joint lesion, muscle spasm or pain may affect the normal lumbar curvature.

Compression

Compression or vertical loading of the spine tends to increase the lordosis. If a weight is held in front of the spine, activity of erector spinae rises to prevent the trunk falling forwards, and there is a subsequent increase in the lordosis.

Footwear

When high-heeled shoes are worn, the body's centre of gravity is displaced forwards; this is associated with an increase in pelvic tilt and thereby an increase in lordosis.

Biomechanical considerations of the lower limbs

Biomechanical alignment of the lower limbs also influences lumbar posture. Bilateral foot deformities that cause a compensatory over-pronation of the feet displace the body weight forwards so that there is an increase in lumbar erector spinae activity which increases the lumbar lordosis. Bilateral foot deformities that cause compensatory over-supination have the opposite effect and tend to decrease the lumbar lordosis.

Bilateral anteverted hips are commonly associated with an increase in lordosis. In the weight-bearing position anteverted hips are medially rotated which displaces the body forwards causing a compensatory increase in lordosis. Bilateral retroverted hips are laterally rotated in weight-bearing and are associated with a decrease in lumbar lordosis.

LORDOSIS AND STABILITY

In the erect posture the sacrum tilts forwards and there is a tendency for L5 to slip forwards on the sacrum, and to a lesser extent for L4 to slide forwards on L5. This tendency to forward displacement is resisted by:

1. *Orientation of the apophyseal joints*. The superior facets of the sacrum face backwards and form a bony locking mechanism with the inferior facets on L5, which face forward (see p. 54, 56). The orientation of the L4/5 apophyseal joints also prevents forward displacement, but above L4 the vertebral bodies are inclined slightly back and there is no tendency, at rest, for the upper lumbar vertebrae to slide forwards.

2. *Ligamentous support:*

a. The *ligaments connecting the bony arches of the vertebrae* prevent forward displacement. Under normal circumstances, in the upright position, the annulus fibrosus is not under strain and does not prevent forward displacement of the vertebral body. If there is a breakdown of the bony mechanism or if the joints are affected by disease or injury as, for example, in spondylolisthesis (see p. 310), the annular fibres may then be placed under strain.

b. The strong *iliolumbar ligament* attaches the thick transverse processes of L5 to the ilium. They help to prevent L5 from sliding forwards.

c. The *anterior longitudinal ligament* and *anterior annulus fibrosus*. When compression forces are applied to the lumbar spine, the lordosis tends to increase so that the posterior ends of the intervertebral discs are compressed while the anterior ends of the vertebral bodies tend to separate. In these circumstances, the anterior longitudinal ligaments and anterior annulus fibrosus are placed under tension to resist the tendency of the vertebral bodies to separate. Eventually, a state of equilibrium is achieved so that the force tending to separate the vertebral bodies is balanced exactly by the anterior ligaments. Any further increase in force is resisted by tension in these ligaments (Bogduk and Twomey, 1987).

The curve of the lumbar spine gives it a certain resilience and helps to protect the spine from compressive forces. If the spine were straight, compressive forces would be transferred through the vertebral bodies to the intervertebral discs alone. In the curved lumbar spine, some of the compressive force is taken by the anterior longitudinal ligaments.

Pelvic tilt

Kendall et al (1993, pp. 416–417) define pelvic tilt as an anterior, posterior or lateral tilt of the pelvis from the neutral position. The neutral position is one in which the anterior superior spines are in the same transverse plane, and the anterior superior spines and the symphysis pubis are in the same vertical plane. Kendall et al describe three deviations from the neutral position of the pelvis:

1. In a position of *anterior tilt* the vertical plane through the anterior superior spines is anterior to the vertical plane through the symphysis pubis.

2. In *posterior tilt* the vertical plane through the anterior superior spines is posterior to the vertical plane through the symphysis pubis.

3. In *lateral tilt* the crest of the ilium is higher on one side than the other.

As the lumbar spine articulates directly with the sacrum, any alteration in the angle of the pelvis inevitably affects the position of the lumbar spine. If the pelvis is tilted forwards, the lumbar lordosis increases; when the pelvis is tilted backwards, the lordosis becomes flattened. If the pelvis is in lateral tilt the lumbar spine may be shifted laterally or have a degree of lateral curvature.

Pelvic tilt is to a great extent determined by muscle action. Erector spinae acts to increase the lordosis, while the abdominal muscles, glutei and hamstrings flatten the lordosis through their action on the pelvis. When psoas acts bilaterally it increases the lordosis.

SCOLIOSIS

Scoliosis is a lateral curvature of the spine in which the vertebrae show transverse plane rotation. A scoliosis in the lumbar spine may be (1) an idiopathic structural scoliosis, or (2) a functional or postural scoliosis.

An *idiopathic scoliosis* appears to develop spontaneously and it is not understood what causes the deformity. Idiopathic scoliosis is more common in girls, and various factors such as abnormal growth and development of the spine, joint laxity, sagittal spinal curvature and neurological factors may play a part (Nachemson and Sahlstrand, 1977). Progression of the scoliosis is believed to be controlled by mechanical factors. The 'Hueter-Volkmann law' (Arkin, 1949) suggests that the increased compression on the concave side of the curvature decreases rate of growth of the vertebrae, while the reduced compression on the convex side accelerates growth. During adolescence, an idiopathic scoliosis of greater than 20° is liable to progress if there is still significant growth potential (Lonstein and Carlson, 1984).

A *functional or postural scoliosis* has been associated with a number of factors such as leg-length inequality, muscle spasm, degenerative changes of the intervertebral discs and apophyseal joints and osteoarthritic changes of the hip and knee. The most common cause of a postural scoliosis is leg-length inequality. In some individuals with a short leg, there is a dipping down of the pelvis on the short side, and a compensatory lumbar curve convex to the short side will be present, with a corresponding thoracic convexity to the long-leg side. In some individuals the convexities and concavities may be reversed (Grieve, 1989).

Minor structural changes are associated with the postural scoliosis of leg-length inequality. On the convex side, early attenuation of the lateral annulus fibrosus may occur, while the joints of that side have thicker subchondral bone plates and thinner articular cartilage than the concave side, suggesting that greater loading occurs on the convex side of the curve (Giles and Taylor, 1984). It is thought that this may be related to the greater effect of the forces of the postural muscles on the convex side which act to prevent the scoliotic column giving way under axial loading.

Although some investigators have demonstrated a correlation between leg-length inequality and low back pain (Giles and Taylor, 1981), others have not found any conclusive evidence of a relationship between back pain and unequal leg length (Troup, 1975; Grundy and Roberts, 1984).

STRUCTURE OF A TYPICAL LUMBAR VERTEBRA (L1–4) (Fig. 1.20)

The five lumbar vertebrae are the largest moveable vertebrae, their large bodies taking more weight and their vertebral arches being more developed than in other regions to sustain greater stresses.

Vertebral body

The body is large and kidney-shaped. It is wider transversely than anteroposteriorly and is slightly deeper in front than behind. Its outer surface is somewhat concave from above downwards, except posteriorly, where it is flatter.

Posterior arch

The body and the posterior arch enclose the *vertebral foramen*, which is normally triangular in this region. It is larger than in the thoracic region, but smaller than in the cervical. Collectively, the vertebral foramina constitute the vertebral canal in which lies the spinal cord/cauda equina.

Figure 1.20   A typical lumbar vertebra.

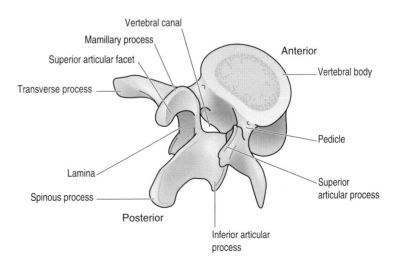

Stenosis or narrowing of the foramen, which is more pronounced in men, can be a congenital abnormality or acquired through degenerative changes such as bony or ligamentous hypertrophy or disc bulging/herniation. This can result in signs and symptoms arising from cauda equina compression, which may not otherwise have manifested in a normal, more spacious foramen.

The posterior arch is formed by the pedicles, laminae and articular processes.

The *pedicles* are short, stout processes projecting backwards from the posterolateral aspect of the vertebral body just below its upper border. The superior border of each pedicle forms the shallow *superior vertebral notch*; the inferior border forms the more pronounced *inferior vertebral notch*. These notches form the inferior and superior boundaries of the *intervertebral foramen*.

The two *laminae* are broad, strong plates of bone which run posteromedially. They meet in the midline to form the *spinous process* which projects posteriorly and is broad and quadrangular. Its tip is bulbous and is sometimes slightly indented. At the junction of the laminae with the pedicles lie two *superior articular processes* and these house the concave *superior articular facets* which face medially and slightly posteriorly. The posterior border of each process is reinforced by a bony elevation called the *mamillary process*. The two *inferior articular processes* arise from the junction of the laminae with the spinous process. They house the convex *inferior articular facets* which face laterally and slightly anteriorly.

The two *transverse processes* are long and thin, and project laterally and slightly posteriorly from the junctions of the superior articular processes with the laminae.

PARTICULAR FEATURES OF THE 5TH LUMBAR VERTEBRA (Fig. 1.21)

The 5th lumbar vertebra usually has the largest body, which is more wedge-shaped (deeper in front than behind) than the other lumbar vertebrae. The L5/S1 disc is correspondingly wedge-shaped and this accounts for the prominence of the lumbosacral angle (see p. 43). The articular processes are wider apart than in other vertebrae, while the transverse processes of L5 are strong and large. The latter arise from the whole of the lateral aspect of the pedicles and part of the vertebral body itself and

Figure 1.21   The 5th lumbar vertebra – superior aspect.

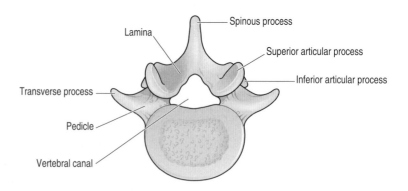

Spinous process

Lamina

Superior articular process

Inferior articular process

Transverse process

Pedicle

Vertebral canal

give rise to the strong iliolumbar ligaments which assist in stabilizing the lumbar spine to the pelvis. The spinous process, however, is usually the smallest of the five, with a blunted tip.

LIGAMENTS OF THE LUMBAR SPINE
(Fig. 1.22)

Anterior longitudinal ligament

The lumbar ligaments form a dense connective tissue sleeve around the vertebrae that extends into the sacral area. The individual ligaments are continuous but different in structure and collagen content.

The anterior longitudinal ligament is a strong band lying anterior to the vertebral bodies and discs. It is firmly attached to the discs and is embedded in the periosteal sheath of the vertebral bodies. Inferiorly the anterior longitudinal ligament is continuous with the anteromedial aspect of the sacroiliac joint capsule. Its longitudinal fibres have several layers: the deeper, shorter fibres joining adjacent vertebrae, and the more superficial layers extending over 2–4 vertebrae. The two crura of the diaphragm attach onto the anterior longitudinal ligament in the upper lumbar spine, and some fibres extend into the ligament in the lower lumbar area.

Figure 1.22   Ligaments in lumbar region. A, Lateral aspect. B, Posterior longitudinal ligament. C, Anterior aspect of ligamenta flava.

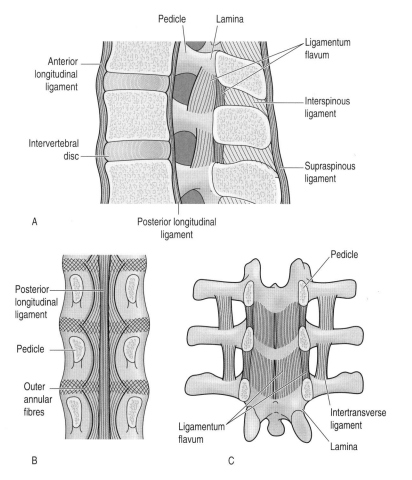

Age-related changes occur in the anterior longitudinal ligament so that it loses its elastic properties and energy dissipation properties. The density of the bone into which the ligament attaches also decreases. As the mineral content of the bone decreases with age there is also a loss of strength of the ligament (Neumann et al, 1993).

The main function of the ligament is to prevent anterior separation of the vertebral bodies during extension. It also helps to stabilize the lumbar lordosis (see p. 43). Forward and backward sliding of the vertebrae is resisted principally by the annulus fibrosus, although the anterior longitudinal ligament also restricts movement. The anterior longitudinal ligament is most vulnerable to injury in rotation (Roaf, 1960).

Posterior longitudinal ligament

Lying posterior to the vertebral bodies and discs in the vertebral canal, the posterior longitudinal ligament generally narrows towards its insertion into the sacrum. The ligament is also embedded in the periosteum of the vertebral bodies and has a denticulate appearance, being broader over the annular fibres of the discs and narrower around the base of the pedicles and the vertebral bodies. The posterior longitudinal ligament is thinner than its anterior counterpart and it helps to prevent separation of the posterior ends of the vertebral bodies. It also works with ligamentum flavum to stabilize the spine in flexion.

Articular capsules

The articular capsules of the apophyseal joints are attached to the margins of the articular facets and are tightly bound to these processes except at the superior and inferior recesses where the capsule forms a fold. The capsule is composed of dense connective tissue which lies orthogonal to the joint line (this is the plane in which the two joints oppose each other) (Willard, 1997). The joint capsule provides a connective tissue link between the ligaments of the neural arch and those of the vertebral bodies. The capsule is invested in a sheet of fascia that is continuous dorsally with the fascia surrounding ligamentum flavum and ventrally with the fascia surrounding the vertebral body. Multifidus muscle reinforces the capsule posteriorly while anteriorly it is strengthened by ligamentum flavum.

Ligamenta flava

Adjacent laminae are connected by ligamenta flava, which are short, thick ligaments fusing in the midline with the contralateral ligament. Superiorly, the ligament is attached to the lower half of the anterior surface of the lamina and the inferior aspect of the pedicle. The ligament divides into medial and lateral portions (Ramsey, 1966). The medial portion attaches to the upper, dorsal surface of the subjacent lamina and posteriorly decreases in elastic fibre content to become the interspinous ligament. The lateral portion passes in front of the apophyseal joint formed by the two vertebrae that the ligament connects, and fibres attach onto the articular capsule.

These ligaments are composed of 80% elastin fibres and 20% collagen fibres. The elastin fibres give the ligament its characteristic yellow appearance and allow a degree of elasticity. Ligamenta flava allow separation of the laminae in flexion and protect the discs by graduating this movement so that an abrupt limit is not reached. The inherent elasticity also assists the movement of returning from flexion to neutral. In the neutral position the ligament is in a state of pre-tension, which helps to prevent it from buckling (Nachemson and Evans, 1968). There is a loss of elastic fibres with age, with resulting decreasing elasticity of the ligament in the elderly and a reduction in the pre-tension state in neutral position. Kashiwagi (1993) describes an increase in collagen fibres and a greater number of high molecular weight proteoglycans occurring with ageing. These events make the ligament more prone to calcification and hypertrophy, which can cause spinal stenosis.

Ligamenta flava have poor regenerative capacity, and damaged areas are replaced by scar tissue (Ramsey, 1966).

Interspinous ligaments

The interspinous ligaments connect adjacent spinous processes from their roots to their apices. They are continuous with the ligamenta flava anteriorly and the supraspinous ligament posteriorly. The interspinous-ligament is continuous with the thoracolumbar fascia posteriorly. The ligament has been described as fan-shaped with the narrow end of the fan blending with ligamentum flavum. In the centre of the ligament, the collagen fibres are parallel to the spinous processes before spreading in a posterocranial and posterocaudad direction to attach to adjacent spinous processes. The fan-like direction of the fibres allows the spinous processes to separate during flexion.

The direction of the central fibres favours the transmission of forces, and it is thought that they transmit the anteroposterior pull of the thoracolumbar fascia, to which the ligament is connected via the supraspinous ligament (Hukins et al, 1990). This could assist in maintaining the pre-tension state of the ligamenta flava and prevent them from buckling into the central vertebral canal. Age-related chondrification of the interspinous ligament occurs in the third decade (Yahia et al, 1990).

Supraspinous ligament

A fibrous cord joining the tips of the spinous processes, the supraspinous ligament ends between L4 and L5. Below the L5 spinous process, fibres from the thoracolumbar fascia intersect. The ligament adheres tightly to the interspinous ligament, creating an interspinous–supraspinous–thoracolumbar ligamentous complex that anchors the fascial planes to the lumbar spinous processes. Traction placed on the thoracolumbar fascia destroys the thoracolumbar sheath before damaging the interspinous–supraspinous–thoracolumbar complex (Willard, 1997).

Both the interspinous and supraspinous ligaments assist in resisting separation of the spinous processes during flexion of the vertebral column, but they do not come into play until about half full flexion. They are relatively weak and are the first structure to be sprained after the limit of flexion is reached (Adams et al, 1980). Rissanen (1960) reported that more than 20% of adult lumbar spines had visibly ruptured interspinous ligaments and that torn attachments to the spinous processes were often seen in those over 30 years of age.

Intertransverse ligaments

Intertransverse ligaments connect adjacent transverse processes and are unlike other ligaments in the lumbar spine in that their collagen fibres are not as densely packed or as regularly orientated. These ligaments have been described as connective tissue sheets (Vallois, 1926) that separate the anterior lumbar muscles from the posterior lumbar musculature.

Laterally, the ligaments divide into two layers: the anterior layer becomes the thoracolumbar fascia, while the posterior layer blends with the aponeurosis of transversus abdominis to form the middle layer of the thoracolumbar fascia (see p. 126). Medially, the ligament divides into ventral and dorsal portions (Lewin et al, 1962). The dorsal leaf attaches to the lateral margin of the lamina of the vertebra that lies opposite the intertransverse space. Inferiorly, it blends with the capsule of the subjacent apophyseal joint. The ventral leaf passes anteriorly around the vertebral body to blend with the lateral margins of the anterior longitudinal ligament. This part of the ligament forms a connective tissue sheet that closes the outer end of the intervertebral foramen. It is pierced by nerve branches to psoas and also the ventral ramus of the spinal nerve and accompanying nerves and veins.

Between the ventral and dorsal leaves is a fat-filled space called the *superior articular recess*. The fat in this recess is continuous with the intraarticular fat of the joint below. This recess accommodates movements of the subjacent apophyseal joint, and the fat acts as a displaceable space filler (see p. 52).

Transforaminal ligaments

Bands of fibres that cross the outer end of the intervertebral foramen have been identified and are known as transforaminal ligaments (Golub and Silverman, 1969). They are not always present and more closely resemble bands of fascia. It is possible that, when present, they may decrease the space available for the emerging spinal nerve. These ligaments may be thickenings of the ventral leaf of the intertransverse ligaments (Bogduk and Twomey, 1987).

Mamillo–accessory ligament

The mamillo-accessory ligament attaches to the tips of the ipsilateral mamillary and accessory processes. In 10% of individuals it may be ossified, forming a small foramen at the mamillo-accessory notch. The ligament covers the medial branch of the dorsal ramus of the spinal nerve.

Iliolumbar ligaments

The iliolumbar ligaments connect the transverse processes of L4 and L5 to the ilium. These ligaments appear to vary in number and form. They have been described as having superior and inferior bands (Williams, 1995), anterior, superior and inferior bands (O'Rahilly, 1986), and five different bands (Shellshear and Macintosh, 1949). Willard (1997) states that although they are highly variable they consistently blend superiorly with the intertransverse ligaments and inferiorly with the sacroiliac ligaments. The ligament has been observed in the fetus at 11–15 weeks (Luk et al, 1986) and therefore does not develop out of the inferior border of the quadratus lumborum muscle as was once thought.

The powerful, complex structure of the iliolumbar ligaments provides stability at the lumbosacral junction, preventing the fifth lumbar vertebral from being displaced forwards. It also is an important structure in restricting movement. Bilateral transection of this ligament increased axial rotation by 18%, extension by 20%, flexion by 23% and lateral bending by 29% (Yamamoto et al, 1990).

The ligaments pass over the L4 and L5 nerve roots and have been implicated in compression of these nerves.

Thoracolumbar fascia

The thoracolumbar fascia has extensive attachments in the lumbar spine into soft tissue, muscle and bone. It plays an important role in stabilization of the spine. A full description of the thoracolumbar fascia is given on page 126.

STRUCTURE OF A TYPICAL LUMBAR APOPHYSEAL JOINT (Fig. 1.23)

Joint capsule

The lumbar apophyseal joints are true synovial joints. They are non-axial and diarthrodial, allowing small gliding movements to occur.

The joint capsule surrounds the dorsal, superior and inferior margins of each apophyseal joint, attaching just beyond the margins of the cartilage. The fibrous capsule is continuous anteriorly with ligamentum flavum and posteriorly it is reinforced with the deep fibres of multifidus. The collagen fibres pass transversely from one articular process to the other. At the superior and inferior ends of the joint, the capsule is loose. This arrangement of fibres allows gliding movement in the sagittal plane, but restricts rotation (see p. 201).

At the inferior and superior ends of the joint there are subcapsular pockets which contain fat. There are two tiny holes in the superior and inferior parts of the capsule through which fat can communicate with the fat in the extracapsular space. Fat within the joint is covered externally by the capsule and, internally, it is lined with synovium.

Figure 1.23   A typical lumbar apophyseal joint – posterolateral aspect.

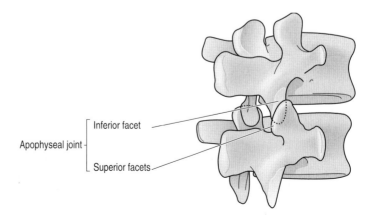

Inferior facet

Apophyseal joint

Superior facets

Intra-articular
structures

There are three types of intra-articular structure within the lumbar apophyseal joints:

1. *Fat pads* are found at the superior and inferior ends of the joint. The superior fat pad is intracapsular, within the recess formed by ligamentum flavum and the inferior articular process. It is lined with synovium and projects downwards approximately 3 mm between the articular processes. The fat pad becomes fibrofatty with ageing. At the inferior end of the joint there is a small gap where ligamentum flavum merges with the fibrous capsule. Here a large extracapsular fat pad communicates with the fat-filled synovial fold which projects upwards between the articular surfaces. On autopsy material this fat pad has been seen to move in and out of the lumbar apophyseal joint during passive movement (McFadden and Taylor, 1990). It is suggested that the fat pad acts as a dampening and lubricating mechanism.

2. *Synovial folds* are the largest intra-articular inclusion. These folds enclose fat, collagen and blood vessels and may project 5 mm into the joint cavity. The synovial folds are innervated and may be a source of pain when irritated by degenerative changes or trauma (Giles and Taylor, 1987). In the young, these folds are able to adapt easily to the changing shape of the joint during movement, assisting lubrication and secreting synovial fluid essential to articular cartilage nutrition (Giles and Taylor, 1982). In older individuals the folds become stiffer, are more triangular in shape and their tips become fibrous where they are compressed between joint margins.

3. The *connective tissue rim* is the smallest identified structure. It is a wedge-shaped thickening of the internal surface of the capsule, filling the space left by the curved margins of the articular cartilage. This structure can increase the surface area of contact when the articular facets are impacted, thereby transmitting some loads (Lewin et al, 1962).

Articular facets

Each lumbar apophyseal joint is formed by the articulation of the inferior facets of one lumbar vertebra with the superior facets of the subjacent vertebra. The articular processes contain cancellous bone but their shell of cortical bone is thicker than that of the vertebral bodies.

The shape and orientation of the lumbar facets varies, thereby affecting the direction and range of movement of a motion segment. The orientation of these joints is an important factor in preventing forward displacement and rotatory dislocation of the intervertebral joint.

If the facets of the joints are viewed from behind, the joint surfaces appear to be straight. However, when viewed from above in the transverse plane, the facets may be seen to be curved or flat (Fig. 1.24). The curved superior articular facets have been described as having a J shape or a C shape. Horwitz and Smith (1940) found that curved joints predominated between the 1st and 2nd, 2nd and 3rd, and 3rd and 4th lumbar vertebrae, but flat joints were more common between the 4th and 5th vertebrae and at the lumbo-sacral junction.

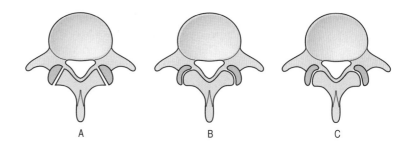

Figure 1.24 Variations in curvature of lumbar apophyseal joints. A, Flat joints. B, C-shaped joints. C, J-shaped joints. (Adapted from Horowitz T, Smith RM 1940 An anatomical, pathological and roentgenological study of the intervertebral joints of the lumbar spine and of the sacroiliac joints. *American Journal of Roentgenology and Radium Therapy* 43: 174–186.)

Orientation of a lumbar apophyseal joint is defined by the angle between the average plane of the joint with respect to the sagittal plane. In joints with flat articular facets, the plane of the joint is parallel to the line of the facets. In curved joints, the average plane is taken as a line through the anteromedial and posterolateral ends of the joint surfaces.

The angle between the plane of the facet joints and the sagittal plane varies between individuals and in any individual it varies at different spinal levels. The larger the angle, the more the joints tend to face in the frontal plane. This is more common at the lower two lumbar levels (Fig. 1.25).

In flat (planar) apophyseal joints, where the superior articular facets face backwards and medially, the facets resist forward displacement. If the upper vertebra moves forward, its inferior facets impinge upon the superior articular facets of the vertebra below. The more the joint is

Figure 1.25 Variations in orientation of lumbar apophyseal joints. A, Joints orientated in the frontal plane strongly resist forward displacement. B, Joints orientated in the sagittal plane are less able to resist forward displacement. C, Joints orientated in the frontal plane are less able to resist rotation. D, Joints orientated in the sagittal plane strongly resist rotation. (Adapted from Bogduk N, Twomey LT 1987 *Clinical Anatomy of the Lumbar Spine.* Churchill Livingstone, Edinburgh, p. 27.)

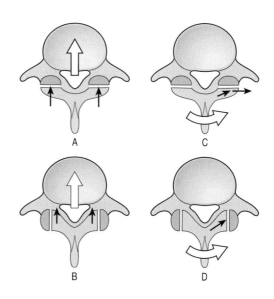

orientated in the frontal plane, the more it resists forward displacement; however, these joints are less able to resist axial rotation.

The more the joint is orientated in the sagittal plane, the more it can resist rotation; however, these joints are less able to resist forward displacement.

In joints with curved articular facets, different parts of the articular surfaces resist different movements. In curved joints, the anteromedial end of the superior facet that faces backwards resists forward displacement. C-shaped joints have a greater surface area and offer greater resistance to forward displacement than J-shaped joints. Both C- and J-shaped joints resist rotation well.

Load-bearing

Opinion is divided as to the degree to which the lumbar apophyseal joints are weight-bearing in the erect posture. It has been reported that the axial load sustained by the apophyseal joints is 28% (Lorenz et al, 1983), 40% (Hakim and King, 1976), 16% (Hutton and Adams, 1980), and 25% (Yang and King, 1984). These differences may be in part due to variations in experimental design and differing appreciation of the apophyseal joints and their behaviour in axial compression. In the normal erect posture, if the articular surfaces are viewed in the sagittal and coronal planes, the facets lie parallel to each other. Bogduk and Twomey (1987) suggest that in axial compression the facets slide relative to one another and, as they do not impact, they are not involved in load-bearing. Studies have yet to address the frequency with which the spine is loaded in positions of flexion and extension, particularly during vigorous sporting activities.

Chondromalacia, with splitting of the articular cartilage on the coronally orientated section of the superior articular facet, and thickening of the subchondral bone are common in young people (Twomey and Taylor, 1987). This indicates that the superior articular facets are subjected to weight-bearing forces.

During full flexion, the force pathway is from the superior articular facet through the pars inter-articularis to the inferior articular facet. The greatest force is sustained by the pars inter-articularis and in adolescents high levels of stress in this area are associated with spondylolysis (a stress fracture) (Taylor and Twomey, 1994b). The forces borne by the lumbar apophyseal joints during a road traffic accident are similar to those sustained in full flexion, and small articular fractures frequently accompany capsule tears and strains (Twomey et al, 1989). If the normal postural alignment of the facet joints is altered, the apophyseal joints may then become involved in the weight-bearing process. This situation may occur if a vertebral body rocks backwards on the subjacent intervertebral disc without also sliding backwards, so that the tips of the inferior articular processes impact onto the superior articular facets of the vertebra below. During vertical compression, some of the load will be transferred through the area of impact, usually the inferior medial portion of the facets. Dunlop et al (1984) demonstrated that the inferomedial portion of the facets is the site where maximal pressure is sustained when the vertebrae are loaded in extension.

Narrowing of the intervertebral discs due to severe sustained axial compression or degenerative changes can cause the inferior facets to impact on the lamina of the vertebra below. In normal extension the fat pad at the inferior recess reduces the stresses on the lamina, but in rapid extension the sudden impingement of the tip of the inferior articular process imposes stress on the lamina below and may be responsible for the sclerotic changes observed there. There may be greater loading on the facets of those individuals with an increased lumbar lordosis. Experimentation has shown that in the lordotic spine during prolonged standing, the impacted joints at each segmental level bear an average 16% of the axial load (Adams and Hutton, 1983), but that the lower joints (L3/4, L4/5, L5/S1) take approximately 19% of the load, while the L1/2 and L2/3 joints bear approximately 11% of the load (Adams and Hutton, 1980).

Adams and Hutton (1983) also estimated that pathological disc space narrowing might result in up to 70% of the axial load being transmitted through the articular processes and laminae.

Joints involved in weight-bearing are more prone to degenerative changes; therefore, if weight-bearing occurs through the apophyseal joints, there is a greater risk of a pathological condition developing.

Tropism (Fig. 1.26)

Articular tropism is asymmetrical orientation of the apophyseal joints so that at one vertebral level the plane of one apophyseal joint is more inclined in the frontal or sagittal plane than the plane of the contralateral apophyseal joint. It is most common at the lowest two lumbar levels (Cyron and Hutton, 1980), and it is reported to occur in one quarter of human spines (Grieve, 1989). Tropism causes imbalanced movement between facets (Kraft and Levinthal, 1951) and probably leads to altered spinal mechanics of the segment (Lippitt, 1984). Premature degenerative changes often occur at vertebral levels where tropism is present (Cyron and Hutton, 1980).

Tropism has been linked with rotational instability that puts the ligaments of the apophyseal joint under strain (Cyron and Hutton, 1980).

Figure 1.26   Tropism of the 5th lumbar vertebra – superior aspect. X–X', plane of sagittally orientated facet. Y–Y', plane of coronally orientated facet.

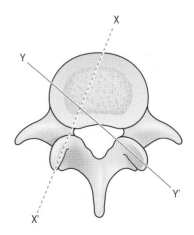

This may lead to a rotation strain of the disc as more stress is placed on the intervertebral disc on the side of the more obliquely orientated apophyseal joint. When flexion occurs in the presence of tropism it will usually do so about some oblique axis X–X' (see Fig. 1.26), so that the capsular ligaments will be equidistant from the axis of rotation. Flexion about X–X' causes maximum stretching of the posterior lateral annulus; hence, posterolateral tears will usually be on the side of the more oblique facet. In studies done by Farfan and Sullivan (1967), there was a high correlation between the side of the more oblique facet and the side of sciatica. In studies of CT scans, Taylor and Twomey (1994b) found joint angle asymmetry of 10° or more in 22% of controls and 28% of back pain patients. In only 3.5% of instances was the difference between the right and left joint angle greater than 20°, and this was observed in 8.8% of controls and 14% of low back pain patients. Taylor and Twomey also noted that this degree of tropism is more common in younger patients than in older patients suggesting a developmental origin for the larger degrees of tropism.

L5/S1 apophyseal joint

In the standing position, the lordotic curve of the lumbar spine places particular stress on the L5/S1 junction. The wedge-shaped disc and body of L5 create a tendency for L5 to slide forward on the sacrum. The inferior process of L5, instead of facing laterally and slightly anteriorly, as in the typical lumbar vertebra, may tend to face more anteriorly, thereby forming a more effective 'hook' to prevent a forward slip.

Nerve supply

Each joint receives a multiple innervation from a dorsal ramus of a spinal nerve and two medial branches of a dorsal ramus. The capsules are richly innervated with encapsulated and free nerve endings, and can, therefore, transmit proprioceptive and nociceptive information.

PALPATION OF THE LUMBAR SPINE (Fig. 1.27)

In 60% of subjects, the iliac crests are level with the L4/5 interspace. In 20%, they are level with the vertebral body of L4, and in the remaining 20% they are level with the body of L5. Using the level of the iliac crests to identify a spinous process is not, therefore, always accurate.

The following bony points may be palpable:

1. *Spinous processes.* These may be palpated with the patient in prone- or side-lying. The small, blunted tip of the L5 spinous process lies in the lumbosacral depression and the therapist's thumbs usually need to be slightly angled caudally in order to palpate its 'posteroanterior' movement. In some individuals the spinous process of L5 may be difficult to find and, in order to confirm palpation findings, the therapist may need to have the patient in side-lying to palpate the interspinous space between L5 and the sacrum by flexing the lumbar spine to feel if gapping occurs.

Figure 1.27   Palpation points in the lumbar spine. A, Lateral aspect. B, Posterior aspect.

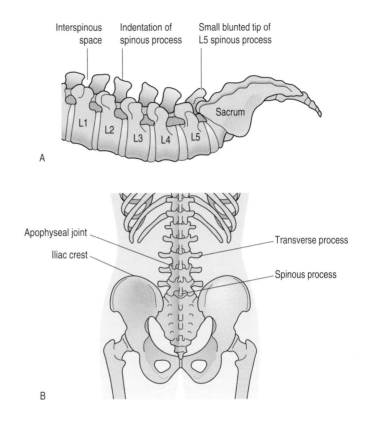

The remaining spinous processes are larger and may be indented, so care needs to be taken to clarify whether the therapist is actually on one of these indentations rather than an interspinous space. Palpating the lateral aspect of the spinous process may help, or gapping the joints as described above.

2. *The interspinous spaces*. In a healthy spine, the interspinous spaces are easily palpable. In patients who have chronic degenerative changes in the lumbar spine, or who have performed excessive exercise over a period of time, the spinous processes may almost appear to be joined together due to chronic ligamentous thickening, and the interspinous spaces are less obvious.

3. *Apophyseal joints*. Except in slim patients, the apophyseal joints may be difficult to palpate in this region. However, if one of these joints has marked degenerative changes with swelling, it can be more easily located. They lie just lateral to the lower third of the spinous process, i.e. the L3/4 apophyseal joint lies level with the lower third of L3's spinous process. At the L5/S1 level, the joints lie slightly more laterally and caudally than above.

4. *Transverse processes*. Approximately 4–5 cm lateral to the spinous processes, the tips of the transverse processes lie level with the interspinous space, i.e. the tip of L3's transverse process lies level with the

L2/3 interspinous space. The length of the transverse processes increases from L1 to L3, then decreases again.

Soft tissue palpation

Immediately under the skin is a layer of superficial fat, and beneath that is the posterior layer of the thoracolumbar fascia. Thickening and reduced mobility of the connective tissues can often be palpated in those with lumbar spine dysfunction. The contractile elements of the superficial erector spinae are only present in the mid and upper lumbar spine. Paravertebrally, in the lower lumbar spine, the thick erector spinae aponeurosis, which has an extensive attachment onto the sacrum, can be palpated. Deep to the erector spinae aponeurosis are the bulk of the multifidus and deep erector spinae muscles bilaterally. Segmental wasting of multifidus may be palpated in those with long-standing low back pain.

References

Adams MA, Hutton WC (1983) The mechanical function of the lumbar apophyseal joints. *Spine* 8: 327.

Adams MA, Hutton WC, Stott JRR (1980) The resistance to flexion of the lumbar intervertebral joints. *Spine* 5: 3, 245.

Andriacchi T, Schultz A, Beltyschko T, Galante J (1974) A model for studies of mechanical interactions between the human spine and rib cage. *Journal of Biomechanics* 7: 497–507

Arkin AM (1949) The mechanism of the structural changes in postural scoliosis. *Journal of Bone and Joint Surgery (Am)* 31A: 519–528.

Bogduk N, Jull G (1985) The theoretical pathology of acute locked back: a basis for manipulative therapy. *Manual Medicine* 1: 78–82.

Bogduk N, Twomey LT (1987) *Clinical Anatomy of the Lumbar Spine*. Churchill Livingstone, Edinburgh, p. 43.

Boreadis AG, Gershon-Cohen J (1956) Luschka joints of the cervical spine. *Radiology* 66: 181.

Brain, Lord, Wilkinson M, eds (1967) *Cervical Spondylosis*. William Heinemann Medical Books, London.

Clark CC (1988) Cervical spondylitic myelopathy: history and physical findings. *Spine* 13: 847.

Cyron BM, Hutton WC (1980) Articular tropism and stability of the lumbar spine. *Spine* 5: 168–172.

Davis PR (1959) The medial inclination of the human thoracic intervertebral articular facets. *Journal of Anatomy* 93: 68.

Dunlop RB, Adams MA, Hutton WC (1984) Disc space narrowing and the lumbar facets. *Journal of Bone and Joint Surgery (Br.)* 66-B: 706.

Dvorak J, Panjabi MM (1987) Functional anatomy of the alar ligaments. *Spine* 12: 183–189.

Edgelow PI (1997) Neurovascular consequences of cumulative trauma affecting the thoracic outlet: a patient-centered treatment approach. In: Donatelli RA (ed.) *Physical Therapy of the Shoulder*. Churchill Livingstone, New York, pp.153–178.

Edmondston SJ, Singer KP (1997) Thoracic spine: anatomical and biomechanical considerations for manual therapy. *Manual Therapy* 2: 132–143.

Farfan HF, Sullivan JD (1967) The relation of facet orientation to intervertebral disc failure. *Canadian Journal of Surgery* 10: 179.

Ferdinand R, Fox DE (1985) Evaluation of lumbar lordosis. A prospective and retrospective study. *Spine* 10: 799.

Fielding JW (1957) Cineroentgenography of the normal cervical spine. *Journal of Bone and Joint Surgery (Am)* 39A: 1280.

Gilad I, Nissan M (1985) Sagittal evaluation of elemental geometrical dimensions of human vertebrae. *Journal of Anatomy* 143: 115.

Giles LGF, Singer KP (2000) *Clinical Anatomy and Management of Thoracic Spine Pain*. Butterworth Heinemann, Oxford, p. 25.

Giles LGF, Taylor JR (1981) Low back pain associated with leg length inequality. *Spine* 6: 510.

Giles LGF, Taylor JR (1982) Intra-articular protrusions in the lower lumbar apophyseal joints. *Bulletin of the Hospital for Joint Diseases* XLII: 248–254.

Giles LGF, Taylor JR (1984) The effect of postural scoliosis on lumbar apophyseal joints. *Scandinavian Journal of Rheumatology* 13: 209.

Giles LGF, Taylor JT (1987) Human zygapophyseal joint capsule and synovial fold innervation. *British Journal of Rheumatology* 26: 93–98.

Gitman L, Kamholtz T (1965) Incidence of radiographic osteoporosis in a large series of aged individuals. *Journal of Gerontology* 20: 32–33

Goh S, Price RI, Leedman PJ, Singer KP (1999) The relative influence of vertebral body and intervertebral disk shape on the thoracic kyphosis. *Clinical Biomechanics* 14: 439–448.

Golub BS, Silverman B (1969) Transforaminal ligaments of the lumbar spine. *Journal of Bone and Joint Surgery (Am)* 51-A: 947.

Grieve GP, ed. (1986) *Modern Manual Therapy*. Churchill Livingstone, Edinburgh, Ch. 8.

Grieve GP (1989) *Common Vertebral Joint Problems*, 2nd edn. Churchill Livingstone, Edinburgh, p. 426.

Grundy PF, Roberts CJ (1984) Does unequal leg length cause back pain? *Lancet* 2: 256–258.

Hadley LA (1957) The uncovertebral articulations and cervical foramen encroachment. *Journal of Bone and Joint Surgery (Am)* 39A: 910.

Hakim NS, King AI (1976). Static and dynamic facet loads. Proceedings of the Twentieth Stapp Car Crash Conference, pp. 607–639.

Hamilton W (1976) *Textbook of Human Anatomy*, 2nd edn. Macmillan, London.

Hansson T, Bigos S, Beecher P, Wortley M (1985a). The lumbar lordosis in acute and chronic low back pain. *Spine* 10: 154–155.

Hansson T, Sandstrom J, Roos B, Jonson R, Andersson GB (1985b) The bone mineral content of the lumbar spine in patients with chronic low-back pain. *Spine* 10: 158–160.

Hellems HK, Keates TE (1971) Measurement of the normal lumbosacral angle. *American Journal of Roentgenology* 113: 642.

Hijioka A, Suzuki K, Nakamura T, Yokoyama M, Kanazawa Y (1994) Light and electron microscopy of hydroxyapatite depositions in the ligamentum flavum. *Spine* 19: 2626–2631.

Hirsch C, Schajowicz F, Galante J (1967) Structural changes in the cervical spine. *Acta Orthopaedica Scandinavica Supplementum* 109: 9.

Horwitz T, Smith RM (1940) An anatomical, pathological and roentgenological study of the intervertebral joints of the lumbar spine and of the sacro-iliac joints. *American Journal of Roentgenology* 43: 173.

Huelke D F, Nusholz GS (1986) Cervical spine biomechanics: a review of the literature. *Journal of Orthopaedics* 109: 42.

Hukins DWL, Kirby MC, Sikoryn TA, Aspden RM, Cox AJ (1990) Comparison of the structure, mechanical properties, and functional lumbar spinal ligaments. *Spine* 15: 787–795.

Hutton WC, Adams MA(1980) The forces acting on the neural arch and their relevance to low back pain. In Engineering Aspects of the Spine. Mechanical Engineering Publications, London, pp. 49–55.

Hytten FE, Leitch J (1971) *The Physiology of Human Pregnancy*, 3rd edn. Blackwell Scientific, Oxford.

Kaplan E (1945) The surgical and anatomic significance of the mammillary tubercle of the last thoracic vertebra. *Surgery* 17: 78–92.

Kashiwagi K (1993) Histological changes of the lumbar ligamentum flavum with age. *Nippon Seikeigeka Gakkai Zasshi* B67: 221–229.

Kendall F, McCreary EK, Provance PG (1993) *Muscles. Testing and Function*. 4th edn. Williams and Wilkins, Baltimore.

Koeller W, Meier W, Hartmann F (1984) Biomechanical properties of the human intervertebral discs subjected to axial dynamic compression. A comparison of lumbar and thoracic discs. *Spine* 9: 725.

Kraft GL, Levinthal DH (1951) Facet synovial impingement. A new concept in the etiology of lumbar vertebral derangement. *Surgery Gynaecology Obstetrics* 93: 439.

Kramer J (1981) *Intervertebral Disc Lesions: Causes, Diagnosis, Treatment and Prophylaxis*. Georg Thieme Verlag, Stuttgart.

Lewin T, Moffet B, Vildik A (1962) The morphology of the lumbar synovial intervertebral joints. *Acta Morphologica Neerlando-Scandinavia* 4: 299–317.

Lippitt AB (1984) The facet joint and its role in spine pain. Management with facet joint injections. *Spine* 9: 746–750.

Lonstein JE, Carlson JM (1984) The prediction of curve progression in untreated idiopathic scoliosis during growth. *Journal of Bone and Joint Surgery (Am)* 66A: 1061–1071.

Lorenz M, Patwardham A, Vanderby R (1983) Load-bearing characteristics of lumbar facets in normal and surgically altered spinal segments. *Spine* 8: 122.

Luk KDK, Ho HC, Leong JYC 1986 The iliolumbar ligament: a study of its anatomy development and clinical significance. *Journal of Bone and Joint Surgery (Br.)* 68: 197–200.

Malmivaara A, Videman T, Kuosma E, Troup JD (1987) Zygapophyseal joint orientation, zygapophyseal and costovertebral joint osteoarthrosis, disc degeneration, vertebral body osteophytosis and Schmorl's nodes in the thoracolumbar junctional region of cadaveric spines. *Spine* 12: 458–463.

Manns RA, Haddaway MJ, McCall IW, Cassar Pullicino V, Davie MW (1996) The relative contribution of disc and vertebral morphometry to the angle of the thoracic kyphosis in asymptomatic subjects. *Clinical Radiology* 51: 258–262.

McFadden KD, Taylor JT (1990) Axial rotation in the lumbar spine and gaping of the zygapophyseal joints. *Spine* 15: 295–299.

Mercer S (1994) The menisci of the cervical synovial joints. In: Boying JD, Palastanga N (eds) *Grieve's Modern Manual Therapy*, 2nd edn. Churchill Livingstone, Edinburgh pp. 69–72.

Milne JS, Lauder IJ (1974) Age effects in kyphosis and lordosis in adults. *Annals of Human Biology* 1: 327–337.

Morris JM, Lucas DB, Bresler B (1961) Role of the trunk in stability of the spine. *Journal of Bone and Joint Surgery (Am)* 43, 327.

Nachemson A, Evans JH (1968) Some mechanical properties of the third lumbar interlaminar ligament (ligamentum flavum). *Journal of Biomechanics* 1: 211.

Nachemson A, Sahlstrand T (1977) Etiologic factors in adolescent idiopathic scoliosis. *Spine* 2: 176–184.

Nakagawa H, Mikawa Y, Watanabe R (1994) Elastin in the human posterior longitudinal ligament and spinal dura mater. *Spine* 19: 2164–2169.

Neumann P, Keller T, Ekstrom L, Hult E, Hansson T (1993) Structural properties of the anterior longitudinal ligament. Correlation with the lumbar bone mineral content. *Spine* 18: 637–645.

Oda I, Abumi K, Duosai L, Shono Y, Kaneda K (1996) Biomechanical role of the posterior elements, costovertebral joints, and rib cage in the stability of the thoracic spine. *Spine* 21: 1423–1429.

O'Rahilly R (1986) *Anatomy: A Regional Study of Human Structure*. WB Saunders, Philadelphia.

Orofino C, Sherman MS, Schechter D (1960). Luschka's joint – a degenerative phenomenon. *American Journal of Orthopedics* 42-A: 853–8.

Palastanga N, Field D, Soames R (1989) *Anatomy and Human Movement*. Heinemann Medical, Oxford, p. 796.

Panjabi MM, Brand RA, White AA (1976) Three dimensional flexibility and stiffness properties of the human thoracic spine. *Journal of Biomechanics* 9: 185–192.

Panjabi MM, Hausfield JN, White AA (1981) A biomechanical study of the ligamentous stability of the thoracic spine in man. *Acta Orthopaedica Scandinavica* 52(4): 315–326.

Patriquin DA (1983) The mechanical aetiology of Tietze's syndrome. British Association of Manual Medicine. Newsletter, 5th November.

Pearcy MJ (1985) Stereo radiography of lumbar spine motion. *Acta Orthopaedica Scandinavica Supplementum* 56: 3–41.

Pettman E (1994) Stress tests of the craniovertebral joints. In: Boyling JD, Palastanga N (eds) *Grieve's Modern Manual Therapy*, 2nd edn. Churchill Livingstone, Edinburgh.

Ramsey RH (1966) The anatomy of the ligamenta flava. *Clinical Orthopaedics and Related Research* 44: 129–140.

Rickenbacher J, Landolt AM, Theiler K (1985) *Applied Anatomy of the Back*. Springer-Verlag, Berlin, pp. 93, 184–186.

Riggs BL, Wahner HW, Melton LJ III, Richelson LS, Judd HL, Offord KP (1986) Rates of bone loss in appendicular and axial skeletons of women: evidence of substantial vertebral bone loss before menopause. *Journal of Clinical Investigation* 77: 1487–1491.

Rissanen PM (1960) The surgical anatomy and pathology of the supraspinous and interspinous ligaments of the lumbar spine with special reference to ligament ruptures. *Acta Orthopaedica Scandinavica Supplementum* 46: 1–100.

Roaf R (1960) A study of the mechanics of spinal injuries. *Journal of Bone and Joint Surgery (Br.)* 42: 810.

Schmorl G, Junghanns H (1971) *The Human Spine in Health and Disease*, 2nd American edn. Grune and Stratton, New York.

Shea KG, Schlegel JD, Bachus KN, Dunn HK, West JR (1996) The contribution of the rib cage to thoracic stability. In: Proceedings: International Society for the Study of the Lumbar Spine, Vermont: p. 50.

Shellshear JL, Macintosh NWG (1949) The transverse process of the fifth lumbar vertebra. In: Shellshear JL, Macintosh NWG (eds) *Surveys of Anatomical Fields*. Grahame, Sydney, pp. 21–32.

Singer KP (1989) The thoracolumbar mortice joint. Radiological and histological observations. *Clinical Biomechanics* 4: 137–143.

Singer KP (1997) Pathoanatomy of the thoracolumbar transitional junction. In: Giles LGF, Singer KP (eds) Clinical Anatomy and Management of low Back Pain. Butterworth Heinemann, Oxford, pp. 183–195.

Singer KP, Edmonson SJ, Day RE, Breidahl WH (1994) Computer-assisted and Cobb angle determination of the thoracic kyphosis: An in-vivo and in-vitro comparison. *Spine* 19: 1381–1384.

Singh I (1978) The architecture of cancellous bone. *Journal of Anatomy* 127, 305–310.

Taylor JR, Twomey LT (1987). The lumbar spine from infancy to old age. In: Twomey LT, Taylor JR (eds) *Physical Therapy of the Low Back*. Churchill Livingstone, New York, Ch. 1.

Taylor JR, Twomey LT (1994a) Functional and applied anatomy of the cervical spine. In: Grant R (ed.) *Physical Therapy of the Cervical and Thoracic Spine*. Churchill Livingstone, New York, pp. 1–25.

Taylor JR, Twomey LT (1994b) Structure and function of the lumbar zygapophyseal (facet) joints. In: Boyling JD, Palastanga N (eds) *Grieve's Modern Manual Therapy*. Churchill Livingstone, Edinburgh, Ch. 8.

Tietze A (1921) Über eine eigenartige Häufung von Fallen mit Dystrophie der Rippenknorpel. *Berliner Klinische Wochenshrift* 58: 829.

Torgerson WR, Dotter WE (1976) Comparative roentgenographic study of the asymptomatic and symptomatic lumbar spine. *Journal of Bone and Joint Surgery (Am.)* 58-A: 850.

Troup JDG (1975) The biology of back pain. *New Scientist* 65: 17.

Twomey LT, Taylor JR, eds (1987) *Physical Therapy of the Low Back*. Churchill Livingstone, New York, Ch. 2, p. 55.

Twomey LT, Taylor JR (1994) Functional and applied anatomy of the cervical spine. In: Grant R (ed.) *Physical Therapy of the Cervical and Thoracic Spine*, 2nd edn. Churchill Livingstone, New York, p. 8.

Twomey LT, Taylor JR, Taylor M (1989) Acute injuries to the lumbar zygapophyseal joints. *Australian Medical Journal* 151: 210–217.

Vallois HV (1926) Arthologie. In: Nicholas A (ed.) *Poirier and Charpy's Traite d'Anatomie Humaine*, Vol. 1. Masson, Paris, p. 68.

Van Roy P, Caboor D, De Boelpaep S, Barbaix E, Clarys JP (1997) Left-right asymmetries and other common anatomical variants of the first cervical vertebra. *Manual Therapy* 2: 24–36.

Von Luschka H (1858) *Die Halbenke des menschlichen Körpers. Eine Monographie*. Reimer, Berlin.

White AA (1969) Analysis of the mechanics of the thoracic spine in man. *Acta Orthopaedica Scandinavica Supplementum* 127: 1–105.

Willard FH (1997) The muscular, ligamentous and neural structure of the low back and its relation to back pain. In: Vleeming A, Mooney V, Dorman T, Snijders C, Stoeckart R (eds) *Movement Stability and Low Back Pain. The Essential Role of the Pelvis*. Churchill Livingstone, pp. 4–14.

Williams PL (1995) *Gray's Anatomy: The Anatomical Basis of Medicine and Surgery*. Churchill Livingstone, Edinburgh.

Williams P, Warwick R (1980) *Gray's Anatomy*, 36th edn. Churchill Livingstone, London, p. 277.

Yahia LH, Garzon S, Strykowski H, Rivard CH (1990) Ultrastructure of the human interspinous ligament and ligamentum flavum. *Spine* 15: 262–268.

Yamamoto I, Panjabi MM, Oxland TR, Crisco JJ (1990) The role of the iliolumbar ligament in the lumbosacral junction. *Spine* 15: 1138–1141.

Yang KM, King AI (1984) Mechanism of facet load transmission as an hypothesis for back pain. *Spine* 9: 557.

Chapter 2

Intervertebral discs

CHAPTER CONTENTS

The intervertebral discs play a vital role in the normal function of the spine, yet their importance in relation to spinal pathology was high-lighted only as recently as 1934 by Mixter and Barr.

Adjacent vertebrae from the 2nd cervical to the sacrum are linked by the annular fibres of the discs, and they may be likened to sophisticated ligaments, the joints that they form being the interbody joints. The gross and microscopic structures of the discs reflect how these fibres fulfil their two main functions, which are to allow and restrain movements at the interbody joints, and to act as the prime component in the transmission of loads from one vertebral body to the next. An account of the development of the intervertebral discs is given in Chapter 9.

GROSS STRUCTURE OF THE INTERVERTEBRAL DISC

The two basic components of the disc are the annulus fibrosus (outer part) and the nucleus pulposus (inner part).

ANNULUS FIBROSUS
(Figs. 2.1 to 2.3)

The annulus fibrosus is a composite structure consisting of concentric layers or lamellae of collagen fibres, encapsulating the nucleus pulposus, and a proteoglycan gel, which binds the collagen fibres and lamellae firmly together to prevent them from buckling. The outer annular fibres are formed from fairly coarse collagen fibres and attach to the outer margins of adjacent vertebral bodies. In a child the outer annular fibres attach to the edge of the cartilage plate; in an adolescent they attach to the ring apophysis; and in an adult they attach to the outer vertebral

Figure 2.1   Concentric bands of annular fibres.

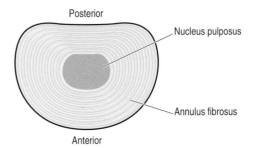

Figure 2.2   Horizontal section through a disc.

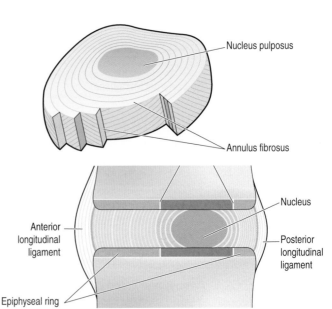

Figure 2.3   Attachment of annular fibres.

ring. There are few cells and little matrix between the collagen fibres of the outer annulus and there is a relatively low content of glycosamino-glycans (GAGs; Taylor et al, 1992). The inner annular fibres completely enclose the nucleus pulposus and are continuous with the lamellar structure of the cartilage end plates.

The annular fibres are parallel to each other and the majority of them run obliquely between the two vertebrae, lying in opposite directions in adjacent lamellae. This laminated arrangement is essential to the biomechanical properties of the fibres and function of the disc: it permits angular movements (flexion-extension, lateral flexion) while providing stability against shear and torsion. Each fibre extends for approximately half of the circumference of the disc, providing some control over rotatory movements. At the end of rotation to one side, half of the total number of annular fibres are stressed – those angled in the direction of the movement – while the other half are relaxed. The laminated structure of the annulus is complex. At any 20° sector of the annulus, at least 40% of the annular layers have been found to be incomplete, the posterolateral area containing the maximum percentage of incomplete layers (Marchand and Ahmed, 1990).

The angle of the annular fibres in relation to the horizontal can vary between 40° and 70°, depending on their position in the annulus. This angle changes on loading (Pearcy and Tibrewal, 1984) and becomes more acute (see Fig. 2.11. p. 78) providing the annulus with an elasticity in compression.

The increased collagen content of the outer lamellae is thought to provide additional strength in torsion as well as in flexion, extension and lateral flexion because greater stress falls on the outer lamellae than on the inner lamellae during these movements (Eyre, 1979).

In the posterior part of the disc, the fibres differ from the rest of the annulus in that they have a more parallel arrangement. Here also the lamellae are thinner, more tightly packed, and have less binding gel. In addition, in the lumbar spine, the anterior and lateral portions of the annulus are approximately twice as thick as the posterior portion. These factors combine to make the posterior annulus a weak area, predisposing it to degenerative change and trauma. Greater protection is afforded to the discs in the upper lumbar spine than in the lower, because the posterior annulus there tends to be thicker and stronger.

Attached to the surface of the outer annular fibres are the anterior and posterior longitudinal ligaments (see pp. 47–48), the latter of which is thinner in the lumbar region than in other spinal regions. The outer annular fibres are almost indistinguishable from the longitudinal ligaments, but the annular fibres attach to adjacent vertebrae while the longitudinal ligaments bridge several segments. Blood vessels pass between the annular fibres and the ligaments and send a few tributaries to the outer annulus (Giles and Singer, 1997).

NUCLEUS PULPOSUS
(See Fig. 2.3)

The nucleus pulposus is a semi-fluid gel comprising 40–60% of the disc. At birth, the gel consists of mucoid material with a few notochordal cells and is distinct from the surrounding annulus. After the first decade, the mucoid material is gradually replaced by fibrocartilage (Sylvén, 1951) and there is less distinction between it and the annulus. At birth the water content of the nucleus is 88%; this reduces to 76% in the young adult. In adults, a normal intervertebral disc still has a relatively high water content.

High-power microscopic examination shows that a small area of the nucleus pulposus has a random collagen network. Low-power microscopic examination shows that there is some organization in the orientation of the collagen bundles. In the upper and lower parts of the nucleus the bundles are parallel to the cartilage end plates; in the area where the annulus and nucleus merge, loose, poorly formed bundles are convex inwards towards the centre of the nucleus. In the centre there are a few loosely arranged vertical bundles (Giles and Singer, 1997).

Being a fluid, the nucleus can be deformed under pressure without a reduction in volume. This essential property enables it both to accommodate to movement and to transmit some of the compressive load from one vertebra to the next.

The position of the nucleus varies in the different regions of the spine. In the thoracic region it lies centrally within the disc, whereas in the cervical and lumbar regions it is positioned more posteriorly.

VERTEBRAL END PLATES (Fig. 2.4)

Thin end plates separate the discs from their adjacent vertebral bodies. At the periphery of the cartilage plate a bony ring apophysis fuses with the centrum and forms the hard bony rim of the vertebral end plate. The larger central hyaline cartilage plate is part of the envelope that surrounds the nucleus. In the young, the end plates consist of both hyaline cartilage and fibrocartilage. Histologically, they are considered to be part of the disc, but during the growth period they are responsible for the growth in depth of the vertebral body. The disc side of the end plate, to which the inner annular lamellae are firmly anchored, is fibrocartilage, the vertebral body side being hyaline cartilage in young discs.

The end plates have two important functions. The first is related to the nutrition of the disc: they form a permeable barrier through which water and nutrients can pass between the nucleus pulposus and the cancellous bone of the vertebral bodies. Secondly, they play a mechanical role in

Figure 2.4   Horizontal section showing the cartilage end plate and epiphyseal ring, which is wider anteriorly.

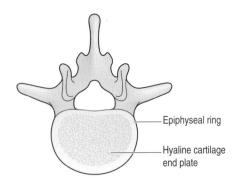

Epiphyseal ring

Hyaline cartilage end plate

preventing the nucleus bulging into the vertebral body (Urban, 1989, written communication). The end plates are approximately 1 mm thick and contribute to the resilience of the motion segment (Giles and Singer, 1997).

During fetal life, the end plates are well vascularized. These blood vessels gradually involute during the first 10–15 years of postnatal life (Taylor and Twomey, 1985), leaving small, weakened areas that make the vertebral body vulnerable to *intra*vertebral disc prolapses from the nucleus. These areas are called Schmorl's nodes (see p. 299). In the adult, approximately 10% of the vertebral end plate is perforated by small vascular buds that are in direct contact with the cartilage plate. There are more vascular contacts centrally than peripherally (Maroudas et al, 1975).

Under high compressive loading, the end plates are the most common site of failure and are, therefore, considered to be the weakest part of the disc.

SHAPE AND HEIGHT OF INTERVERTEBRAL DISCS

Cross-sections through a disc and its adjacent vertebral bodies show that the shape of the disc corresponds to that of the vertebral bodies. It is approximately elliptical with the anteroposterior axis being the minor axis. This particular shape provides some protection against annular failure in flexion, indicating the potential danger of this movement. If the disc had a circular cross-section it would have fewer posterior annular fibres to resist flexion.

The shape of the posterior surface of the disc is variable. It can be flat, rounded or re-entrant (concave; Fig. 2.5). Flattened and re-entrant discs have a greater number of posterior fibres than discs with a rounded posterior surface and are therefore better able to withstand the posterior stretch that occurs in flexion (Hickey and Hukins, 1980). Such discs are more easily damaged by torsional stresses, however, as these tend to be concentrated at the points of maximum curvature. The shape of the posterior surface of the disc is an important factor in determining the pattern of radial fissure formation (see p. 312), particularly in the lower lumbar spine. A study performed on 71 cadaveric discs taken from the lower two

Figure 2.5   Cross-sections of intervertebral discs showing variations in shape of posterior surface.

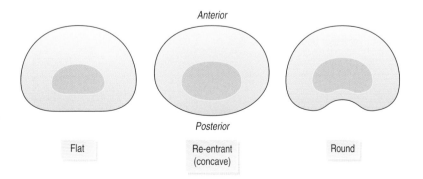

lumbar levels found that the posterior surfaces of 49 were flat, 21 were rounded and 1 was re-entrant (Farfan et al, 1972).

Disc height varies in the different regions of the spine and may also vary in different parts of the same disc. In the cervical and lumbar regions, the discs are wedge-shaped, being deeper anteriorly than posteriorly, thus helping to form the lordotic curves of these regions. The lumbosacral disc shows the greatest wedging with an anterior height approximately 6–7 mm greater than the posterior height (Schmorl and Junghanns, 1971). In the thoracic region the discs are of nearly uniform thickness.

The discs are thickest in the lumbar region, where they are required to bear a greater portion of the body weight, and thinnest in the upper thoracic region. The latter is normally a stiff area of the spine where spondylosis commonly occurs.

Disc height also varies according to factors such as:

Age: There is a progressive loss of height in the spine with increasing age (Wood and Badley, 1983). This is due to loss of height of both the discs and vertebral bodies.

Congenital anomalies: Joints with imperfect segmentation such as lumbarization or sacralization commonly have discs of reduced height, which appear to be developmental rather than degenerative in origin (Farfan, 1973).

Pathology: Marked degeneration in a disc, or prolapsed nuclear material, causes loss of disc height.

Diurnal variation: Overall body height decreases between 15 and 20 mm over a day (de Puky, 1935), principally due to loss of disc height. Prolonged loading of the spine has the same effect. In these instances, normal disc height will return following unloading of the spine (see pp. 79–81).

The height of the disc is an important factor controlling movement at the interbody joint: thicker discs allow more flexion-extension and lateral flexion. It has been proposed that the *ratio* of disc height to vertebral body height (Fig. 2.6) may influence the movement possible in the sagittal plane (Kapandji, 1974). The cervical region is the most mobile with a ratio of disc/body height of 2:5. The lumbar region is slightly less mobile with a ratio of 1:3, and the thoracic region is the least mobile with a ratio

Figure 2.6   Ratio of disc height to vertebral body height.

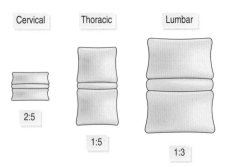

Cervical   Thoracic   Lumbar

2:5

1:5

1:3

of 1:5. Cadaveric studies have failed to identify any correlation between disc/vertebral body height and sagittal mobility in the thoracic spine (White, 1969).

MICROSCOPIC STRUCTURE OF THE INTERVERTEBRAL DISC (Fig. 2.7)

The matrix of the disc principally consists of collagen fibres embedded in a proteoglycan/water gel with some elastic fibres. Also contained within it are chondrocytes and fibroblasts, whose functions are to maintain and repair it. The mean cell density of the disc is low: cells occupy only 1–5% of the tissue volume. The annulus and nucleus both have these constituents, but in different concentrations.

PROTEOGLYCANS

Proteoglycans are found in many of the tissues of the body, but not connective tissues. They are large molecules that have the property of attracting and retaining water. Hence, the amount of proteoglycans in the nucleus (65%) is much greater (particularly in early life) than in the annulus (20%). They are formed of polysaccharide chains consisting mostly of sulphated glycosaminoglycans (GAGs) linked to a central protein core and they are densely packed between collagen fibrils. The two major GAGs in the disc are chondroitin sulphate (CS) and keratin sulphate (KS). CS has twice the water-binding capacity of KS. The proteoglycans in the

Figure 2.7 Schematic view of microscopic structure of intervertebral disc

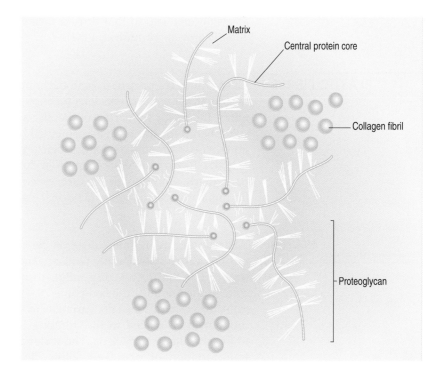

annulus are similar to those in the nucleus, although there are slight structural differences.

The fixed negative charges on CS and KS lead to an excess of cations in the matrix. This, and to a lesser extent the size of the proteoglycans, gives the disc a high osmotic pressure which maintains its fluid content and ensures that it remains inflated even under conditions of high vertical loading. The proteoglycan content of the disc decreases with maturation and degeneration and the ratio of KS to CS increases: fluid is then lost more rapidly under a given load.

COLLAGEN FIBRES

Collagen is the main structural protein of the body. At least 14 genetically distinct types of collagen have been identified. A characteristic fibrillar collagen molecule is formed from three polypeptide chains joined together in a triple helix. The molecules are arranged in a quarter-stagger pattern to form the collagen microfibril (Urban and Roberts, 1994). Inter- and intramolecular cross-links give collagen the property of high tensile strength.

Seven types of collagen have been identified in the disc, but only Types I and II are present in significant proportions. Types I and II are different both chemically and physically, reflecting the particular functions of the annulus (in sustaining tension) and the nucleus (in sustaining compression). Type I collagen (skin and tendon collagen) predominates in the outer annular fibres. This type of collagen gives the annulus considerable *tensile* strength. The fibres are relatively inextensible and will only stretch up to 3% of their length, but increased extensibility on loading is given to the annulus by virtue of the change in angle between fibres in adjacent lamellae, so that during flexion it may effectively 'extend' by 30% (Pearcy and Tibrewal, 1984).

ELASTIC FIBRES

Elastic fibres are present in both the annulus and nucleus with a concentration at the annulus–nucleus junction. Despite the presence of elastic fibres, the elastic properties of the disc are principally due to the hydrostatic nature of the nucleus combined with the ability of the collagen fibres in the annulus to change their orientation. The elastic fibres may help the disc to recover its shape after deformation. This function may be particularly important as the disc, especially the nucleus, becomes more fibrous with age and loses its normal elasticity (Ayad and Weiss, 1987).

WATER

Water is the main constituent of the disc. The water content of the nucleus varies considerably with age and state of health of the disc. It is over 85% in the juvenile disc, falling to approximately 70% in the mature disc. In the annulus, the content is 70–75%, and this remains fairly constant throughout life. This variation in water content across the disc is thought to be related to the differing concentrations of proteoglycans in the annulus and nucleus. The water is mostly extracellular, enabling transportation of dissolved solutes to the chondrocytes. The water content of the disc also varies in response to changes in loading (see pp. 79–81).

The water-binding capacity of the nucleus is of paramount importance in maintaining its elasticity. The rate at which water can pass in and out of the disc is influenced by the concentration of proteoglycans and by changes in intradiscal pressure.

INTRADISCAL PRESSURE

The intervertebral discs have an intrinsic pressure of approximately 0.7 kg/cm^2, even when they are unloaded (Nachemson and Evans, 1968). This 'prestressed' state of the disc provides it with some intrinsic stability. It is due to the compressive effect of the ligamentum flavum, which consists principally of elastic fibres and is at a distance from the motion centre of the disc. When the disc is subjected to external loading, such as body weight or lifting, the resting pressure of the disc rises. The amount of loading depends on a number of factors such as the position of the body (due to the effects of the force of gravity and muscular contraction) and whether or not a weight is being lifted or carried in the hands or on the back. When a vertical load is applied to the disc, the pressure in the nucleus is 50% higher than that applied externally, i.e. a load of 10 kg/cm^2 gives a pressure of 15 kg/cm^2 inside the disc (Nachemson, 1966). Forces acting in the annulus are related to those acting in the nucleus (Nachemson, 1965). The vertical stress in the annulus was calculated to be 50% of the applied external load per unit area, while the tangential, tensile strain was 4–5 times the applied external load, at least in its outer parts.

Intradiscal pressure also rises simply by flexion of the motion segment, whether or not it is loaded, which is surprising since its volume remains the same. In autopsy specimens, when the discs were tilted forward by 8°, the intradiscal pressure was increased by 1.5 kg/cm^2, which corresponds to approximately 20 kg of external load (Nachemson, 1965). This increase is the same whatever load is borne by the disc and is, therefore, more significant proportionately for smaller loads than for larger ones. It is also important to consider the effect of specific exercises for patients with disc disorders. On average, a disc flexed by 5.5° has a nuclear pressure 50% greater than a disc extended by 3° (calculated from Nachemson et al, 1979, by Adams and Hutton, 1983).

EFFECT OF THE POSITION OF THE BODY ON INTRADISCAL PRESSURE

Sitting

In a series of in vivo investigations, Nachemson and Morris (1964) and Nachemson (1966) measured the intradiscal pressures in the 2nd–4th lumbar discs with the subjects in various positions and performing different exercises (Fig. 2.8). The relationship between the positions is of more significance than the absolute values.

The highest intradiscal pressures were recorded in the upright unsupported sitting position, with pressures varying between 100 kg and 180 kg. The load on the disc was shown to be directly related to the body

Figure 2.8 Relative change in pressure (or load) in the 3rd lumbar disc. A, in various positions. B, in various muscle strengthening exercises. (Adapted from Nachemson A 1976. The lumbar spine: an orthopaedic challenge. *Spine* 1: 59–71.)

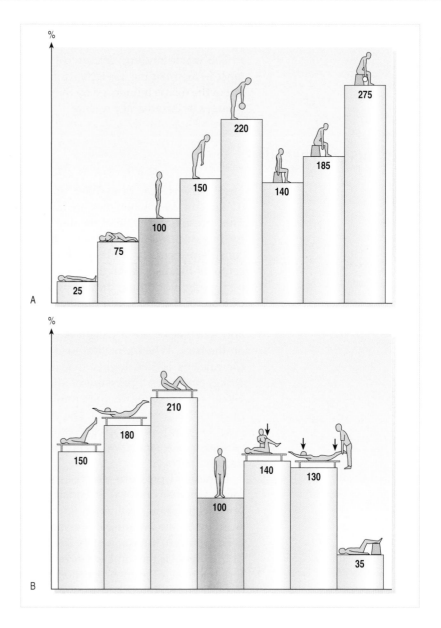

weight above the level of the disc measured, and it was approximately three times that of the body weight above it. The lower the position of the disc in the vertebral column, the greater the load became. Nearly 60% of body weight is above the L4/5 disc (Ruff, 1950).

The relatively high intradiscal pressure in the sitting position is partly due to the activity of the vertebral portion of psoas major, which has a stabilizing influence on the lumbar spine but at the same time exerts a compressive force. Psoas activity contributes a considerable load in addition to gravitational forces. In the sitting position on a horizontal surface, the lumbar spine is usually in some degree of flexion, increasing the intradiscal pressure as well as transferring the load from the apophyseal joints onto the discs.

In Nachemson's experiments, when the subjects leaned forward 20°, the load on the disc was increased by 40–60 kg. Although psoas activity was reduced, activity in erector spinae increased considerably in order to prevent the trunk from falling further forward and thereby had a compressive effect on the discs. The method used did not permit measurements of intradiscal pressure at angles exceeding 20°.

There are many postures that can be assumed when sitting, and the intradiscal pressure varies accordingly. These are considered, together with the effect of intradiscal pressure of lever arms and using a backrest, in Chapter 10, 'Posture'.

Standing

In the upright standing position, a decrease from the pressure in the sitting position of approximately 30% was observed, and values from 80 kg to 150 kg were noted. Leaning forward by 20° in the standing position further increased intradiscal pressure.

Reclining

Problems with the method used for the in vivo measurements did not permit complete relaxation of the subjects in the reclining position. Even so, the stress on the discs decreased by about 50% as compared with the sitting position, values between 35 and 85 kg being obtained.

Holding weights

When subjects held weights of 10 kg in the forward-leaning sitting position, the total amount of load varied between 230 and 270 kg. Similarly, in the forward standing position, when holding the same weights, loads of up to 250 kg were recorded. A combination of rotation and flexion also subjected the lumbar spine to considerable load, especially when a weight was held (Nachemson, 1987).

Exercises

During certain exercises, intradiscal pressures were greatly increased (see Fig. 2.8B), for example when the subjects performed sit-ups with their knees bent, *active* back hyperextension in prone-lying and bilateral straight-leg raising in lying. It is essential to consider the effect of specific exercises and their influence on intradiscal pressure in patients who are recovering from acute lumbar disc pathology.

It is possible that disruption of the annular fibres could give rise to pain because of increases in intradiscal pressure and subsequent tensile stresses on the annulus. Patients who say that their pain is absent in reclining, but comes on when standing and is much worse when sitting and during certain exercises, may be describing the effects of stressing an annular tear.

Corsets

Wearing an inflatable corset decreased the load on the disc by approximately 25%. To achieve the same effect on a patient, the corset would need to be well fitting and tight.

NUTRITION OF THE INTERVERTEBRAL DISCS (Fig. 2.9)

Apart from its outermost annular fibres, the disc is avascular after the age of 10. For its nutrition, it subsequently relies on the diffusion of nutrients such as glucose, sulphate and oxygen. These reach the disc by two routes: from the blood vessels surrounding the periphery of the annulus fibrosus (the annular route), and from the capillary plexuses beneath the end plates (the end plate route). The nucleus receives most of its nutrition through the end plate route.

Certain areas of the disc have a higher permeability: the periphery of the annulus and the inner one-third of the end plates in the region of the nucleus and inner annular fibres. There is a region 4.4–6 mm from the posterior border of the disc which has a deficient supply of nutrition from all sources (Maroudas et al, 1975). Overall, the anterior annulus receives a better nutrient supply than the posterior annulus (Adams and Hutton, 1986); this fact could help to explain why degenerative changes occur less frequently in the anterior part of the disc. The outer annulus is more or less in equilibrium with the blood oxygen but the interior part of the disc is anaerobic and has a low oxygen concentration (Holm and Nachemson, 1982). The interior of the disc has a high lactic acid content and low pH, which may lead to a high activity of degradative enzymes (Urban and Roberts, 1994). It has been suggested that this environment

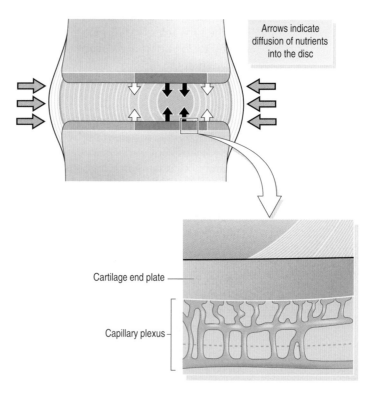

Figure 2.9   Nutrition of the intervertebral disc.

Arrows indicate diffusion of nutrients into the disc

Cartilage end plate

Capillary plexus

is a potentially precarious metabolic state for the internal disc and that instabilities could lead to cell death and disc degeneration.

The chondrocytes are found in greater proportions close to the end plates and in the outer layers of the annulus, near the available blood supply. Chondrocytes in the centre of the disc are further away from the blood vessels, and diffusion alone can barely supply them with nutrients (Maroudas et al, 1975).

Diffusion is more effective for transporting small molecules (Urban et al, 1982), while experiments performed on cadaveric lumbar discs have suggested that *fluid flow* may play some part in the transport of larger molecules such as proteins (Adams and Hutton, 1983). Fluid flows into and out of the disc in response to changes in posture and loading.

EFFECT OF POSTURE ON FLUID FLOW

Certain postures have been shown to affect fluid flow in the intervertebral discs, probably due to differences in loading in a particular posture (Adams and Hutton, 1983). The erect posture favours diffusion into the anterior half of the disc compared to the posterior half. The fully flexed lumbar spine posture favours diffusion into the posterior annulus by thinning it and thus increasing the surface area of the posterior annular fibres and by decreasing the distance from the nucleus to the periphery of the annulus. This is offset by a decrease in the supply to the end plate route because flexion increases the distance from the end plates to the midplane nucleus. Adams and Hutton's experiments showed that flexion reduced the thickness of the posterior annulus by 37% on average, which would bring the whole of the 'deficient' region mentioned above to within 4.4 mm of the surface, and ensure a sufficient supply of nutrients to all cells in the posterior annulus.

If the blood supply at the periphery is altered it may affect the nutrition of the disc and hence changes in posture may indirectly affect the disc's nutrition. Experiments on porcine intervertebral discs have shown that cigarette smoking adversely affects the circulation outside the disc by nicotine-induced vascular constriction, as well as cellular uptake rates and metabolic production within the disc (Holm and Nachemson, 1988). The inevitable consequence over a longer period of time will be deficient nutrition leading to degenerative metabolic processes. These effects, found in animals after a single exposure to smoking, do not necessarily represent the effects of long-term smoking in humans.

Experiments on dogs showed that after several months' exercise training, the transport of nutrients into the disc was increased. This may have been due to changes in the blood circulation surrounding the discs (Holm and Nachemson, 1982).

It is useful to consider the factors affecting disc nutrition when giving prophylactic advice on back care to patients who have early disc pathology. Inadequate metabolite transport has been linked with disc degeneration (Nachemson et al, 1970; Holm and Nachemson, 1982) and it may be feasible that alternating periods of activity and rest, and frequent changes of posture, could boost the fluid exchange in the discs and consequently improve disc nutrition. Although the flexed posture has been shown to improve nutrition to the disc, it also increases the intradiscal pressure by approximately 50% compared with the lordotic posture (calculated from Nachemson et al, 1979) and this may be significant in some cases where disc pathology is more advanced. Exercises may also play an important part in improving disc nutrition, possibly by increasing the blood supply to its periphery, provided that the exercises are carefully selected and do not exacerbate the patient's symptoms. Long-term lack of exercise has been shown to have a permanent effect on transport of nutrients into the disc and this subsequently affects the health of the tissue (Holm and Nachemson, 1982, 1983).

EFFECTS OF MOVEMENTS ON THE INTERBODY JOINTS

Movements in the interbody joints occur in conjunction with those in the other joints in the motion segments and can never be isolated from them. Movements of the interbody joints are accompanied by movements in the apophyseal joints in all regions of the spine; in addition, in the cervical spine, the uncovertebral joints and, in the thoracic spine, the costovertebral and costotransverse joints. Normal functional movement is usually a combination of physiological ranges rather than 'pure' movement in one plane only.

FLEXION

During flexion, the anterior fibres are compressed and tend to bulge, while the posterior fibres are under tensile stress.

The movement of the nucleus has been of particular interest, partly due to the number of posterior herniations of the nucleus in the lumbar spine attributed to flexion injuries. Kapandji (1974) proposed that the nucleus acted as a ball-bearing and was driven away from the side of the movement so that, on flexion, it was driven posteriorly (Fig. 2.10A). Bogduk and Twomey (1987) also described the posterior movement of the nucleus as it attempted to 'escape' from the anterior compression that deformed it. Dolan (1989, written communication) stated that in flexion the posterior annulus was stretched and thinned, so that the distance between the nucleus and outer annular fibres was decreased and the nucleus was relatively closer to the posterior margin of the disc (Fig. 2.10B).

Intradiscal pressure rises even if the interbody joint is flexed without being loaded. Functional flexion movements can be accompanied by muscular activity and this can increase intradiscal pressure still further (see p. 71).

The effects of *repeated* flexion are of particular practical significance. Although a patient may describe an isolated flexion movement causing injury to the lumbar spine, in many cases the offending movement was probably the last in a succession of repeated flexion movements. Studies on cadaveric discs have shown that repeatedly stressing the disc in compression and flexion distorted the annular fibres and nucleus (see Fig. 9.8, p. 313). The nucleus appeared to deform posterolaterally (Adams and Hutton, 1985).

Figure 2.10   Different theories of nuclear position during flexion. A, Kapandji. B, Dolan. X–X' = distance (nucleus to outer fibres) decreases with flexion.

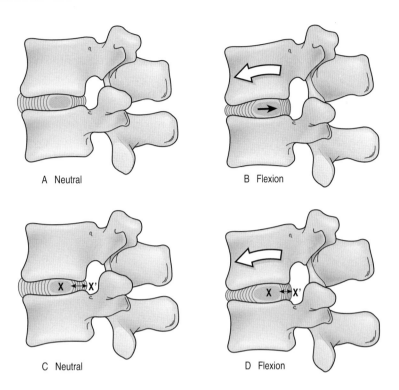

A Neutral

B Flexion

C Neutral

D Flexion

EXTENSION

The reverse occurs during extension, in that the anterior annulus is stretched and there is a tendency for the nucleus to deform forwards. Intradiscal pressure is lower than in flexion, but the effect of muscular activity must also be considered.

The proposed anteroposterior deformation of the nucleus during movements in the sagittal plane has been the basis of an exercise regime described by McKenzie (1981) to relieve pain and restore function in patients with certain types of disc pathology.

LATERAL FLEXION

Lateral flexion has received little attention but it is an important component of many functional movements, for example when flexing and bending to one side to pick up an object from the floor. During the movement of lateral flexion, the annular fibres are compressed and tend to bulge on the side to which the movement occurs, while those on the opposite side have their attachments separated. In the younger individual there may be some deformation of the nucleus in a similar manner to that which occurs in flexion. Intradiscal pressure also rises (Nachemson, 1987).

SLIDING

A small amount of sliding (1–2 mm) occurs at the interbody joints as an accessory movement in flexion, extension and lateral flexion. In flexion, *forward sliding* occurs and is resisted by the apophyseal joints and the annular fibres; in particular, half of the lateral annular fibres which are orientated in the direction of movement are stretched longitudinally

(Bogduk and Twomey, 1987). The anterior and posterior fibres offer relatively less resistance to forward sliding, because their orientation is not in the principal direction of the movement.

ROTATION

Half of the annular fibres lie in the direction of rotation, while the other half lie in the opposite direction. Therefore, during rotation to one side, only half of the annular fibres have their points of attachment separated, while the other half have them brought closer together. Rotation puts more strain on the outer annular fibres than the inner (Klein and Hukins, 1983) and the higher collagen concentration in the outer lamellae (Eyre, 1979) provides additional tensile strength. The inner fibres are the most oblique and, during rotation, they compress the nucleus, thereby raising intradiscal pressure.

DISTRACTION

Distraction of a motion segment can occur if a person hangs by the arms (for instance during gymnastic exercises) or during some therapeutic traction, if accurately applied. During annular distraction, every annular fibre has its points of attachment separated, disc height increases and intradiscal pressure decreases.

EFFECTS OF VERTICAL LOADING ON THE SPINE (Fig. 2.11)

The intervertebral discs are always under a vertical load due to the weight of the body and the compressive effects of muscle activity. Any

Figure 2.11 Effects of vertical loading on the spine.

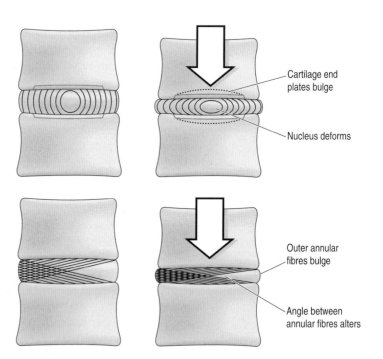

Cartilage end plates bulge

Nucleus deforms

Outer annular fibres bulge

Angle between annular fibres alters

weight carried in the arms or on the back (e.g. a backpack) will further increase the vertical loading.

When the spine is loaded, the nucleus pulposus and annulus fibrosus work in coordination to transmit weight from one vertebra to the next. The nucleus, being incompressible, tries to deform radially but is resisted by the strong annular fibres, causing pressure in the nucleus to rise. Any resultant stresses are distributed radially to the annulus and end plates. In a normal disc these stresses are the same in all directions. The extent of the deformation varies from disc to disc and no consistent pattern of deformation has been identified with respect to age, sex or degree of degeneration (Shirazi-Adl et al, 1984).

The direction of the annular fibres allows the resultant stresses to be absorbed. The angle that the fibres make with the horizontal becomes more acute (Pearcy and Tibrewal, 1984) – see Figure 2.11. While the inner fibres are compressed, the outer fibres are put under tension, but the annulus bulges only slightly. A load of 100 kg causes a lateral expansion of only 0.75 mm in a normal disc (Hirsch and Nachemson, 1954). However, increased bulging of the annulus occurs after prolonged loading (Köller et al, 1981). This occurs more readily in degenerated discs, since they lose more height than non-degenerated discs (see p. 307). Tensile stresses 4–5 times higher than the applied load are borne by the posterior annular fibres (Nachemson, 1965).

There is some deformation of the cancellous bone during vertical loading, and bulging of the end plates into the vertebral bodies may occur (Roaf, 1960) – see Figure 2.11. Some of the compressive energy is dissipated by blood flowing out of the cancellous bone of the vertebral bodies into the perivertebral veins, providing some protection against fracture. The perivertebral veins are unusual in that they do not have any valves, so that when the load is removed, some blood flows from the veins back into the vertebral bodies. The cancellous bone may fracture if it is subjected to a sudden application of vertical loading. This might occur because there is insufficient time for blood flow to dissipate energy or for the posture to be altered to absorb the shock (Klein and Hukins, 1983). Similarly, during cyclic loading, the energy-dissipating mechanism eventually fails if the period of loading is less than the time taken for the blood to flow back into the cancellous bone. It has been suggested that vibrations with a frequency of around 5 Hz could be damaging (Pope et al, 1980).

If a high vertical load is applied to the spine, damage usually results in collapse of the end plates (rather than herniation of the disc), suggesting that the end plates are the weakest part of the disc in compression.

When a vertical load is maintained, fluid passes out from the disc at a slow and decelerating rate. This movement of fluid is known as 'creep'. The fluid passes into the vertebral bodies and surrounding tissues until the disc is in equilibrium with the applied load; the heavier the load, the faster the rate of creep. The extent of the initial deformation for each load largely depends on the structure and integrity of the collagen network, but the rate and magnitude of the creep deformation is related more to the proteoglycan content of the disc.

Over the period of one day, the body height can decrease by 15–20 mm (de Puky, 1935), principally due to loss of fluid from the discs. This is relatively more marked in children and least in elderly people. Conversely, increases in height of approximately 5 cm have been reported in astronauts who were weightless for 3 months. Many factors influence disc height loss in each individual, such as number of hours of sleep, the time of getting up, the time of day, the magnitude and duration of loads applied to the spine, postures adopted, previous loads and the condition of the disc. Disc height loss has been found to be related to the experience of discomfort and also to the perception of exertion during physical exercises (Eklund and Corlett, 1987).

As the disc loses height and bulges, the vertical and transverse dimensions of the intervertebral foramen are reduced, leaving less room for its contents, including the nerve root. The apophyseal joint surfaces are brought closer together and, in the lumbar spine at least, their tips begin to resist some of the intervertebral compressive forces (Dunlop et al, 1984). These effects can give rise to symptoms if pathology is present.

The loss of disc height affects the normal biomechanics of the spine (Adams and Hutton, 1983). The approximation of the facets of the apophyseal joints is thought to reduce the range of axial rotation, since they normally limit this movement, and the range of extension may similarly be reduced. Conversely, the extra slack in the disc and ligaments is thought to decrease spinal stiffness in flexion, thereby increasing the range of flexion. This has clinical significance in that measurements of a patient's movements, if done at the start of a working day, are likely to differ from those done at the end of the afternoon if, for example, the spine has been subjected to reasonably heavy loading.

The rate at which fluid is lost from the disc tends to be slower than the rate at which it is imbibed; hence fluid lost during 16 h of daytime activity is replaced during 8 h of rest. At night, a rapid recovery of height occurs, approximately 70% of lost height being regained within 4 h (Fig. 2.12; Tyrell et al, 1985). On rising, the disc may be in a state of hyperhydration for the first few hours; this is relevant to the clinical observation that many patients report that their back 'went' after a trivial incident in the first couple of hours after rising. It was found that when the fluid content of a cadaveric disc was artificially raised by saline injection it became more resistant to bending stresses (Andersson and Schultz, 1979). Adams et al (1987) suggested that perhaps the same effect happens in life, so that in the early morning a forward bending movement may subject the lumbar ligaments and discs to damaging bending stresses, even though the movement would be easier and safe later in the day.

Unloading the spine during the day, even for short periods, results in a substantial recovery in disc height; this can have practical implications for managing those with disc problems. Some rest positions result in more fluid imbibition than others; the lying position takes the load off the spine and encourages fluid intake, but flexing the lumbar spine has been shown to have a beneficial effect on the nutrition of the disc by aiding the transport of metabolites (Adams and Hutton, 1986). Resting in a

Figure 2.12 Height gained and lost during a 24–hour period from a midline baseline set at 3.5 mm. (From Tyrell AR, Reilly T, Troup JDG 1985. Circadian variation in stature and the effects of spinal loading. *Spine* 10: 163, with permission.)

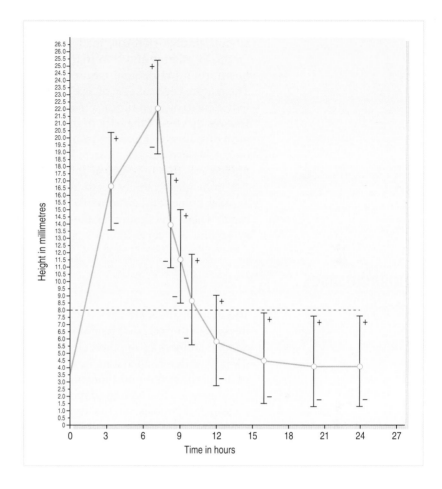

posture such as Fowler's position could aid nutrition and therefore the normal functioning of the disc.

CERVICAL DISCS

The cervical intervertebral discs are different in structure to the lumbar discs. At birth, the nucleus pulposus is present but is made of soft fibro-cartilage (Taylor and Twomey, 1994) and even at an early stage there is more collagen in the cervical nucleus than the lumbar nucleus. The nucleus pulposus becomes less evident with age and by the age of 40 it is virtually indistinguishable from the annulus. The adult disc is collagenous, dry and has areas of hyaline cartilage and even some tendon-like material. The proteoglycan content of the cervical disc is low (Giles and Singer, 1998). The cervical disc bears less axial loading and this is borne out by its structure with a lower water and proteoglycan content. An adult cervical disc is therefore less likely to prolapse because the nucleus is unlike the more fluid and deformable lumbar disc (Taylor and Twomey, 1994; Giles and Singer, 1998).

Between the ages of 9 and 14, bilateral clefts develop in the postero-lateral annulus fibrosus, medial to the uncinate processes. The clefts gradually enlarge and start to track medially until they meet in the midline, forming horizontal fissures across the back of the disc (Fig. 2.13). The mature cervical disc of a person aged 60 has little proteoglycan content, dense collagen fibres, a marked loss of volume of disc material and fissures that bisect the back of the disc. The changes that occur in the cervical disc are considered to result from its biophysical properties and the biomechanical stresses incurred during the large range of physiological movements that the cervical spine enjoys (Milne, 1991).

Pathological changes occur in the posterior annulus so that transverse annular bulges and osteophytic bars protrude posteriorly into the spinal canal. These can compress the spinal cord and give rise to signs and symptoms of a cervical myelopathy.

THORACIC DISCS

The thoracic discs are narrower than the lumbar and cervical discs, and the lack of thoracic disc height is one of the factors that contribute to the relative stiffness of the thoracic region. The thoracic discs are generally slightly wedge-shaped and are a little deeper posteriorly than anteriorly, particularly in the mid-thoracic region. The shape of the thoracic discs, together with the wedge-shaped thoracic vertebrae, gives the thoracic region its kyphosis. In the upper segments the disc has an elliptical shape, in the middle region it is a rounded triangle, and in the lower thoracic spine the disc takes on a larger elliptical shape that is flattened posteriorly. The structure of the thoracic disc with its low disc height and greater cross-sectional area enables it to fulfil the functions of bearing axial loading and providing support for limited thoracic mobility (White and Panjabi, 1990).

NERVE SUPPLY OF THE INTERVERTEBRAL DISCS

For many years there was a debate about whether or not the intervertebral discs are innervated. The innervation of the lumbar intervertebral

Figure 2.13 Posterior fissure across cervical intervertebral disc. (From Grant R, ed. 1999. *Physical Therapy of the Cervical and Thoracic Spine.* Churchill Livingstone, Edinburgh, p.18, with permission.)

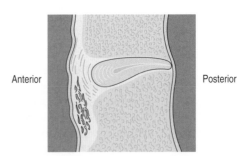

Anterior   Posterior

discs has now been confirmed and there is also evidence of innervation of the cervical discs (Bogduk, 1994).

Unmyelinated nerve endings were reported to be present in the immature intervertebral discs of the fetus and neonate (Tsukada, 1938, 1939) and it was Roofe (1940) who first found nerve endings in the outer annular fibres of mature lower lumbar discs. This was followed by controversy about whether or not *normal* mature discs were innervated, most studies being done on lumbar discs (Wiberg, 1949; Pederson et al, 1956).

Many researchers found evidence of innervation in the superficial layers of the annulus of mature discs (Malinsky, 1959; Hirsch et al, 1963; Jackson et al, 1966; Yoshizawa et al, 1980; Bogduk et al, 1981). The nerve endings were reported to be unevenly distributed, being more abundant in the lateral regions of the disc, less so in the posterior region and even less in the anterior region. No significant increase in nerve elements was observed in degenerated discs, nor were there any significant nerve endings in the areas where ingrowth of granulation tissue could be found.

The sources of these nerve endings are the lumbar sinuvertebral nerves, branches of the lumbar ventral rami and the grey rami communicantes (Bogduk et al, 1981). Each lumbar sinuvertebral nerve supplies the disc at the particular level at which it enters the vertebral canal and, in addition, the disc above. Outside the vertebral canal, the lumbar discs are innervated laterally by the grey rami communicantes, and posterolaterally by the grey rami communicantes and the ventral rami (Bogduk and Twomey, 1987).

A study on human fetuses (Groen et al, 1990) showed that the entire vertebral column is covered by an extensive network of microscopic plexuses that lie anterior and posterior to the vertebral bodies and intervertebral discs. Anteriorly, the plexuses arise from the sympathetic trunks and the grey rami communicantes. Posteriorly, the plexuses stem from the grey rami communicantes. Nerve elements from the anterior and posterior vertebral plexuses penetrate both the vertebral bodies and intervertebral discs. This study revealed that the sinuvertebral nerves in the lumbar and cervical regions constitute only a small number of the nerves that innervate the discs. The sinuvertebral nerves are larger and visible by microdissection but the majority of filaments innervating the discs are too small to be found by dissection and can only be identified in microscopic studies (Bogduk, 1994).

The function of these nerve endings remains unknown. Three possibilities have been proposed: (1) since there are similarities between the structure of the annulus fibrosus and that of a ligament, the nerve endings, like those in other ligamentous structures, could serve a proprioceptive function; (2) those that are associated with blood vessels could have either a vasomotor or vasosensory function (Malinsky, 1959); (3) it is possible that the nerve endings have a nociceptive function, which would mean that, even in the absence of herniation, the disc could be a primary source of pain.

Clinical studies support the view that the disc can be a source of pain. Pain has been reproduced by the injection of hypertonic saline into the L4/5 and L5/S1 disc (Hirsch et al, 1963) and also by discography (Holt,

1968; Walsh et al, 1990). This pain can be eliminated by injections of local anaesthetic into the disc (Bogduk, 1984). Walsh et al (1990) found that only patients with back pain complained of pain during discography; asymptomatic patients did not report pain. This study has shown that lumbar discography can be a highly specific diagnostic test as provocation discography is only positive in those individuals who have underlying symptomatic disc changes.

There is no clinical or manual test that can identify disc pathology as being the source of the patient's symptoms but it is essential for the therapist to understand that pathological changes within a disc may give rise to symptoms, and that low back pain when the disc is implicated is not necessarily due to pressure from a herniated disc on innervated structures.

References

Adams MA, Hutton WC (1983) The effects of posture on the fluid content of lumbar intervertebral discs. *Spine* 8: 665.

Adams MA, Hutton WC (1985) The effect of fatigue on the lumbar intervertebral disc. *Journal of Bone and Joint Surgery (Br.)* 65: 199.

Adams MA, Hutton WC (1986) The effect of posture on diffusion into lumbar intervertebral discs. *Journal of Anatomy* 147: 121.

Adams MA, Dolan P, Hutton WC (1987) Diurnal variations in the stresses on the lumbar spine. *Spine* 12: 130.

Andersson GB, Schultz AB (1979) Effects of fluid injection on the mechanical properties of the intervertebral disc. *Journal of Biomechanics* 12: 453.

Ayad S, Weiss JB (1987) Biochemistry of the intervertebral disc. In: Jayson MIV (ed.) *The Lumbar Spine and Back Pain*, 3rd edn. Churchill Livingstone, Edinburgh.

Bogduk N (1994) The innervation of the intervertebral discs. In: Boyling JD, Palastanga N (eds) *Grieve's Modern Manual Therapy. The Vertebral Column.* 2nd edn. Churchill Livingstone, Edinburgh, Ch. 12, pp. 149–161.

Bogduk N, Twomey L (1987) *Clinical Anatomy of the Lumbar Spine.* Churchill Livingstone, Edinburgh, pp. 58–71.

Bogduk N, Tynan W, Wilson AS (1981) The nerve supply to the human lumbar intervertebral disc. *Journal of Anatomy* 132: 39–56.

de Puky P (1935) The physiological oscillation of the length of the body. *Acta Orthopaedica Scandinavica* 6: 338.

Dunlop RB, Adams MA, Hutton W (1984) Disc space narrowing and the lumbar facet joints. *Journal of Bone and Joint Surgery (Br.)* 66: 706.

Eklund JAE, Corlett EN (1987) Shrinkage as a measure of the effect of load on the spine. *Spine* 9: 189.

Eyre DR (1979) Biochemistry of the intervertebral disc. *International Review of Connective Tissue Research* 8: 227.

Farfan HF (1973) *Mechanical Disorders of the Low Back.* Lea & Febiger, Philadelphia.

Farfan HF, Huberdeau RM, Dubow HI (1972) Lumbar intervertebral disc degeneration. The influence of geometrical features on the pattern of disc degeneration – a post-mortem study. *Journal of Bone and Joint Surgery (Am.)* 54: 492.

Giles LGF, Singer KP (1997) *Clinical Anatomy and Management of Low Back Pain.* Butterworth Heinemann, Oxford, Ch. 4, pp. 49–71.

Giles LGF, Singer KP (1998) *Clinical Anatomy and Management of Cervical Spine Pain.* Butterworth Heinemann, Oxford, p. 31.

Groen GJ, Baljet B, Drukker J (1990) Nerves and nerve plexuses of the human vertebral column. *American Journal of Anatomy* 188: 282–296.

Hickey DS, Hukins DWL (1980) Relation between the structure of the annulus fibrosus and the function and failure of the intervertebral disc. *Spine* 5: 106.

Hirsch C, Inglemark BE, Miller M (1963) The anatomical basis for low back pain. *Acta Orthopaedica Scandinavica* 33: 1.

Hirsch C, Nachemson A (1954) New observations on mechanical behaviour of lumbar discs. *Acta Orthopaedica Scandinavica* 23: 254.

Holm S, Nachemson A (1982) Nutritional changes in the canine intervertebral disc after spinal fusion. *Clinical Orthopaedics and Related Research* 169: 243.

Holm S, Nachemson A (1983) Variation in the nutrition of the canine intervertebral disc induced by motion. *Spine* 8: 866–874.

Holm S, Nachemson A (1988) Nutrition of the intervertebral disc: acute effects of cigarette smoking. An experimental animal study. *Upsala Journal of Medical Sciences* 93: 91.

Holt AP (1968) A question of lumbar discography. *Journal of Bone and Joint Surgery (Am.)* 50: 720–725.

Jackson HC, Winkelmann RK, Bickel WH (1966) Nerve endings in the human lumbar spinal column and related structures. *Journal of Bone and Joint Surgery (Am.)* 48-A: 1272.

Kapandji IA (1974) *The Physiology of the Joints, Vol. 3: The Trunk and the Vertebral Column.* Churchill Livingstone, Edinburgh.

Klein JA, Hukins DWL (1983) Functional differentiation in the spinal column. *Eng. Med.* 12: 83.

Köller W, Funke F, Hartmann F (1981) Das Verformungsverhalten vom lumbalen menschlichen Zwischwirbelscheiben unter langeinwirkender axialer dynamischer Druckkraft. *Zeitschrift fur Orthopadie* 119: 206.

Malinsky J (1959) The ontogenetic development of nerve terminations in the intervertebral discs of man. *Acta Anatomica* 38: 96.

Marchand F, Ahmed AM (1990) Investigation of the laminate structure of lumbar disc annulus fibrosus. *Spine* 14: 166.

Maroudas A, Stockwell RA, Nachemson A, Urban J (1975) Factors involved in the nutrition of the human intervertebral disc. *Journal of Anatomy* 120: 113–130.

McKenzie RA (1981) *The Lumbar Spine. Mechanical Diagnosis and Therapy.* Spinal Publications, Waikanae.

Milne N (1991) The role of the zygapophyseal joint orientation and uncinate processes in controlling motion in the cervical spine. *Journal of Anatomy* 178: 189–201.

Mixter WJ, Barr JS (1934) Rupture of the intervertebral disc with involvement of the spinal canal. *New England Journal of Medicine* 211: 210.

Nachemson A (1965) The effect of forward leaning on lumbar intradiscal pressure. *Acta Orthopaedica Scandinavica* 35: 314.

Nachemson A (1966) The load on lumbar discs in different positions of the body. *Clinical Orthopaedics and Related Research* 45: 107.

Nachemson A (1987) Lumbar intradiscal pressure. In: Jayson MIV (ed.) *The Lumbar Spine and Back Pain*, 3rd edn. Churchill Livingstone, Edinburgh, pp. 191–203.

Nachemson A, Morris JM (1964) *In vivo* measurements of intradiscal pressure. Discometry, a method for the determination of pressure in the lower lumbar discs. *Journal of Bone and Joint Surgery (Am.)* 46: 1077–1092.

Nachemson A, Lewin T, Maroudas A, et al (1970) *In vitro* diffusion of dye through the end-plates and the annulus fibrosus of human intervertebral discs. *Acta Orthopaedica Scandinavica* 41: 589.

Nachemson A, Schultz A, Berkson M (1979) Mechanical properties of human lumbar spine motion segments: influences of age, sex, disc level and degeneration. *Spine* 4: 1.

Nachemson AL, Evans JH (1968) Some mechanical properties of the third human lumbar interlaminar ligament (ligamentum flavum). *Journal of Biomechanics* 1: 211–220.

Pearcy MJ, Tibrewal SB (1984). Lumbar intervertebral disc and ligament deformations measured *in vivo*. *Clinical Orthopaedics and Related Research* 191: 281.

Pedersen HE, Blunck CFJ, Gardner E (1956) The anatomy of the lumbosacral posterior rami and meningeal branches of spinal nerves (sinu-vertebral nerves). *Journal of Bone and Joint Surgery (Am.)* 38: 377–391.

Pope MH, Wilder DG, Frymoyer JW (1980) Vibrations as an aetiologic factor in low back pain. In: *Engineering Aspects of the Spine*. Institute of Mechanical Engineers Conference Publications, London, pp. 11–16.

Roaf R (1960) A study of the mechanics of spinal injuries. *Journal of Bone and Joint Surgery (Am)* 420B: 810.

Roofe PG (1940) Innervation of annulus fibrosus and posterior longitudinal ligament. *Archives of Neurology and Psychiatry*. 44: 100.

Ruff S (1950) Brief acceleration less than one second. In: *German Aviation Medicine, World War II*. US Government Printing Office, Washington, DC, 1: 584.

Schmorl G, Junghanns H (1971) *The Human Spine in Health and Disease*, 2nd American edn. Grune & Stratton, New York.

Shirazi-Adl SA, Shrivastava SC, Ahmed AM (1984) Stress analysis of the lumbar disc-body unit in compression: a three dimensional nonlinear finite element study. *Spine* 9: 120–133.

Sylvén B (1951) On the biology of nucleus pulposus. *Acta Orthopaedica Scandinavica* 20: 275.

Taylor JR, Twomey LT (1985) Vertebral column development and its relation to adult pathology. *Australian Journal of Physiotherapy* 31: 83.

Taylor JR, Twomey L (1994) Functional and applied anatomy of the cervical spine. In: Grant R (ed.) *Physical Therapy of the Cervical and Thoracic Spine*. Churchill Livingstone, Edinburgh, Ch. 1, 1–25.

Taylor JR, Scott JE, Bosworth TR, Cribb AM (1992) Human intervertebral disc acid glycosaminoglycans. *Journal of Anatomy* 180: 137–141.

Tsukada K (1938) Histologische Studien über die Zwischenwirbelscheibe des Menschen: histologische Befunde des Foetus. Mitteilungen Medicine Akademiseyen Kioto 24: 1172.

Tsukada K (1939) Histologische Studien über die Zwischenwirbelscheibe des Menschen: Alters-veränderungen. Mitteilungen Medicine Akademiseyen Kioto 25: 207.

Tyrell AR, Reilly T, Troup JDG (1985) Circadian variation in stature and the effects of spinal loading. *Spine* 10: 161.

Urban JP, Roberts S (1994) Chemistry of the intervertebral disc in relation to functional requirements. In: Boyling JD, Palastanga N (eds) *Grieve's Modern Manual Therapy. The Vertebral Column*. 2nd edn. Churchill Livingstone, Edinburgh, Ch. 13, pp. 163–175.

Urban JPG, Holm S, Maroudas A, et al (1982) Nutrition of the intervertebral disc: effect of fluid flow on solute transport. *Clinical Orthopaedics and Related Research* 170: 296.

Walsh TR, Weinstein JN, Spratt KF, et al (1990) Lumbar discography in normal subjects. *Journal of Bone and Joint Surgery (Am.)* 72: 1081–1088.

White AA (1969) Analysis of the mechanics of the thoracic spine in man. An experimental study of autopsy specimens. *Acta Orthopaedica Scandinavica Supplementum* 127: 1–105.

White AA III, Panjabi MM (1990) *Clinical Biomechanics of the Spine*, 2nd edn. J.B. Lippincott, Philadelphia.

Wiberg G (1949) Back pain in relation to the nerve supply of the intervertebral disc. *Acta Orthopaedica Scandinavica* 19: 211.

Wood PHN, Badley EM (1983) An epidemiological appraisal of bone and joint disease in the elderly. In: Wright V (ed.) *Bone and Joint Disease in the Elderly*. Churchill Livingstone, Edinburgh, pp. 1–22.

Yoshizawa H, O'Brien JP, Thomas-Smith W, Trumper M (1980) The neuropathology of intervertebral discs removed for low-back pain. *Journal of Pathology* 132: 95–104.

Chapter **3**

Muscles of the vertebral column

The trunk and pelvic musculature play a fundamental role in the normal functioning of the spine. During the last twenty years there has been a greater understanding of the role of muscles and fascia in movement and control of the vertebral column and pelvis: assessment of muscle function is an essential element in the management of spinal disorders. Although mobilization or manipulation may help in the short term to relieve a patient's symptoms, manual treatment alone is unlikely to provide long-term relief or prevent a recurrence of the problem.

MUSCLE FUNCTION

> The muscles of the vertebral column can have the following functions:
>
> 1. Contract concentrically to produce or accelerate movement
> 2. Contract isometrically or eccentrically to decelerate movement or provide stability
> 3. Direct forces through tissues that are designed to absorb and transfer those forces such as the intervertebral discs and articular cartilage
> 4. Act as shock absorbers themselves
> 5. Provide afferent proprioceptive feedback to the central nervous system for coordination and regulation of muscle function.

Muscles are highly sensitive structures that react to all parts of the motor system. While muscles themselves may be a source of local pain, the presence of pain or dysfunction in any element in the motion segment with the same segmental nerve supply causes a response – such as spasm and/or referred tenderness – in the muscles controlling that segment, e.g. experimental stimulation of the C5/6 interspinous ligament elicited spasm in the supraspinatus, infraspinatus and biceps muscles (Feinstein, 1977).

It is important to consider not only the movements produced by individual muscles but also how the spinal muscles work together to control and stabilize the spine. Biomechanical abnormalities in any region of the spine can eventually give rise to secondary dysfunction elsewhere. For instance, when there is leg length inequality, compensation often occurs in the vertebral column, particularly in the lumbar region, but it may also result in secondary compensatory malalignment of head and neck posture. The secondary problem may be more troublesome to the patient than the first, but treating the cervical spine alone would achieve only limited and temporary results.

MUSCLE STRUCTURE (Fig. 3.1)

Skeletal muscle is highly complex and specialized. It consists of muscle cells, muscle-specific extracellular matrix, nerves and vessels.

Skeletal muscle cells (fibres) are cylindrical and range from 10 μm to approximately 100 μm in diameter – less than the diameter of a human hair (Lieber, 1992). The muscle cell is ensheathed by collagenous tissue known as the endomysium, and bundles of fibres are organized into muscle fascicles and surrounded by the stronger collagenous perimysial tissue. Bundles of fascicles are organized into muscles and are surrounded by epimysial connective tissue. The layers of connective tissue fuse together at either end of the muscle to form the highly specialized connective

Figure 3.1   Muscle structure. The muscle (A) is composed of bundles of muscle fibres (B). Each myofibril (C) is made up of sarcomeres (D) arranged end to end. Within each sarcomere, myosin (E) and actin (F) filaments interdigitate.

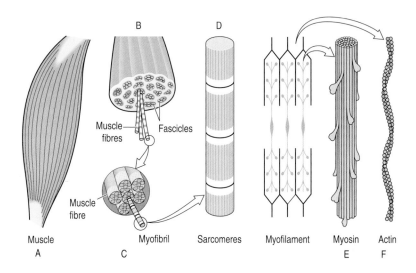

tissue tendons. The complex connective tissue matrix may play an important role in transferring forces from muscle fibres to the tendons.

A myofibril is the largest functional unit of contractile filaments. It is approximately 1 μm in diameter. Myofibrils are arranged parallel to each other to make up a muscle fibre; a single muscle fibre may consist of thousands of myofibrils. The myofibrils are interwoven so that their arrangement is similar to the weave of a rope (Peachy and Eisenberg, 1978). Myofibrils can be subdivided into their component units, known as sarcomeres. Sarcomeres are arranged end to end and the total number of sarcomeres depends on the length and diameter of the myofibrils.

The sarcomere is the functional unit of muscle contraction and is made up of myofilaments. Myofilaments are constructed from a number of proteins: the two important proteins, actin and myosin, comprise 84% of the total (McArdle et al, 1986). The myosin-containing filaments are relatively thick and they interdigitate with the thinner actin-containing filaments to form a hexagonal lattice (Lieber, 1992). The myosin contains cross-bridges that link to the actin, and it is the active interdigitation of these two proteins that allows the actin to slide over the myosin. The Z line is attached to the sarcolemma of the muscle cell, helping to secure it. The distance from one Z line to the next is defined as sarcomere length. Force is transmitted from the sliding of actin and myosin to the Z line and then to the connective tissue matrix of the muscle into the tendon and then in to bone. Sarcomeres have the ability to change length and vary the state of stiffness of the myofilaments; the myosin-containing filament generates tension during muscle contraction while the actin-containing filament regulates tension generation.

MUSCLE CONTRACTION

Many of the skeletal muscles are, at any one time, in a state of reflex contraction known as muscle tone. This applies particularly to muscles that are opposing the effects of gravity. Muscle contraction occurs as a result of interactivity between the nervous, muscular and skeletal systems.

MOTOR UNIT

Skeletal muscle fibres are innervated by axons that have their cell bodies in the anterior horn of the spinal cord. Each axon has many terminal branches which innervate different muscle fibres. The smallest group of muscle fibres employed voluntarily or in a reflex action is called a motor unit; it constitutes of a single motor neurone together with the muscle fibres that it innervates. These muscle fibres are often spread widely within a muscle, which means that even when only a few motor units are active, the force is generated diffusely. Each muscle is made up of several thousand motor units, each with its own anterior horn cell in the spinal cord, and the ratio of muscle fibres to nerve varies in different muscles. In normal circumstances, only a proportion of the motor units are active at the same time. This proportion may, of course, increase when a muscle group is exercised, or it may decrease. A decrease in motor unit activity may be seen clinically in a patient who presents with paresis of muscles supplied by one spinal nerve following irritation or compression of the nerve by, for example, a herniated intervertebral disc. As most muscles are supplied by more than one spinal nerve, paresis rather than paralysis tends to occur.

The amount of tone present in striated muscle at any one time depends not only on the integral state of the motor units, some of which will be contracting, some relaxing, and some quiescent, but also on the impulse frequency in the neurone supplying each motor unit, and on the tension of the muscle's connective tissues.

EXCITATION COUPLING

The process by which a neural activation signal results in muscle contraction is known as excitation coupling. This is a sequence of events, each of which is essential for muscle contraction to occur; if there is impairment of any step in the excitation coupling process, contraction does not normally occur.

Depolarization of the peripheral nerve that innervates a muscle causes an *action potential*. The axon may be depolarized by a signal from the CNS, trauma or an externally applied electrical stimulating device. Once generated, the action potential travels distally down the motor neurone until it reaches the neuromuscular junction. At the muscle–nerve interface the nerve terminates at a small indentation on the muscle fibre surface known as the synaptic cleft. The nerve endings contain acetylcholine, a chemical neurotransmitter that causes muscle fibre excitation. Following depolarization of the peripheral nerve, acetylcholine is released into the synaptic cleft and diffuses across it to combine with receptors in the postsynaptic membrane of the muscle fibre. The permeability of the muscle fibre to sodium and potassium is altered so that changes in the intracellular and extracellular ion concentrations cause the muscle cell membrane to be depolarized.

After depolarization has occurred at the postsynaptic membrane, the action potential is conducted deep into the muscle fibre by the transverse tubule system (T-system; Fig. 3.2). The myofibrils are surrounded by a

Figure 3.2 Transverse tubules and sarcoplasmic reticulum. (From Porterfield J, DeRosa C 1997 *Mechanical Low Back Pain. Perspectives in Functional Anatomy.* 2nd edn. Saunders, Philadelphia, p. 57 Figure 3.5, with permission.)

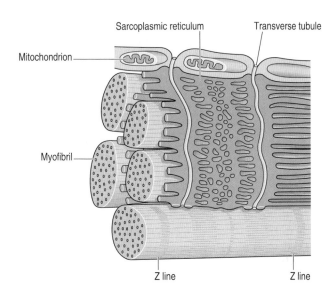

sleeve-like structure called the sarcoplasmic reticulum; lateral sacs within the sarcoplasmic reticulum contain calcium. The action potential within the T-system signals the sarcoplasmic reticulum to release calcium. Calcium ions are rapidly released into the myofibrils and bind to troponin, the actin filament regulatory protein. The activated troponin changes shape, pulling tropomyosin, another regulatory protein which lies end to end along the actin molecule, away from the myosin binding site, resulting in attachments developing between the actin and myosin; these are known as cross bridges. The interaction between actin and myosin during the cross bridge cycling generates force.

At the attachment of actin and myosin there is a breakdown of the enzyme adenosine triphosphate (ATP) to adenosine diphosphate (ADP), releasing the energy stored in ATP. This energy release provides a force that causes movement of the myosin cross-bridge. As the actin slides over the myosin, the myofibril shortens. The force generated by the actin–myosin sliding is transmitted to the connective tissue matrix of the muscle, into the tendon, and then into bone. If calcium levels in the myofilaments drop below a critical level, inhibition of the thin filaments (actin) occurs and actin–myosin interaction is prevented.

THE MECHANORECEPTOR ROLE OF MUSCLE SPINDLES AND GOLGI TENDON ORGANS

The muscle spindles and Golgi tendon organs (muscle and muscle–tendon units) are important mechanoreceptors that convey sensory information to the central nervous system. They provide information regarding the status of the muscle and are essential for the conscious appreciation of proprioception and kinaesthesia.

Each neuromuscular spindle consists of intrafusal and extrafusal muscle fibres. Intrafusal muscle fibres are innervated by both sensory and gamma motor neurons. Excitation by the gamma motor neuron causes contraction of the intrafusal fibres, shortening the muscle spindle. This contraction distorts the spindle, which applies tension to the sensory ending in the spindle, resulting in an afferent discharge to the central nervous system. This, in turn, increases contraction of the extrafusal fibres so that there is a decrease in muscle spindle activity. Two different types of muscle spindle fibres produce different types of contraction: slow contractions are produced by 'bag' fibres and fast contractions by 'chain' fibres. Different rates of contraction provide afferent information about the status of the muscle to the central nervous system.

Excitation of the alpha neurone causes the extrafusal muscle fibres to contract, and this tends to decrease activity in the muscle spindle. In some cases of voluntary movement, the activity in the alpha motor neurone may precede that in the gamma motor neurone, the spindle thereby detecting the degree of muscle contraction.

The gamma efferent system acts as a fine mechanism for adjusting the degree of contraction of the voluntary muscles. Changes in gamma motor neurone activity reset the muscle spindles and the main muscle mass alters its degree of contraction to the new equilibrium position.

The Golgi tendon organs are connective tissue capsules situated at the muscle–tendon junction. There are between 15 and 20 skeletal muscle fibres to each capsule and the Golgi tendon organs respond to stretching of the muscle, contraction of the muscle, or both. The Golgi tendon organs become distorted when the muscle stretches or contracts; this causes the axons to fire, providing an afferent discharge to the central nervous system. Information from the Golgi tendon organs goes to the cerebellum and assists in regulation of motor output.

MUSCLE SPASM

Hypertonus – or spasm – of a muscle can either result from injury to the muscle itself or occur as a reflex response to nociceptor irritation of joints and associated tissues. The severity of the spasm generally depends on the intensity of pain. It initially plays a protective role in splinting a painful lesion, and may be present over several segments or span a whole vertebral region. In itself, spasm may be asymptomatic if short-lived. However, its presence may increase the compressive forces on the structures of the motion segment, the intervertebral disc in particular, thereby giving rise to greater pain and dysfunction.

Another mechanism whereby muscle spasm causes pain is through tension on its attachments to periosteum; a patient with a lumbar lesion giving rise to erector spinae spasm may complain of thoracic pain caused by the muscle's attachments into the rib angles. Muscle spasm may also be the primary mechanism involved in referred pain, e.g. piriformis spasm associated with a sacroiliac lesion causing buttock and trochanteric pain (Kirkaldy Willis and Hill, 1979). If the spasm persists, implying a continuing source of deep pain, it results in a decrease in blood flow to the muscle, leading to anoxia and the accumulation of metabolic waste products which would normally be dispersed during relaxation. Fatigue and eventually pain in the muscle itself occur. Finally, internal changes take place in the muscle causing contracture.

An asymmetrical distribution of spasm may result in the classic deformity of a 'sciatic' scoliosis. Psoas spasm may occur because of a herniated intervertebral disc, creating a sciatic side shift. Another example is the unilateral spasm of sternocleidomastoid seen in some patients presenting with an acute 'wry neck'.

SPINAL REFLEXES

A spinal reflex is an involuntary response to a stimulus involving nerve pathways restricted to the spinal cord. Sensory nerves from the same and adjacent segments of the spinal cord give off branches which synapse with the anterior horn cells. Often there are one or more internuncial neurones along the route. Such synapses give rise to spinal reflexes which can cause motor contraction even in the absence of higher control from the brain.

The stretch reflex is a simple spinal reflex involving only two neurones and one synapse. When a muscle is stretched, the stretch receptors in the muscle spindle are stimulated, and nerve impulses enter the spinal cord via the IA afferent nerves. These nerves synapse with the anterior horn cells supplying the same muscle, which responds with a short, involuntary contraction. The anterior horn cells are also under the influence of higher centres, and under normal circumstances the inhibitory component of the extrapyramidal system 'damps down' any spinal reflexes.

Maintenance of the upright posture depends on activation of the stretch reflex. The tendency is for the body to sway slightly the whole time. As it sways forwards, the muscles at the back of the legs are stretched, the muscle spindles are stimulated and, due to the stretch reflex, they contract, thereby bringing the body backwards. This then stretches the muscles at the front of the legs, and the stretch reflex is stimulated, bringing the body forwards. Balance is, therefore, maintained by the alternate contraction and relaxation of these muscles.

In clinical practice, the stretch reflex is used to test conduction of certain spinal nerves, e.g. the knee jerk is used to test the nerves supplying the quadriceps muscle. When the quadriceps tendon is tapped suddenly, the muscle spindles lying in the muscles are stimulated and the monosynaptic reflex causes the muscle to contract so that the knee is extended. The stretch reflex may be absent or depressed if the spinal nerve supplying the muscle is damaged due to a pathological process, e.g. osteophytic encroachment or disc prolapse. Inhibition from higher centres may be so great that it is difficult to elicit a knee jerk. This central inhibition can be reduced if the subject concentrates on some other voluntary movement, e.g. clasping his hands and then pulling outwards, whilst the test is being performed.

The mechanism of the stretch reflex may be used during treatment to stimulate voluntary contraction of a muscle. This principle is the basis of one of the proprioceptive neuromuscular techniques described by Voss et al (1985).

SLOW AND FAST MUSCLE FIBRES

A number of classification systems for muscle fibre types have been proposed, based on physiological, histochemical and biomechanical properties (Brooke and Kaiser, 1970; Peter et al, 1972). A literature review combined the classification schemes of previous studies and described three muscle fibre types (Rose and Rothstein, 1982).

Type I   These are slow oxidative, slow twitch fibres that have large amounts of oxidative enzymes and small amounts of glycolytic enzymes. These fibres are red, have a well-developed metabolism and are resistant to fatigue. They are adapted to produce a relatively slow, but repetitive, type of contraction which generates the sustained 'tonic' forces characteristic of postural muscles.

Type IIB   These are fast glycolytic, fast twitch fibres that are well supplied with glycolytic enzymes and are poorly endowed with oxidative enzymes, indicating a high capacity for anaerobic metabolism. These fibres are paler in colour and are called 'white'; they obtain energy primarily by glycolytic respiration, but are easily fatigued. These form the greater part of muscles that are primarily responsible for movement.

Type IIA   These are fast oxidative glycolytic, fast twitch and fatigue resistant fibres. They contain intermediate amounts of oxidative and glycolytic enzymes, indicating the use of both aerobic and anaerobic metabolism. These fibres have cytological characteristics that fall between type I and type IIB fibres.

Slow twitch fibres (type I) are recruited first, followed by intermediate fibres (type IIB); type IIA fibres are recruited when maximal contraction is needed. The distribution of different fibre types varies between individuals and among different muscle groups in the same individual (Elder et al, 1982).

TYPES OF MUSCLE CONTRACTION

There are two types of muscle contraction:

1. Isometric (from *iso-* = equal, and *-metric* = measurement) contraction occurs when a muscle contracts at a fixed length, creating tension at its attachments but performing no external work (work being the product of force and the distance through which the force acts). Serratus anterior, with the upper and lower fibres of trapezius, works isometrically to assist in stabilization of the scapula during activities of the upper limb

such as typing. This type of muscle activity is usually termed static muscle work, as no external movement occurs.

2. Isotonic contraction occurs when there is an increase in intramuscular tension and a change in length of the muscle, either by shortening or lengthening, thereby performing work. This type of muscle activity is often called dynamic muscle work.

If the muscle contracts isotonically in *shortening* to produce movement, drawing its attachments closer together, it performs concentric muscle work (*concentric = towards* the centre). The erector spinae muscles work concentrically in the standing position during extension of the trunk from a flexed to a neutral position.

If the muscle contracts isotonically in *lengthening*, the muscle attachments draw apart as it works to oppose the action of a force greater than that of its own contraction. It performs excentric or eccentric muscle work (*excentric = from* the centre). For example, the erector spinae work eccentrically from the erect standing posture when the trunk is slowly flexed. In this instance, these muscles are opposing the force of gravity.

The speed of action may influence which muscles work in a particular movement; for instance, in the last example, if the trunk is flexed at a more natural speed, the activity of erector spinae is then absent except at the initiation and the end of movement.

When planning a reconditioning programme for spinal muscles, consideration should be given to all of the different types of work they have to perform during everyday activities of the patient. Simply exercising the erector spinae muscles concentrically fulfils only part of their normal function, and does not enhance their ability to work eccentrically.

STATIC AND DYNAMIC MUSCLE WORK

There are basic differences between static and dynamic muscle work.

Static work

During static work, there is a rise in pressure within the muscles that compresses the blood vessels, decreasing the amount of blood flowing into them in proportion to the force of contraction (Grandjean, 1971). When the applied force amounts to 60% of the maximum force, the blood supply is stopped completely; the muscle then does not receive oxygen or nutrients from the blood and it has to consume its reserves. In addition, waste products are not carried away but accumulate, causing acute pain from muscular fatigue. During a static effort of 15–20% of a maximum voluntary contraction, the blood supply to the muscle is thought to be normal. Static work with efforts of 50% and more of the maximum force can last for a minute at the most, while efforts of less than 20% will allow longer-lasting static muscular contraction. Static muscle work which demands a substantial effort in working life is, therefore, obviously unendurable and detrimental.

Static muscle work is less efficient (greater consumption of energy for smaller efforts) than dynamic muscle work.

Dynamic work

In dynamic muscle work, contraction of a muscle is rhythmically followed by relaxation. Contraction causes an expulsion of blood from the muscle, and the subsequent relaxation allows a renewed flow of blood into the muscle. This increases the blood circulation to such an extent that the muscle receives up to twenty times more blood during dynamic work than during static activity. During dynamic work, the muscle receives a good supply of nutrients and oxygen to provide energy, and waste products are readily removed. So long as a suitable rhythm is chosen, dynamic work can be executed for a long time without fatigue.

RANGE OF MUSCLE WORK

Muscle fibres have the ability to shorten to almost half their resting length. Consequently, the arrangement of fibres within a muscle determines how much it can shorten when it contracts (Palastanga et al, 1989). The muscular system is so arranged that habitual contractions involve only limited length changes in comparison with the overall length of the muscle.

The maximum excursion of a muscle that is possible, i.e. the amount of shortening and lengthening, is called the full range of muscle work. The terms inner, outer and middle range indicate in which part of the range the muscle contraction takes place.

Inner range is that nearest the point at which the muscle is shortest.
Outer range is that nearest the point at which the muscle is longest.
If a muscle is very weak, a contraction is usually initiated more easily from stretch and, therefore, in its outer range.
Middle range lies between the two. This is the range in which muscles are most often used in everyday life and in which they are as a rule most efficient.

GROUP ACTIONS OF MUSCLES

Functionally, muscles work together in groups, although each muscle may have a specific role to play in relation to the action of the whole group. The integrated action of many groups is necessary for efficient movement to occur. The groups are named according to their function.

When muscles act to initiate and maintain a movement, they are classed as *prime movers* (or *agonists*). Muscles which would oppose such a movement are called *antagonists*. Except at the initiation and end of a movement, the antagonists usually remain quiescent, while the prime movers produce movement.

When testing spinal movements, it is important to remember that nearly all of them are either opposed or assisted by the force of gravity. This has a profound effect upon the play of muscles during a particular movement. The activity of prime movers is always replaced by gravity whenever this is appropriate – in such cases the conventionally described role of muscles is often reversed.

Both prime movers and antagonists may contract together to hold a joint in one position, thereby acting as *fixators*. These muscles work to stabilize the joint, often providing an immobile base from which other prime movers can act more efficiently. At the same time, the transarticular compression is increased.

When muscles pass over more than one joint, or with multiaxial joints, unrestrained contraction of the prime movers may produce additional unwanted movements. The contraction of *synergist* (*syn* = with) muscles acting as partial antagonists to the prime movers eliminates these unwanted movements. For example, during trunk rotation, when abdominals contract to produce movement, they produce flexion simultaneously; multifidus, by producing an extension moment (together with a small amount of rotation), balances the flexion moment generated by the abdominals, thereby acting synergistically during rotation.

MUSCLE FUNCTIONAL CLASSIFICATION

Muscles have also been classified according to their function. The concept of mobilizer and stabilizer muscles was proposed by Rood (Goff, 1972) and developed further by Janda (1983) and Sahrmann (2000), who differentiated between one-joint stabilizer and two-joint mobilizer muscles.

Characteristics of stabilizer and mobilizer muscles (after Goff, Janda and Sahrmann)

Stabilizer muscles
- Mono-articular
- Muscle attachments are segmental
- Deep muscles: short levers and a small movement arm
- Superficial muscles: aponeurosis with a broad insertion that distributes load and force

Mobilizer muscles
- Bi-articular/multi-articular
- Superficial
- Long levers, large movement arms
- Muscles designed for speed and a large range of movement

Comerford and Mottram (2001) propose a functional classification based on whether a muscle is a local stabilizer, global stabilizer or global mobilizer.

Functional classification of muscles (Comerford and Mottram, 2001)

Local stabilizer muscles

These muscles control segmental movement in all joint positions and in all directions of movement. Normally, they fire continuously to provide a low-level force that increases muscle stiffness, controlling intersegmental physiological movement and preventing unwanted translational movement. They are particularly important in the neutral position of the joint where there is minimal support from joint capsule and ligaments. Activity in these muscles can increase with the anticipation of loading or movement, providing control and support. An example of a local stabilizer is multifidus (transversospinalis).

Global stabilizer muscles

These muscles act eccentrically to provide control of the inner and outer ranges of joint motion. They are able to shorten concentrically into full physiological inner range positions, lengthen eccentrically to control a functional load, and isometrically hold a position. They are important in controlling rotation in functional movements. An example of a global stabilizer is the deep erector spinae.

Global mobilizer muscles

These muscles act primarily as mobilizers but require sufficient length to allow full physiological and translatory movement without causing compensatory counterstrain elsewhere in the movement system. They assist in providing functional stability in situations of high loading such as pulling, pushing, ballistic shock absorption and lifting. These muscles are effective in the sagittal plane but do not provide significant control of rotation.

Dysfunction is specific to each of these muscle types. Dysfunction of the local stabilizer muscles occurs as a result of alteration of the normal motor recruitment, leading to decreased segmental control (Richardson et al, 1999). Dysfunction of the global stabilizer muscles occurs from increased functional muscle length or decreased low-threshold recruitment (Gossman et al, 1982). Dysfunction of the global mobilizer muscles arises from a loss of functional extensibility or excessive low-threshold activity (Comerford and Mottram, 2001).

MUSCLE DYSFUNCTION

In order for muscles to function efficiently, they must maintain their normal length and be supple and flexible, with an adequate blood and nerve supply. Any condition that deprives muscles of these essential elements will lead to impairment of function, i.e. dysfunction.

EFFECTS OF POSTURE

During the mature lifespan of the individual, changes that occur in the soft tissues are largely adaptations to environmental factors (Editorial, 1979). The functional resting length of a muscle changes and adapts to the length at which the muscle is habitually used or positioned (Richardson and Sims, 1991; Wiemann et al, 1998). Kendall et al (1993) described adaptive shortening as tightness occurring in muscles that remain in a shortened position. This occurs mainly in two-joint muscles. Kendall et al define stretch weakness as a weakness that occurs when a muscle remains in an elongated position beyond its normal resting length. Stretch weakness is seen more commonly in mono-articular muscles.

Mechanical stresses, such as those imposed by prolonged asymmetrical postures, have a marked effect on the muscles and soft tissues, causing fibroblasts along the lines of stress to multiply more rapidly and produce more collagen. These extra collagen fibres take up space in the connective tissue of the muscle and begin to encroach on the space normally occupied by nerves and blood and lymphatic vessels. As a result of this trespass, the muscle loses its elasticity and may become painful when required to do work. In the long term, the collagen begins to replace the active fibres of the muscle. Since collagen is fairly resistant to enzyme breakdown, these changes tend to be irreversible.

EFFECTS OF OVERUSE, MISUSE OR DISUSE

Sustained muscle activity, as in strenuous exertion, leads to temporary swelling of the muscle, but this passes off unnoticed except in cases where the surrounding fascia is too tight, e.g. in the anterior tibial syndrome.

Excessive use of muscle will lead to hypertrophy; lack of use to atrophy. Certain occupations and activities, such as those involving the persistent use of one arm as opposed to the other, as in operating machinery, can cause muscles to be overused. The effect may not necessarily be felt in the arm itself, but in the muscles that stabilize the scapula and vertebral column for the use of the arm, because of the fatiguing static contraction imposed on them. Excessive use of a particular muscle may also give rise to muscle imbalance.

Clinical signs of muscle atrophy are a decrease in the cross-sectional area (CSA) of the muscle and decreased muscle strength and endurance. Reduced muscular support will increase the load on the joints and lead to abnormal movement patterns. Muscle atrophy can occur secondary to muscle pathologies (Wheeler, 1982), denervation (Lieber, 1992), disuse (Booth and Gollnick, 1983; Lieber, 1992) and malnutrition. A reduction in the CSA of lumbar multifidus has been demonstrated in both acute and chronic low back pain pathology (Stokes et al, 1992; Hides et al, 1994, 1996; Kader et al, 2000). Changes have also been reported in the CSA of psoas in a patient with chronic low back pain (Cooper et al, 1992).

Reductions in muscle flexibility may occur in sportsmen when defective training methods are used, and they are associated with a failure to take powerful joint movements to their extreme.

ALTERED MOTOR
RECRUITMENT

Habitually using certain muscle groups within a small and abnormally restricted amplitude of their available extensibility ranges can lead to them being in a state of overactivation, and hence they eventually shorten. Their antagonists respond by inhibition, weakness and lengthening. Janda (1983, 1985, 1994) described muscles as 'postural' (shortened two-joint muscles) and 'phasic' (weakened one-joint muscles). Muscles with a predominantly postural function shorten or tighten, while their antagonists, the phasic muscles, become weaker and tend to lengthen.

Muscle imbalance (from Janda, 1976)

Postural muscles – tend to tighten
Sternocleidomastoid
Pectoralis major (clavicular and sternal parts)
Trapezius (superior part)
Levator scapulae
The flexor groups of the upper extremity
Quadratus lumborum
Erector spinae
Iliopsoas
Tensor fasciae latae
Rectus femoris
Piriformis
Pectineus
Adductor longus, brevis and magnus
Biceps femoris
Semitendinosus
Semimembranosus
Gastrocnemius
Soleus
Tibialis anterior

Phasic muscles – tend to lengthen and weaken
Scaleni and the prevertebral cervical muscles
Extensor groups of the upper extremity
Pectoralis major, the abdominal part
Trapezius, the inferior and middle part
Rhomboids
Serratus anterior
Rectus abdominis
Internal and external obliques
Gluteal muscles (minimus, medius, maximus)
The vasti muscles (medialis, lateralis, intermedius)
Tibialis anterior
The peroneal muscles

Abnormal movement patterns develop as a consequence of altered motor recruitment, and subsequent changes in the quality and control of movement can be observed. Janda (1996) studied recruitment and sequencing differences in functional movements and compared recruitment sequences in pathological and non-pathological subjects. He identified consistent patterns of 'normal' recruitment in the non-symptomatic subjects and identified characteristic abnormal patterns of recruitment in symptomatic subjects.

There is normally an imbalance between the strength of the trunk extensors and flexors. The extensors are invariably dominant, the ratio being approximately 5:3 (Suzuki and Endo, 1983). A change in this ratio of normal trunk muscle balance may be a risk factor for low back pain.

Altered motor recruitment can be caused by denervation, abnormal neural sensitization, reflex inhibition due to pain or secondary stress, or it may be imposed by ligamentous failure. Poor posture and suboptimal movement habits can also result in altered recruitment and muscle imbalances: for example, a sedentary lifestyle could lead to tightening of psoas and weakening of the glutei. Recruitment may also be affected by impaired control from the limbic system which regulates muscle tone (Bannister, 1985) and which, in turn, can be influenced by emotional states.

Motor recruitment and good control of movement also depends on adequate proprioceptive stimuli from muscles, joints, ligaments, skin, etc., as dysfunction in these structures reflexly affects motor control. Light corsets, backrests and adhesive strapping may well owe some of their effectiveness to proprioceptive stimulation of the skin.

TRIGGER POINTS

Spindle-shaped thickenings in muscle tissue are common, especially in the postural muscles. They used to be referred to as fibrositis – a misleading term because of the absence of inflammation in the muscle fibres – and are now known as trigger points. These are sustained contractions of isolated groups of muscle fibres; they lie in the line of the fibres and can be moved at right angles to them. They are tender on palpation.

There are several theories concerning their aetiology. The most likely causes are irritation of the nerve supply to the muscle, causing localized muscle spasm, or a reflex response to irritation of deeper structures supplied by the same segment. Treatment directed at the cause is indicated in the early onset of these points; if they become chronic, then local treatment is also necessary.

JOINT DISEASE OR TRAUMA

The spinal muscles and joints are functionally interdependent. It therefore follows that dysfunction in either of them will sooner or later have an effect on the other. It has been shown that muscle dysfunction commonly accompanies degenerative joint disease (Jowett and Fidler, 1975). The presence of pain or a lesion in any element in the articular system influences the responses of the muscles controlling it, leading to abnormal patterns of movement which, in turn, contribute to muscle dysfunction.

The reverse mechanism, where muscle dysfunction precedes the joint problem, can also occur. In individuals who are generally anxious and have excessive muscular tension, the compressive force across the joint surfaces is increased, and pain or strain eventually results from abnormal movement patterns.

When joints become stiff through trauma or disease, eventually the soft tissues surrounding them adapt by shortening. In some cases this acts as a protective mechanism: for instance, if an intervertebral joint is mechanically unstable with excessive translatory movements, the soft tissues surrounding it will eventually tighten (Kirkaldy Willis and Hill, 1979) and provide a certain amount of stability by limiting the available excursion of the joint.

In most cases, adaptive muscle shortening is undesirable. A management programme should ensure that essential flexibility and strength of the muscles controlling the motion segment are regained as far as possible in order to restore motor coordination and function.

EFFECTS OF NERVOUS TENSION

Nervous tension has a profound effect on the body in terms of chemical alterations and also on the musculature. Whatever the cause of the tension – be it anxiety, depression, frustration or the general stresses of life – it expresses itself in muscular tension. The most common site for this is in the cervical muscles at their attachment to the skull. Tension in the splenius capitis, semispinalis capitis, and trapezius gives rise to headache, neck ache and shoulder ache. If the tension is maintained, pain is produced by the accumulation of metabolites in the muscle. These metabolites can then be a source of irritation, perpetuating the contraction and thereby establishing a vicious cycle. Sustained tension can eventually lead to joint restriction.

Neck pain due to tension can be relieved by manual treatment, but this may be of only temporary value unless the cause is also treated.

CERVICAL MUSCLES

The cervical region is the most mobile in the spine. As well as producing and controlling the movements, the neck muscles have the important function of balancing the head on the neck and controlling posture. Many of the neck muscles are small, deeply situated and impossible to palpate in isolation.

Contraction of the posterior cervical muscles increases the normal lordotic cervical curve, thereby increasing a tendency towards buckling of the spine (Jull, 1997). The anterior deep cervical muscles have an important function in postural and segmental control by stiffening and stabilizing the neck, particularly the mid-cervical segments. The superficial neck muscles such as sternocleidomastoid have a major function in torque production, while the deeper muscles such as longus capitis and longus colli show lesser but continuous (tonic) activity concomitant in a postural, supporting role (Conley et al, 1995).

There is evidence that recruitment deficiency and endurance fatigue of the upper and deep neck flexors is an important factor in patients with neck pain and cervicogenic headaches (Watson and Trott, 1993; Beeton and Jull, 1994; Jull et al, 1999). A study of patients suffering from whiplash-associated disorder showed that compared to asymptomatic controls they were less able to control staged recruitment of the deep neck flexors, were consistently less able to sustain activation of these muscles and were more likely to substitute with superficial neck muscles (Jull, 2000).

The posterior neck muscles are also important in control of the head and neck position, particularly in mid range (Winters and Peles, 1990). Patients with chronic neck pain have been shown to have atrophy of the deep suboccipital extensors (Hallgren et al, 1994; McPartland et al, 1997). McPartland et al suggested that dysfunction of the deep segmental neck extensors reduces mechanical support. There is a consequent loss of normal inhibition of nociceptor interneurons at the dorsal horn due to the reduced proprioceptive input and this predisposes to neural sensitization and a chronic pain state.

The neck muscles contain a high proportion of afferent fibres – 80% – compared with most other striated muscles, which contain 50% (Abrahams, 1977). This makes them much more sensitive. Impaired function of the limbic system, such as that brought about by anxiety states, primarily affects these muscles (Bannister, 1985) and they react by going into spasm. This can cause a variety of symptoms, not only in the neck but also in the face and head. It is thought that this is one of the factors responsible for syndromes such as the tension headache. The area on the occiput that provides attachment for some of the neck muscles is a common site of pain and tenderness, which can be caused by spasm of the muscles pulling on the periosteum. Referred pain in the face, such as over the region of the temporomandibular joint, has also been noted clinically, due to spasm of cervical muscles. Movements of the jaw, as in chewing, are associated with static activity of the deep muscles in the upper cervical spine, and dysfunction in one will automatically affect the function of the other.

The widespread use of computers and visual display units (VDUs) in the workplace has resulted in an increase in neck problems due to the sustained static contraction of the neck muscles. Assessment of those with neck problems must include a detailed analysis of the individual's workstation and working position and also take into account the length of time the individual may work at a VDU. It is essential that people who work at VDUs for prolonged periods have regular breaks to help reduce the sustained static load on the neck.

In the following sections, the muscles are described in groups according to the prime movements they produce, without regard for their relative positions in the neck, after the style of Palastanga et al (1989). During examination of a patient it should be remembered that the force of gravity may replace prime mover muscular activity, in which case the activity in the muscles will alter accordingly.

Muscles which flex the neck

- Longus colli
- Sternocleidomastoid
- Scalenus anterior

Longus colli

Longus colli (Fig. 3.3) is the deepest of the anterior muscles and lies on the front and sides of the upper thoracic and cervical vertebral bodies. It has three sets of fibres:

1. *Inferior oblique fibres* from the anterior aspects of the 1st, 2nd and 3rd thoracic vertebral bodies pass upwards and laterally to the anterior tubercles of the transverse processes of the 5th and 6th cervical vertebrae.

2. *Vertical fibres* from the anterior part of the bodies of the upper three thoracic and lower three cervical vertebrae pass to the anterior part of the bodies of the 2nd, 3rd and 4th cervical vertebrae.

3. *Superior oblique fibres* from the anterior tubercles of the transverse processes of the 3rd, 4th and 5th cervical vertebrae pass upwards and medially to the anterior tubercle on the anterior arch of the atlas.

Nerve supply.   The ventral rami of C3, 4, 5 and 6.

Actions.   The main action of longus colli is flexion of the neck. Contraction of the muscle causes anterior sagittal rotation of the cervical vertebrae because the muscle lies anterior to the centre of rotation for flexion and extension. In addition, contraction increases the compressive force on the cervical vertebrae. Due to their anterior position, these muscles are particularly vulnerable to injury during forced hyperextension of the cervical spine, such as in whiplash disorders. The longus colli and capitis are

Figure 3.3   Longus colli and longus capitis-anterior view. (From Porterfield JA, DeRosa C 1994 *Mechanical Neck Pain. Perspectives in Functional Anatomy.* Saunders, Philadelphia, p. 74, Figure 3.24B, with permission.)

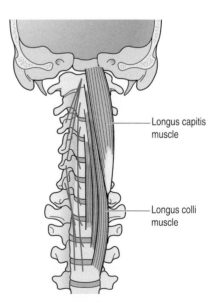

Longus capitis muscle

Longus colli muscle

immediately proximal to two important structures: the vertebral arteries and the cervical sympathetic chain.

The inferior and superior oblique fibres of one side assist in laterally flexing the neck, and the inferior oblique fibres in rotating it to the opposite side.

Sternocleidomastoid

Sternocleidomastoid (Fig. 3.4) has two heads: the *sternal head* is attached to the upper part of the manubrium sterni; the *clavicular head* is attached to the upper surface of the medial third of the clavicle. The sternal head passes upwards, laterally and backwards; the clavicular head passes almost vertically upwards, behind the sternal head, blending with its deep surface. The sternocleidomastoid is attached by a short tendon into the lateral surface of the mastoid process of the temporal bone (especially the clavicular fibres) and lateral half of the superior nuchal line of the occipital bone (sternal fibres).

Nerve supply. The motor supply of sternocleidomastoid is by the spinal part of the accessory (eleventh cranial) nerve. It receives sensory fibres from the anterior rami of C2 and C3.

Actions. *Unilateral* contraction of sternocleidomastoid laterally flexes the head on the neck, rotating it to the opposite side, and laterally flexes the cervical spine to the same side.

The oblique course of sternocleidomastoid from the sternum to the mastoid allows it to have a number of different actions. Because the superior part of the muscle lies behind the centre for rotation of flexion and extension and the inferior part of the muscle lies anterior to this centre of rotation, the sternocleidomastoid is able to extend the upper cervical spine, particularly the occiput on the atlas, and flex the lower cervical spine.

Figure 3.4 Superficial neck muscles – left lateral aspect.

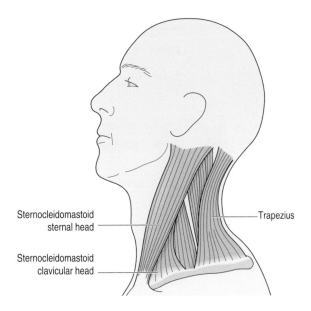

Sternocleidomastoid sternal head

Sternocleidomastoid clavicular head

Trapezius

If the head and neck are fixed, the muscle acts *bilaterally* to assist in elevating the thorax in forced inspiration.

Sternocleidomastoid lies at some distance from the centre of rotation of the cervical vertebrae and, along with trapezius, the muscle acts as anterior and lateral guy wires to support the head and neck. The orientation of the lower portion of the muscle helps to resist forceful extension or posterior movement of the cervical spine, and this muscle is therefore often injured during an acceleration/deceleration trauma that forcefully extends the neck.

Spasm of sternocleidomastoid is a significant feature of several deformities seen in the neck. In *spasmodic torticollis* ('wry neck') shortening of this muscle is the deforming force, often accompanied by spasm of the clavicular portion of trapezius. In the deformity of *atlanto-axial rotatory fixation*, where there is fixation of the atlas on the axis in a rotatory position, the elongated sternocleidomastoid is in spasm (Fielding and Hawkins, 1978).

Sternocleidomastoid is superficial and can be easily palpated through the skin. In those patients with chronic head and neck pain where there is poor recruitment and endurance of the deep neck flexors, there is usually increased activity in sternocleidomastoid in functional postural positions that can be both seen and palpated.

Muscles which flex the head and neck

- Sternocleidomastoid (see p. 105)
- Longus capitis (see Fig. 3.3)

Longus capitis

Longus capitis is a long muscle attached below to the anterior tubercles of the transverse processes of the 3rd, 4th, 5th and 6th cervical vertebrae and passing upwards and medially to attach to the basilar part of the occipital bone.

Nerve supply. The ventral rami of C1–3.

Actions. Longus capitis flexes the head on the neck, and the upper cervical spine.

Muscles which flex the head on the neck

- Rectus capitis anterior

Rectus capitis anterior

Rectus capitis anterior is a short muscle lying deep to longus capitis. It is attached to the anterior aspect of the lateral mass of the atlas up to its transverse process, and passes upwards and medially to attach to the basilar part of the occipital bone.

Nerve supply. The ventral rami of C1 and C2.

Actions.   Rectus capitis flexes the head on the neck. It may also act as a postural muscle in stabilizing the atlanto-occipital joint. Rectus capitis has a large number of muscle spindles and it's principal function may be proprioception for occipital motion rather than a prime mover (Porterfield, 1995).

Muscles which laterally flex the neck

- Scalenus anterior
- Scalenus medius
- Scalenus posterior
- Splenius cervicis
- Levator scapulae (see p. 114-115)
- Sternocleidomastoid (see p. 105)

Scalenus anterior   Scalenus anterior (Fig. 3.5) is attached to the anterior tubercles of the transverse processes of the 3rd–6th cervical vertebrae. Its fibres run almost vertically downwards to attach to the scalene tubercle on the 1st rib, near the groove for the subclavian artery.

Nerve supply.   The ventral rami of C4–6.

Actions.   Unilateral contraction of scalenus anterior causes lateral flexion of the cervical spine to the same side, with a small amount of rotation to the opposite side. Bilateral contraction of the muscles produces flexion of the neck; the lever arm of the anterior scalene muscle is less than that of sternocleidomastoid and it is therefore less effective as a neck flexor. If

Figure 3.5   The scalene muscles – anterolateral aspect.

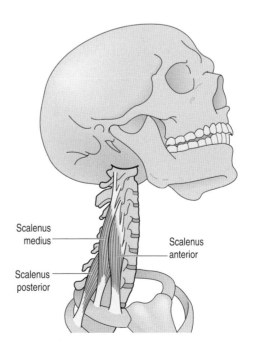

Scalenus medius

Scalenus anterior

Scalenus posterior

the upper attachment is fixed, scalenus anterior assists in elevating the 1st rib.

Scalenus medius   Scalenus medius (see Fig. 3.5) is the largest of the scalene muscles. Proximally, it is attached to the transverse process of the axis, often that of the atlas, and from the posterior tubercles of the transverse processes of the lower five cervical vertebrae. The fibres run downwards and laterally to attach to the superior surface of the 1st rib just posterior to the groove for the subclavian artery.

Nerve supply.   The ventral rami of C3–8.

Actions.   Unilateral contraction of scalenus medius produces lateral flexion of the cervical spine to the same side. If the upper attachment is fixed, it helps to elevate the 1st rib.

Scalenus posterior   Scalenus posterior (see Fig. 3.5) is the smallest of the scalene muscles. Proximally it is attached to the posterior tubercles of the transverse processes of the 4th–6th cervical vertebrae. Its fibres run downwards and laterally to attach to the outer surface of the 2nd rib.

Nerve supply.   The ventral rami of C6–8.

Actions.   Unilateral contraction of scalenus posterior produces lateral flexion of the lower part of the cervical spine to the same side. If its upper attachment is fixed, it helps to elevate the 2nd rib.

Clinical considerations

Scalenus anterior and scalenus medius, together with the 1st rib, form the *scalene triangle*, through which the ventral roots of C5–T1 spinal nerves and the subclavian artery pass. These vessels are vulnerable to compression or irritation and may be affected by the presence of a cervical rib, a band of fascia, variations in muscle attachments, or hypertrophy of the muscles, causing symptoms in the upper limb which simulate those from nerve root irritation and compression (see pp. 25-26).

The scalene muscles are active during inspiration, even during quiet breathing. In chronic respiratory conditions, the 1st rib may be elevated due to muscle spasm.

As a group, the scalene muscles are laterally placed and act as important guys for the cervical spine in the frontal plane.

Scalenus anterior and levator scapulae act together as a force couple due to their orientation, which creates an anterior–posterior pull on the cervical spine (Fig. 3.6). Contraction of levator scapulae imparts a posterior shear force to the cervical spine, while contraction of scalenus anterior creates an anterior shear force. The orientation of these muscles in opposite directions helps to provide a check to anterior and posterior shear forces and enhance stability of the neck.

Figure 3.6   The levator
scapulae and anterior scalene
force couple. (From Porterfield
JA, DeRosa C 1994 *Mechanical
Neck Pain. Perspectives in
Functional Anatomy.* Saunders,
Philadelphia, p. 73, Fig 3.23,
with permission.)

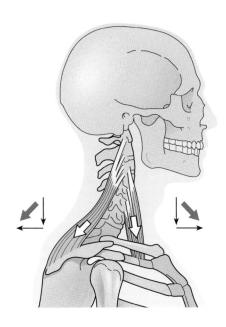

Splenius cervicis

Splenius cervicis (Fig. 3.7) is attached distally to the spinous processes of
the 3rd–6th thoracic vertebrae. Its fibres pass upwards and laterally to
attach to the posterior tubercles of the transverse processes of the upper
three cervical vertebrae.

Figure 3.7   Trapezius, levator
scapulae and splenius cervicis.

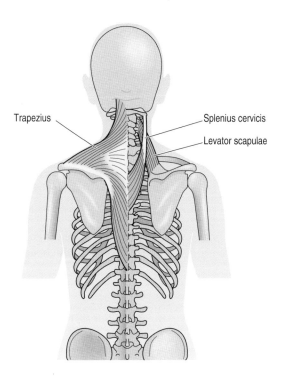

Nerve supply. The dorsal rami of C5–7.

Actions. Unilateral contraction of splenius cervicis laterally flexes and slightly rotates the neck to the same side. Bilateral contraction extends the neck.

Muscles which laterally flex the head and neck

- Sternocleidomastoid (see pp. 105-106)
- Splenius capitis
- Trapezius (see pp. 113-114)
- Erector spinae (see pp. 134-140)

Splenius capitis

Splenius capitis lies deep to sternocleidomastoid and trapezius. Distally, it is attached to the lower half of ligamentum nuchae, the spinous processes of the 7th cervical vertebra and upper four thoracic vertebrae. Its fibres run upwards and laterally to attach just below the lateral third of the superior nuchal line, and on the mastoid process of the temporal bone.

Nerve supply. The dorsal rami of C3–5.

Actions. Unilateral contraction of splenius capitis produces extension of the head and neck, usually combined with lateral flexion of the neck and rotation of the face to the same side. Bilateral contraction produces extension of the head and neck. There is little or no activity in splenius capitis in the upright, balanced postural position (Nolan and Sherk, 1988).

Muscles which laterally flex the head on the neck

- Rectus capitis lateralis

Rectus capitis lateralis

Rectus capitis lateralis is a short muscle attaching distally to the upper surface of the transverse process of the atlas. Its fibres pass upwards to attach to the jugular process of the occipital bone.

Nerve supply. The ventral rami of C1 and C2.

Actions. Unilateral contraction of rectus capitis lateralis produces lateral flexion of the head to the same side.

Muscles which extend the neck

- Levator scapulae (see pp. 114-115)
- Splenius cervicis (see pp. 109)

Muscles which extend the head and neck

- Trapezius (see pp. 113-114)
- Splenius capitis (see p. 110)
- Erector spinae (see pp. 134-140)

Muscles which extend the head on the neck

- Rectus capitis posterior major
- Rectus capitis posterior minor
- Obliquus capitis superior

With obliquus capitis inferior, these muscles are known as the *suboccipital muscles*.

Rectus capitis posterior major

Rectus capitis posterior major (Fig. 3.8) is attached distally to the spinous process of the axis and proximally to the lateral part of the inferior nuchal line of the occipital bone.

Nerve supply.   The dorsal ramus of C1.

Actions.   Unilateral contraction of rectus capitis posterior major may rotate the head to the same side, but its main function is likely to be stabilization of the atlanto-occipital joint. The muscle has a long lever arm, and on bilateral contraction is well placed to produce extension of the head on the neck.

Rectus capitis posterior minor

Rectus capitis posterior minor (see Fig. 3.8) is attached distally to the tubercle on the posterior arch of the atlas and proximally to the medial part of the inferior nuchal line of the occipital bone.

Figure 3.8   The suboccipital muscles – posterolateral aspect.

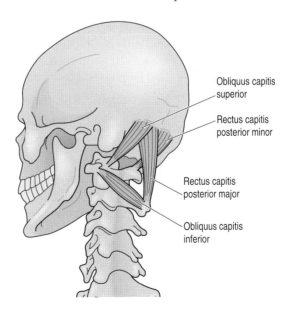

Obliquus capitis superior

Rectus capitis posterior minor

Rectus capitis posterior major

Obliquus capitis inferior

Nerve supply.   The dorsal ramus of C1.

Actions.   Rectus capitis posterior minor extends the head on the neck and stabilizes the atlanto-occipital joint.

Obliquus capitis superior

Obliquus capitis superior (see Fig. 3.8) is attached distally to the transverse process of the atlas, and proximally between the superior and inferior nuchal lines of the occipital bone lateral to semispinalis capitis.

Nerve supply.   The dorsal ramus of C1.

Actions.   Obliquus capitis superior produces extension of the head on the neck and lateral flexion to the same side. It has an important role in stabilization of the atlanto-occipital joint.

Muscles which rotate the neck

- Semispinalis cervicis (see p. 131)
- Multifidus (see pp. 132–134)
- Scalenus anterior (see pp. 107–108)
- Splenius cervicis (see p. 109)

Muscles which rotate the head and neck

- Sternocleidomastoid (see pp. 105–106)
- Splenius capitis (see p. 110)

Muscles which rotate the head on the neck

- Obliquus capitis inferior
- Rectus capitis posterior major (see pp. 111–112)

Obliquus capitis inferior

Obliquus capitis inferior (see Fig. 3.8) is the largest of the suboccipital muscles. It is attached distally to the spinous process of the axis and adjacent lamina, and proximally to the transverse process of the atlas.

Nerve supply.   The dorsal ramus of C1.

Actions.   Obliquus capitis inferior rotates the head to the same side. Bilateral contraction produces extension at the atlanto-axial joint.

Clinical considerations

The suboccipital muscles act to fine-tune movements of the head. These muscles are highly innervated: the number of muscle fibres per neurone is small, each neurone supplying approximately 3–5 fibres. The muscles are capable of rapid changes in tension, and they are able to control head posture with a fine degree of precision.

Continues

Continued

> The suboccipital region is particularly prone to degenerative change, and the muscles have a strong tendency to tighten, resulting in the upper cervical spine being held in extension. In such instances, a compensatory flexion deformity often occurs in the lower cervical spine. Significant atrophy of the suboccipital muscles has been found in patients with chronic neck pain (Hallgren et al, 1994; McPartland et al, 1997).
>
> In patients with cervical dysfunction and headaches, palpation of the soft tissues that insert onto the posterior aspect of the occiput often reproduces head and neck pain; the tissues can also feel thickened and tight and be exquisitely tender. A number of soft tissues insert onto the occiput, including fascia, trapezius, splenius capitis, semispinalis capitis and the suboccipital muscles, so that accurate identification of a single structure is fraught with difficulty. Nevertheless, manual treatment of soft tissue tightness and tissues that are painful on palpation in this area can be very effective as part of the overall treatment plan.

Muscles which elevate the shoulder girdle

- Trapezius (upper fibres)
- Levator scapulae

Trapezius

Trapezius (see Figs 3.4, 3.7) is the most superficial muscle in the cervico-thoracic spine. In the cervical spine trapezius arises from the medial third of the superior nuchal line of the occipital bone, the external occipital protuberance and the ligamentum nuchae as far as C7. In the thoracic spine, trapezius arises from the spinous process of the thoracic vertebrae, but there is a decreasing frequency of fascicles from T6 to T12 (Johnson et al, 1994).

The superior fibres pass downwards and laterally to attach to the lateral third of the clavicle; the middle fibres pass almost horizontally to attach to the medial margin of the acromion and the deltoid tubercle of the scapula; and the inferior fibres blend into an aponeurosis which is attached to the medial and lower part of the deltoid tubercle on the spine of the scapula.

Nerve supply. Trapezius receives its motor supply from the accessory (eleventh cranial) nerve, and sensory branches from the ventral rami of C3 and C4.

Actions. The superior fibres of trapezius do not have a direct action on the scapula because they attach to the clavicle, but they can move the scapula indirectly through the acromioclavicular joint. These fibres have a transverse orientation and can draw the clavicle and scapula backwards in actions such as pulling and rowing. The direction and attachment of the nuchal fibres do not allow them to elevate the scapula directly but they can elevate the scapula through another mechanism (Johnson et al,

1994). In the upright postural position, the clavicle is orientated upwards and laterally, the axis of upward rotation being the sternoclavicular joint or the costoclavicular ligament. The resulting force from the orientation of the nuchal fibres of trapezius, which pass above the axis of upward rotation of the clavicle, creates a medially directed moment onto the clavicle, which draws the clavicle and scapula up by rotating the clavicle. This action creates a compressive force at the sternoclavicular joint.

Trapezius works with serratus anterior to rotate the scapula for functional use of the upper limb. When serratus anterior contracts, it draws the scapula laterally around the chest wall, but this displacement is resisted by the lower fibres of trapezius. The lower fibres sustain a constant length to maintain the position of the deltoid tubercle, which becomes the axis of rotation. The upper fibres of trapezius exert an upward moment about this axis and work with serratus anterior to rotate the scapula laterally. The transverse orientation of the fibres ensures that activity in cervical trapezius does not increase compressive loads on the neck, but helps to transfer the weight of the upper limb onto the sternoclavicular joint.

The superior fibres of trapezius work with levator scapulae to maintain the shoulder position when a heavy load is carried in the hand. When the arm is unloaded, there is often little or no activity in the trapezius (Bearn, 1961).

When the scapula is fixed, the upper fibres of trapezius may laterally flex the neck to the same side and rotate it to the opposite side. Bilateral contraction produces extension of the head and neck.

Clinical considerations

Spasm, tension or trigger points in the upper fibres of trapezius are common in patients with neck problems. This muscle has a limited capacity to withstand sustained static loading, which can occur during activities such as working at a VDU.

The trapezius is an important stabilizer of the scapula for functional activities of the upper limb. In order to fulfil this function, longus capitis and longus colli help to fixate the head and neck to prevent an extension moment occurring during movements of the upper limb. In patients who have decreased activation of the anterior neck muscles (e.g. following an extension acceleration injury), longus capitis and longus colli are unable to adequately fixate the neck so that trapezius cannot pull from a stabilized occiput. This can result in the patient being unable to raise the arms in a pain-free manner and having reduced functional control of the arm.

Levator scapulae   Levator scapulae (see Fig. 3.7) lies deep to sternocleidomastoid in its upper part and trapezius in its lower part. It is attached proximally to the transverse process of the atlas and axis and the posterior tubercles of the transverse processes of the 3rd and 4th cervical vertebrae. Its fibres run downwards and laterally to attach to the medial border of the scapula between its superior angle and the medial end of the spine of the scapula.

Nerve supply.   The ventral rami of C3 and 4, and from C5 through the dorsal scapular nerve.

Actions.   Working with trapezius, levator scapulae helps to stabilize the scapula during movements of the arm. When its proximal attachment is fixed, it assists in elevating the scapula. When its distal attachment is fixed, it laterally flexes the cervical spine and rotates it to the same side. Bilateral contraction produces a posterior shear force on the neck which is resisted anteriorly by the anterior scalene muscles. The effect of gravity on the normal cervical lordosis and the forward head position that develops with poor posture increase the anterior shear force upon the neck; levator scapulae is orientated to act as a dynamic restraint to this force (see Fig. 3.6; Porterfield, 1995) and the muscle has to maintain continuous activity to oppose anterior shear in the upright postural position.

The position of the scapula is not fixed and is determined by a number of factors including the degree of curvature of the thoracic kyphosis and the control of muscles such as trapezius, rhomboid major and serratus anterior. A suboptimal resting position of the scapula will inevitably affect the resting length of levator scapulae and its ability to help stabilize the cervical spine.

MUSCLES OF RESPIRATION

- Diaphragm
- Intercostales
- Transversus thoracis
- Levatores costarum
- Serratus posterior superior
- Serratus posterior inferior
- Subcostales

These muscles all have some attachments to the ribs and, hence, are concerned in their movements and consequently, respiration.

Diaphragm   The diaphragm is a musculotendinous sheet separating the thoracic from the abdominal cavity. Peripherally, its muscular fibres attach to the back of the xiphoid process, the internal surfaces of the cartilages and adjacent parts of the 7th–12th ribs, interdigitating with transversus abdominis. The diagram also arises from the medial and lateral arcuate ligaments and from the lumbar vertebrae by two crura.

The medial arcuate ligament is a thickening of the fascia covering psoas major; it is attached medially to the body of the 2nd lumbar vertebra and laterally to the transverse process of the 1st lumbar vertebra.

The lateral arcuate ligament is a thickening of the anterior layer of the thoracolumbar fascia covering quadratus lumborum; it is attached medially to the transverse process of the 1st lumbar vertebra and laterally to the middle of the 12th rib.

The crura are attached to the anterolateral surfaces of the upper two (on the left) or three (on the right) lumbar vertebral bodies and their discs, and form an arch over the aorta.

These muscular fibres arch upwards and converge into a central strong aponeurosis or tendon, forming a dome-shaped sheet that separates the thorax from the abdominal cavity. Openings in the diaphragm include those for the aorta, vena cava, oesophagus, splanchnic nerves and sympathetic trunks.

Nerve supply. The diaphragm is supplied with motor and sensory fibres from the phrenic nerve (C3–5). Additional sensory fibres to the periphery are supplied by the lower six intercostal nerves.

Actions. The diaphragm is the main muscle of inspiration. On contraction of the muscle, the lower ribs are at first fixed, and the central tendon is drawn downwards and forwards, compressing the abdominal viscera which are prevented from bulging outwards by abdominal muscle tone. The central tendon then becomes the fixed point for the action of the diaphragm, which on further contraction elevates the lower ribs. The anterior ends of the vertebrosternal ribs are pushed forwards and upwards, elevating the sternum and upper ribs (see pp. 199–200).

The diaphragm also has an important part to play in increasing intra-abdominal pressure by resisting upward movement of the abdominal viscera on contraction of the abdominal muscles. It thereby assists in all expulsive actions such as coughing, sneezing, laughing, and prior to expulsion of faeces and urine, and of the fetus from the uterus. By this mechanism, it also supports the lumbar spine in lifting.

The position of the diaphragm varies considerably with the position of the body. It is in its highest position in supine-lying, and during breathing in this position it performs large excursions of movement. In the standing position the dome is lower, and it reaches its lowest level in the sitting position. During normal respiration in sitting, the respiratory excursion of the diaphragm is relatively small. Three factors influence the position of the diaphragm in the thorax:

1. The elastic retraction of the lung tissue, which tends to pull the diaphragm upwards.

2. The viscera exert a pressure on the undersurface of the diaphragm. In sitting and standing it is a negative pressure so that the diaphragm is pulled or sucked downwards. In a lying position it is a positive pressure, so that the diaphragm moves upwards.

3. Intra-abdominal tension due to the abdominal muscles. In standing, the abdominal muscles are in a state of contraction, and they are relaxed in sitting. Hence the diaphragm is pushed higher in standing than sitting.

Intercostales (Fig. 3.9)   The intercostales are three thin layers of muscle lying between adjacent ribs.

Intercostales externi is the outermost and thickest muscle layer. Its fibres pass from the lower border of the rib above to the upper border of the rib below, running obliquely downwards and medially anteriorly, and downwards and laterally posteriorly. Its attachments extend from the tubercles of the ribs posteriorly to the cartilages of the ribs anteriorly, where the muscle is replaced by the external intercostal membrane.

Intercostales interni is the middle muscle layer. Its fibres pass from the floor of the costal groove and costal cartilage of the rib above to the upper border of the rib below, running obliquely downwards and laterally anteriorly, and downwards and medially posteriorly, at right angles to those of the intercostales externi. Its attachments may extend from the sternum to the costal angles posteriorly, where the muscle is replaced by the internal intercostal membrane.

Intercostales intimi is the deepest muscle layer. It runs from the internal aspects of two adjacent ribs in approximately the central two quarters. These muscles may be poorly developed or absent in the upper thoracic spine, but elsewhere in the thoracic spine they are better developed. The direction of muscle fibres is similar to that of the intercostales interni, from which they are separated by the intercostal nerves and vessels.

Nerve supply.   The intercostales are supplied by the ventral rami of adjacent intercostal nerves.

Actions.   The intercostales are unlikely to be involved in moving the ribs. They contract simultaneously and it is thought that they provide

Figure 3.9   The intercostal muscles.

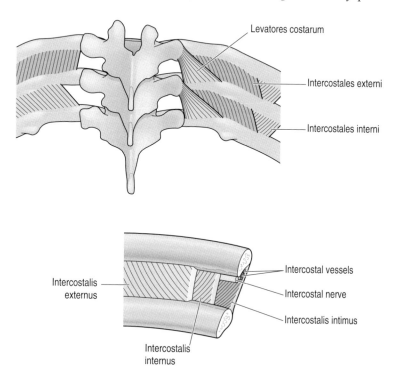

Levatores costarum

Intercostales externi

Intercostales interni

Intercostalis externus

Intercostal vessels

Intercostal nerve

Intercostalis intimus

Intercostalis internus

strong elastic supports that prevent the intercostal spaces from being separated during respiration. The anterior portions of intercostales interni help to prevent separation of the sternocostal and interchondral surfaces, while the intercostales externi help to maintain integrity at the costovertebral articulations.

Transversus thoracis (sternocostalis)

Transversus thoracis is located on the internal surface of the anterior part of the thorax. It is attached to the lower third of the deep surface of the sternum, xiphoid process and adjacent costal cartilages of the 4th–7th ribs. Its upper fibres pass upwards and laterally, while its lower fibres pass horizontally to attach to the inner surfaces of the costal cartilages of the 2nd–6th ribs.

Nerve supply. Transversus thoracis depresses the costal cartilages, aiding expiration.

Levatores costarum (see Fig. 3.9)

The levatores costarum (12 on each side) are small, strong bundles of muscle which lie between the 7th cervical and 11th thoracic vertebrae. Each muscle runs from the tip of the transverse process of the vertebra above to the rib of the next level below between the tubercle and angle. Each of the four lower muscles also has a second fasciculus attaching to the second rib below its origin.

Nerve supply. Levatores costarum are supplied by the dorsal rami of the adjacent thoracic nerves.

Actions. Because the levatores costarum are inserted near the fulcra of the ribs they are unlikely to create much movement of the ribs. Acting from the ribs, these small muscles can produce a slight degree of rotation and lateral flexion of the vertebral column.

Serratus posterior superior

Serratus posterior superior is a thin, quadrilateral muscle lying anterior to the rhomboids. Medially, it is attached to the lower part of the ligamentum nuchae, the spinous processes of the 7th cervical and upper three thoracic vertebrae and their supraspinous ligaments. The fibres pass downwards and laterally to be attached by four fleshy digitations lateral to the angles of the 2nd–5th ribs.

Nerve supply. Serratus posterior superior is supplied by the ventral rami of the 2nd–5th intercostal nerves.

Actions. Serratus posterior superior elevates the ribs and it is therefore an inspiratory muscle.

Serratus posterior inferior

Serratus posterior inferior is a thin, quadrilateral muscle lying deep to latissimus dorsi. Medially, it is attached to the spinous processes of the 11th and 12th thoracic and 1st and 2nd lumbar vertebrae and their supraspinous ligaments via the thoracolumbar fascia. The fibres pass upwards and laterally to attach by four digitations into the lower four ribs, just lateral to their angles.

Nerve supply. The ventral rami of the 9th–12th thoracic spinal nerves.

Actions.   Serratus posterior inferior draws the lower ribs downwards and backwards, elongating the thorax. It fixes the lower ribs and assists the inspiratory action of the diaphragm by resisting the tendency of the lower ribs to be drawn upwards and forwards. It is therefore a muscle of inspiration.

Subcostales   Subcostales are usually best developed in the lower thoracic region. Each muscle passes from the internal surface of one rib near its angle to the internal surface of the second and third rib below. The direction of the fibres is the same as that of the internal intercostales.

Nerve supply.   The ventral rami of the adjacent intercostal nerves.

Actions.   It is thought that it acts with the intercostales interni to help prevent separation of the ribs near the rib angle.

LUMBAR MUSCLES

The intersegmental nature of the deep back muscles (rotatores, multifidus, interspinales and intertransversarii), which connect adjacent vertebrae at appropriate angles, enables them to assist effectively in stabilizing the vertebral column. Because of their larger size, the superficial muscles of the back are better adapted to counterbalance external loads and achieve the overall spinal posture and movement. The quality of performance of the superficial muscles depends on the integrated action of the deeper muscles.

Individuals with or without back pain may lack control of their deep local muscles so that they have poor segmental control during even light everyday activities. The lack of segmental control could result in microtrauma of the tissues which eventually results in sufficient damage to trigger the nociceptors, leading to low back pain.

Most of the back muscles are arranged more or less longitudinally, and on contraction they have a compressive effect on spinal structures in proportion to the strength of the contraction. Intradiscal pressure is particularly sensitive to differing strengths of muscle contraction, as demonstrated by increases recorded in certain postures, exercises and lifting (see pp. 71–73).

Patients with chronic low back pain often exhibit patterns of muscle imbalance such as weakness of abdominal and gluteal muscles combined with tightness of erectores spinae and psoas major. The abdominal muscles have been shown to fatigue more easily than the back extensors, and this is more marked in patients with back pain (Suzuki and Endo, 1983).

When weakness of one muscle group exists, movement patterns alter in an attempt to accommodate it, so that unwanted compensatory movements occur. For example, if gluteus maximus is weak, the pattern of hip extension is altered, and there is compensatory increased activity in the hamstrings and erector spinae.

Muscle spasm, which initially has a protective function, can also be the primary mechanism involved in referred pain, e.g. spasm of piriformis associated with a sacroiliac lesion causing buttock and trochanteric pain (Kirkaldy Willis and Hill, 1979).

Muscles which produce flexion of the trunk

- Psoas major
- Psoas minor
- Obliquus externus abdominis
- Obliquus internus abdominis
- Rectus abdominis

Iliacus and psoas major (iliopsoas)

Iliacus and psoas major are normally considered together as they have a common tendon that attaches onto the femur (Fig. 3.10). Psoas is a long, deep muscle situated on the lateral aspect of the lumbar spine and the pelvic brim. It is attached proximally to the anterior surfaces of the transverse processes of all the lumbar vertebrae, the lumbar intervertebral discs and margins of their adjacent vertebral bodies (the highest being from the lower margin of the 12th thoracic vertebra, the lowest from the upper margin of the 5th lumbar vertebral body), and from fibrous arches between the above digitations, connecting the upper and lower margins of the vertebral bodies.

The muscle descends along the pelvic brim, passing posterior to the inguinal ligament and anterior to the capsule of the hip joint, having received, on its lateral side, nearly all of the iliacus fibres. It converges into a tendon which is attached to the lesser trochanter of the femur.

Iliacus is attached to the iliac fossa and inner lip of the iliac crest. The muscle fibres converge with psoas to form a tendon that attaches onto the lesser trochanter.

Figure 3.10 Psoas and iliacus.

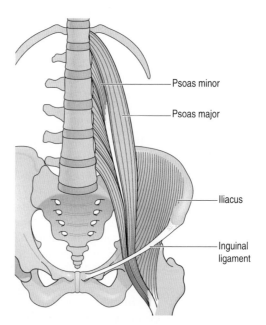

Psoas minor

Psoas major

Iliacus

Inguinal ligament

Nerve supply. The ventral rami of L1–3. The lumbar plexus is situated posteriorly in the substance of the muscle.

Actions. Acting from above, psoas major flexes the hip when the foot is off the ground. Iliopsoas is also a weak lateral rotator of the hip: in the frontal plane, the lesser trochanter is slightly posterior on the medial surface of the femur so that when iliopsoas contracts, the lesser trochanter is pulled forwards, resulting in lateral rotation of the femur.

In the standing position, when the feet are on the floor so that it is a closed kinetic chain, the leg is fixed and the force occurs at the pelvis in the case of the iliacus muscle and in the lumbar spine in the case of psoas. The contraction of iliacus causes an anterior torsion of the ilium, whereas contraction of psoas creates an anterior shear of the lumbar vertebrae creating lumbar extension.

Acting from below when the thighs are fixed, psoas major muscle also has a powerful effect on flexion of the hip. In the initial trunk curl phase of the 'sit-up' exercise, the abdominal muscles contract and shorten, flattening the back so that the pelvis tilts posteriorly. Once the spine is flexed, the hip flexion phase follows and iliopsoas contracts to lift the trunk and pelvis, pulling the pelvis into anterior tilt.

Electromyographic studies have shown that psoas is active in many different postures and movements and it is probably acting in a stabilizing capacity (Nachemson, 1966). Psoas activity creates a compressive force on the intervertebral disc so that contraction of the muscle increases intradiscal pressure. The increase in compression enhances the stability of the lumbar spine in anti-gravity positions.

During quiet sitting, there is no activity in psoas major, but vigorous activity has been demonstrated in these muscles in controlling deviations of the trunk from the rest position, especially in lateral flexion of the trunk to the opposite side and leaning backwards (Keagy et al, 1966). Marked activity has also been demonstrated when the foot is raised from the floor, as in lifting the foot to press the clutch pedal when driving.

During quiet standing there is little activity in psoas major, but it is active in the swing phase in walking.

Spasm of psoas may be one of the contributing factors in the deformity of a 'sciatic scoliosis' seen in some patients with intervertebral disc derangements or other pathology in the lumbar spine. The lumbar spine is held in a degree of lateral flexion and, usually, forward flexion, with a rotatory component. Significant asymmetry in the cross-sectional area of psoas major was found in patients with unilateral sciatica on the side of the pathology (Dangaria and Naesh, 1998).

Adaptive shortening of iliopsoas is commonly seen in individuals with low back and pelvic dysfunction. In the upright standing position, if iliopsoas is short it will create an anterior torsion on the ilia while the lumbar spine is pulled forward and downward creating an extension moment in the lumbar spine. This increases the compressive force on the spine and hence the intradiscal pressure; the lumbar apophyseal joints are also subjected to greater weight-bearing demands.

Psoas minor

Psoas minor (see Fig. 3.10) is inconstant. When present, it lies anterior to psoas major within the abdomen. It is attached to the T12/L1 intervertebral disc and adjacent vertebral body margins and ends in a long tendon which is attached to the pectin pubis.

Nerve supply.   The ventral ramus of L1.

Actions.   Psoas acts as a weak flexor of the lumbar spine.

Obliquus externus abdominis

Obliquus externus abdominis (Fig. 3.11) is the most superficial of the abdominal muscles and is situated on the anterolateral aspect of the abdominal wall. It is the strongest of the diagonal muscles. It is attached proximally to the external surface and inferior borders of the lower eight ribs and their costal cartilages, interdigitating with serratus anterior above and latissimus dorsi below.

The muscle fibres from the lower two ribs pass almost vertically downwards to attach to the anterior half of the iliac crest. Its upper and middle fibres pass downwards and medially to end in an aponeurosis which is broader below than above. The aponeuroses from both sides fuse in the midline at the linea alba, which runs from the tip of the xiphoid process of the sternum to the symphysis pubis. The lower border of the aponeu-

Figure 3.11   The abdominal muscles.

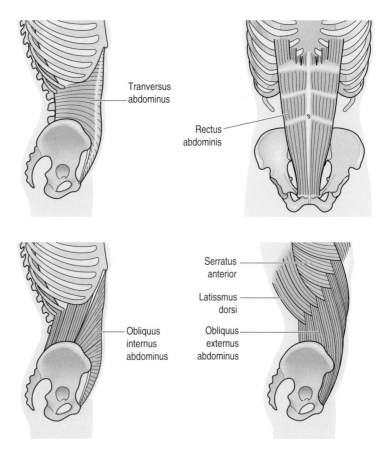

Tranversus abdominus

Rectus abdominis

Obliquus internus abdominus

Serratus anterior

Latissmus dorsi

Obliquus externus abdominus

rosis forms the inguinal ligament, extending from the anterior superior iliac spine to the pubic tubercle. An extension from the medial part of the inguinal ligament to the medial end of the pectin pubis is called the lacunar ligament.

Nerve supply. The ventral rami of T7–12.

Actions. Obliquus externus abdominis flexes the spine by bringing the thorax closer to the pelvis. It also flexes the lumbosacral junction by posteriorly rotating the pelvis. Obliquus externus abdominis rotates the thorax to the contralateral side by working with the fibres of obliquus internus abdominis on the opposite side. Unilateral contraction of obliquus externus abdominis with obliquus internus abdominis on the same side laterally flexes the vertebral column. The arrangement and direction of the inferior and medial fibres of obliquus externus abdominis helps to control the downward and forward movement of the pelvis in the standing position (Kendall et al, 1993).

Obliquus internus abdominis

Obliquus internus abdominis (see Fig. 3.11) lies deep to obliquus externus abdominis. Distally and laterally, it is attached to the lateral two thirds of the inguinal ligament, the anterior two thirds of the iliac crest and the thoracolumbar fascia.

Its posterior fibres pass upwards and laterally to attach to the inferior borders of the lower three or four ribs and are continuous with the intercostales interni; its middle fibres pass upwards and medially to attach to an *aponeurosis* (see below); the fibres from the inguinal ligament pass downwards and medially and, with the lower part of the aponeurosis of transversus abdominis, form the conjoint tendon which attaches to the crest of the pubis and medial part of the pectin pubis.

The aponeurosis: In its upper two thirds, the aponeurosis splits into two laminae at the lateral border of rectus abdominis. The laminae pass around rectus abdominis and reunite in the linea alba. The anterior lamina blends with the aponeurosis of obliquus externus abdominis, while the posterior lamina blends with the aponeurosis of transversus abdominis. The upper part of the aponeurosis attaches to the cartilages of the 7th–9th ribs. In the lower third, the aponeuroses of obliquus externus abdominis and transversus abdominis pass in front of rectus abdominis to the linea alba.

Nerve supply. The ventral rami of T7–12 and L1.

Actions. Obliquus internus abdominis contributes to the support of the abdominal viscera and increases intra-abdominal pressure. It produces ipsilateral rotation of the trunk together with obliquus externus abdominis on the opposite side. Bilateral contraction of obliquus internus abdominis flexes the trunk and helps to stabilize the pelvis during leg movements (Floyd and Silver, 1950). Contraction of obliquus internus abdominis with obliquus externus abdominis on the same side produces ipsilateral lateral flexion.

The posterior fibres of obliquus internus abdominis insert into the lateral raphe of the thoracolumbar fascia and, along with transversus abdominis, it is thought that this muscle contributes to the local support system of the spine (Bergmark, 1989). However, this attachment is not present in some individuals and it would therefore be unable to contribute to segmental stability in these people (Bogduk and Macintosh, 1984).

The horizontal direction of the lower fibres of transversus abdominis and obliquus internus abdominis across the iliac crests assists in compressing and stabilizing the sacroiliac joint (Snijders et al, 1995).

Rectus abdominis

Rectus abdominis (see Fig. 3.11) is a long muscle running vertically on the front of the abdomen, separated from its fellow by the linea alba. It is attached distally by two tendons: to the pubic crest laterally, and to ligamentous fibres covering the front of the symphysis pubis. Proximally, it attaches to the 5th, 6th and 7th costal cartilages. Laterally, it may extend to the 3rd and 4th costal cartilages and, medially, it occasionally attaches to the costoxiphoid ligaments and the side of the xiphoid process.

At three levels, transverse fibrous bands, known as tendinous intersections, cross the muscle fibres. They are normally situated at the level of the umbilicus, at the level of the xiphoid process, and midway between the xiphoid process and the umbilicus. There may be incomplete intersections below the umbilicus.

The muscle is enclosed between the aponeuroses of the obliqui and transversus abdominis.

Nerve supply. The ventral rami of T6/7–12.

Actions. When the pelvis is fixed, rectus abdominis will flex the trunk towards the pelvis; when the trunk is fixed, rectus abdominis flexes the pelvis towards the trunk. This muscle helps to control pelvic tilt and, in the standing position, weakness of rectus abdominis allows an increase in anterior pelvic tilt.

Muscles which raise intra–abdominal pressure

- Obliquus externus abdominis (see pp. 122-123)
- Obliquus internus abdominis (see pp. 123-124)
- Rectus abdominis (see above)
- Transversus abdominis

Transversus abdominis

Transversus abdominis (see Fig. 3.11) is the innermost flat muscle of the abdominal wall and has horizontally arranged fibres. It is attached laterally to the lateral third of the inguinal ligament, the anterior two thirds of the iliac crest, the thoracolumbar fascia between the iliac crest and the 12th rib, and the internal aspects of the lower six costal cartilages, where it interdigitates with the diaphragm.

The muscle fibres pass horizontally around the abdominal wall to attach to an aponeurosis which blends with the linea alba. In the upper three quarters the muscle blends with the posterior lamina of the aponeurosis of obliquus internus abdominis and passes behind rectus, whereas, in the lower quarter, it passes in front of rectus. The upper muscular fibres of transversus abdominis passing behind rectus are sometimes continuous in the midline with the transversus of the opposite side.

The lower fibres, which attach to the inguinal ligament, arch downwards and join with those of obliquus internus abdominis to attach to the pubic crest and pectin pubis forming the conjoint tendon.

Nerve supply.   The ventral rami of T7–12 and L1.

Actions.   Bilateral contraction of transversus abdominis draws in the abdominal contents, resulting in an increase in intra-abdominal pressure. The circumferential direction of the muscle fibres ensures that transversus abdominis is particularly well placed to increase intra-abdominal pressure without producing a concurrent flexion of the spine, as would occur if the other abdominal muscles were dominant in this action.

It is unclear whether contraction of transversus abdominis produces axial rotation of the trunk. DeTroyer et al (1990) found little or no activity in transversus abdominis with resisted rotation in sitting, but Cresswell et al (1992) reported activity in transversus abdominis on the side to which the spine was rotated. It has been hypothesized that transversus may not act to rotate the spine, but instead resists rotation, or returns the spine to neutral from a rotated position through its attachment laterally to the thoracolumbar fascia (Richardson et al, 1999).

Transversus abdominis may contribute to lumbar intersegmental stability through the creation of lateral tension in the thoracolumbar fascia. The fascia acts on the transverse processes of the lumbar vertebrae and, as transversus abdominis contracts, it increases tension in the fascia and hence may limit translation and rotation of the vertebrae (Hodges and Richardson, 1997).

Combined actions of the abdominal muscles

Although the eight abdominal muscles (four on each side) work as a group during some activities, each also plays a specific role and this must be considered when assessing abdominal strength and control and when devising muscle reconditioning programmes.

The muscles form a firm elastic wall which helps to draw in the abdominal cavity to help keep the abdominal viscera in place. The obliquus internus abdominis and transversus abdominis are particularly important for this purpose.

The combined effort of the abdominal muscles has the effect of raising intra-abdominal pressure. This occurs as the contracting muscles pull via their aponeuroses on the rectus sheath and compress the abdominal viscera. Transversus abdominis and obliquus internus abdominis play a more significant role in this respect than obliquus externus abdominis and the recti. The increase in intra-abdominal

Continues

Continued

pressure plays an important part in expulsive efforts: the increased pressure on the bladder assists micturition; on the rectum, defaecation; on the stomach, vomiting; and, during childbirth, the compressive force of the abdominal muscles helps to expel the fetus from the uterus. The significance of raised intra-abdominal pressure in lifting is discussed on pages 339–340.

The abdominal muscles also assist in expiration, coughing and sneezing. When the diaphragm relaxes it is pushed upwards by pressure on the viscera from contraction of the abdominal muscles; this increases the intrathoracic pressure so that, when the glottis is opened, air is expelled from the lungs. If the pelvis and spine are fixed, the act of coughing is further reinforced by obliquus externus abdominis depressing the lower ribs and compressing the lower part of the thorax.

Electromyographic studies have shown that there is some activity in the abdominal muscles during most trunk movements in the standing and sitting positions (Floyd and Silver, 1951; Campbell and Green, 1955; Carman et al, 1972). Depending on the location of the centre of gravity, in normal standing there is either slight constant or intermittent activity in the abdominal muscles in approximately 25% of individuals; the remaining 75% show similar activity in erector spinae (Floyd and Silver, 1951). Activity is increased if considerable resistance is applied to the trunk and during extension from the upright position.

In the curl-up action from a supine to a sitting position, the recti are most important, and they contract as soon as the head is raised. Further flexion activates the obliques, but to a lesser extent. If the thorax is fixed, the recti and obliques tilt the pelvis backwards and flex the lumbar spine.

Thoracolumbar fascia (Fig. 3.12)

The thoracolumbar fascia is a non-contractile tissue that contributes to the functional stability of the lumbopelvic region. Mobility and stability of the lumbopelvic region are dependent on the interplay between the thoracolumbar fascia, fascia lata and abdominal fascial systems. When the skin and subcutaneous fat are removed from the posterior aspect of the lumbar spine, the next structure encountered is the thoracolumbar fascia. The thoracolumbar fascia covers the back muscles over the sacral region and extends through the thoracic region to the nuchal line. Several powerful muscles attach to the fascia and affect the tension within it. The fascia also helps to transfer load from the trunk to the pelvis and lower limbs. In the lumbar region the fascia can be divided into posterior, middle and anterior layers (Bogduk, 1997).

Many descriptions of the thoracolumbar fascia refer to the posterior layer as the superficial layer and the middle layer as the deep layer

Figure 3.12 The
thoracolumbar fascia –
transverse section

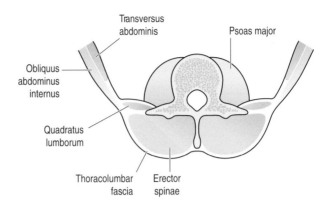

(Porterfield and DeRosa, 1998). It is these two layers that are most important in influencing the biomechanics of the lumbopelvic region.

The thick, fibrous posterior (superficial) layer is further subdivided into superficial and deep laminae. The superficial and deep laminae connect at the level of L4–5. The middle layer and the deep and superficial laminae of the posterior layer fuse together to form a dense thickening called the 'lateral raphe' (Bogduk and MacIntosh, 1984). The raphe is lateral to erector spinae and lies above the iliac crest. Transversus abdominis and the internal oblique muscles attach into the lateral raphe.

Posterior layer of the
thoracolumbar fascia

Superficial lamina of the posterior layer (Fig. 3.13). Most of the fibres of the superficial lamina derive from the aponeurosis of latissimus dorsi and attach to the spinous processes and supraspinous ligaments cranial to L4. Caudad to L4, the superficial lamina is more loosely attached and the fibres cross the midline and attach to the sacrum, posterior superior iliac spine and iliac crest of the contralateral side. In a study of 10 embalmed human specimens (Vleeming et al, 1995) it was found that the level at which fibres crossed the midline varied and in some specimens was as high as L2–3. Inferolaterally the superficial lamina blends with the fascia of gluteus maximus, and superolaterally the thoracolumbar fascia is continuous with the fascia of the contralateral latissimus dorsi. Hence, these two muscles are mechanically linked and together are able to increase tension in the posterior layer of the thoracolumbar fascia. It is proposed that this mechanism plays an important role in stabilizing the lumbosacral and sacroiliac regions (Vleeming et al, 1995).

Deep lamina of the posterior layer (Fig. 3.14). The deep lamina of the posterior layer of the thoracolumbar fascia attaches medially to the interspinous ligaments and the fibres run in an inferolateral direction to attach onto the posterior superior iliac spine, iliac crest and long dorsal sacroiliac ligament. Some fibres blend with the deep fascia of erector spinae. At sacral levels the fibres of the superficial and deep laminae of the thoracolumbar fascia blend together. In the lumbar region the deep lamina attaches to the lateral raphe and is therefore indirectly linked to the internal oblique and transversus abdominis muscles.

Figure 3.13 The superficial lamina of the thoracolumbar fascia. (From Vleeming A, Snijders CJ, Stoeckart R, Mens JMA 1997 The role of the sacroiliac joints in coupling between spine, pelvis, legs and arms. In: Vleeming A, Mooney V, Dorman T, Snijders C, Stoeckart R, eds. *Movement, Stability and Low Back Pain. The Essential Role of the Pelvis.* Churchill Livingstone, Edinburgh, Ch. 3, pp. 61–62.)

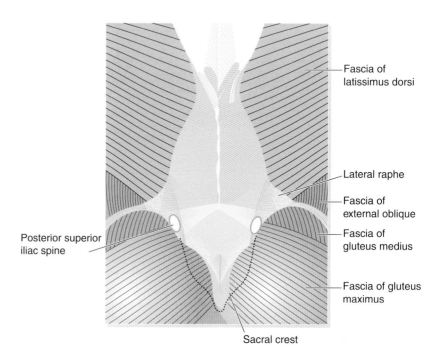

Fascia of latissimus dorsi

Lateral raphe

Fascia of external oblique

Fascia of gluteus medius

Fascia of gluteus maximus

Posterior superior iliac spine

Sacral crest

Figure 3.14 The deep lamina of the thoracolumbar fascia. (From Vleeming A, Snijders CJ, Stoeckart R, Mens JMA 1997 The role of the sacroiliac joints in coupling between spine, pelvis, legs and arms. In: Vleeming A, Mooney V, Dorman T, Snijders C, Stoeckart R, eds. *Movement, Stability and Low Back Pain. The Essential Role of the Pelvis.* Churchill Livingstone, Edinburgh, Ch. 3, pp. 61–62.)

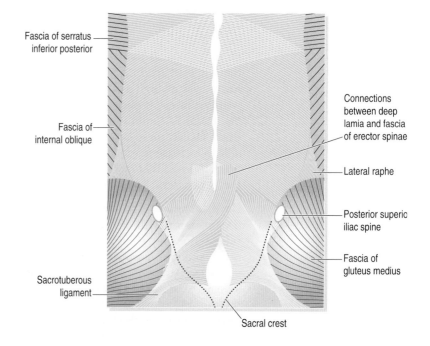

Fascia of serratus inferior posterior

Fascia of internal oblique

Connections between deep lamia and fascia of erector spinae

Lateral raphe

Posterior superic iliac spine

Fascia of gluteus medius

Sacrotuberous ligament

Sacral crest

Middle layer of the thoracolumbar fascia

The middle (deep) layer of the thoracolumbar fascia attaches medially to tips of the lumbar transverse processes and is continuous with the intertransverse ligaments. Laterally it gives rise to the aponeurosis of transversus abdominis. It lies posterior to quadratus lumborum and compartmentalizes the erector spinae muscles.

Anterior layer of the thoracolumbar fascia

The anterior layer is attached medially to the anterior surfaces of the lumbar transverse processes and intertransverse ligaments, and inferiorly to the iliolumbar ligament and adjacent iliac crest; superiorly it forms the lateral arcuate ligament. It covers the anterior surface of quadratus lumborum, lateral to which it blends with the other layers of the thoracolumbar fascia.

Functions of the thoracolumbar fascia

The thoracolumbar fascia fulfils a critical biomechanical role in the stability of the lumbar spine and pelvis. The muscles that attach to the fascia and those muscles that are ensheathed by fascia can affect tension within the thoracolumbar fascia. An increase in tension in the thoracolumbar fascia can occur during muscle contraction by two mechanisms. Firstly, some muscles exert a tensile force on the fascia by 'pulling' on the connective tissue as they contract: muscles having this effect are transversus abdominis, obliquus internus abdominis, gluteus maximus and latissimus dorsi. Those muscles encased by a layer of fascia exert a 'pushing' force. During contraction, the muscle belly broadens within the fascial stocking, acting to increase tension of the fascial walls (Porterfield and DeRosa, 1998). The muscles that have a 'pushing' effect are the superficial erector spinae, deep erector spinae and multifidus.

Tension in the thoracolumbar fascia can also be increased by motion of the arms, legs and trunk. Posterior rotation of the pelvis causes an increase in flexion at the lumbosacral junction and hence increases tension in the thoracolumbar fascia. Lumbar spine flexion also passively increases tension in the thoracolumbar fascia. Competitive weightlifters may flex or 'round out' the lumbosacral area and it is suggested that this affords some protection by increasing tension in the thoracolumbar fascia and posterior ligamentous structures, thereby contributing to stability in the low lumbar area (Dolan et al, 1994).

Latissimus dorsi has an extensive attachment to the spinous processes from T7 caudad to the sacrum and the thoracolumbar fascia. It also attaches to the iliac crest. Superiorly the muscle inserts onto the lesser tubercle of the humerus and the intertubercular groove. The pelvic attachment of latissimus dorsi is via the thoracolumbar fascia. Latissimus dorsi has a long moment arm length and therefore potentially affects lumbopelvic mechanisms with less effort than other tissues (McGill and Norman, 1986). The position of the humerus is able to influence tension within the thoracolumbar fascia. When the arm is in an elevated position there is a stretch on latissimus dorsi with a subsequent increase in tension of the thoracolumbar fascia. This increase in tension is further enhanced by other movements such as posterior rotation of the pelvis. Tension in the thoracolumbar fascia can be a summation of passive tension from humerus and pelvic positioning and active tension from the contraction of muscles that attach to the fascia. Active tensioning occurs through contraction of latissimus dorsi, which increases tension within the thoracolumbar fascia, and this is increased further by contraction of gluteus maximus.

Porterfield and DeRosa (1998) suggest that this mechanism aids stabilization of the spine and pelvis during functional activities such as lifting. During lifting, if the pelvis rotates posteriorly and the arm moves away from the body into flexion to grasp the load to be lifted, the thoracolumbar fascia is tightened passively. Latissimus dorsi then contracts to bring the object closer to the body with a resultant increase in tension within the thoracolumbar fascia. Active tension is further enhanced by contraction of gluteus maximus. A load can be lifted without a change in the angle between the body and the arm so that latissimus dorsi does not act to bring the load closer to the centre of gravity of the individual performing the lift. In this situation there is increased demand on the spinal extensors as they have to contract strongly to overcome the inertia of the stationary load.

The coupled action of latissimus dorsi and gluteus maximus has a line of force that acts perpendicular to the sacroiliac joint and increases the compressive force on the sacrum and ilium, thereby improving stability. This mechanism may also give some stability to the lumbosacral region.

Willard (1997) suggests that the thoracolumbar fascia helps to assist in the alignment of the lumbar vertebrae. The soft tissues of the neural arch form a sheath-like structure over the vertebrae. The ligamentum flavum is continuous with the interspinous and supraspinous ligaments. In the human, the interspinous ligament is a fan-shaped structure with the narrow end blending with the ligamentum flavum and containing elastic fibres. The distal end fans out towards the tips of the spines where it thickens to form the supraspinous ligament, which in turn is anchored to the thoracolumbar fascia. In the centre of the interspinous ligament the collagen fibres are mainly orientated so that they are parallel with the spinous processes. This orientation aids the transmission of forces from the pull of the thoracolumbar fascia through the supraspinous ligament, to the interspinous ligament and subsequently the ligamentum flavum (Hukins et al, 1990). This force helps to prevent the ligamentum flavum from buckling and folding into the central vertebral canal and assists in alignment of the vertebrae by reducing shear forces.

Studies in cadavers (Fairbank et al, 1980) and mathematical analysis led to the proposal that the thoracolumbar fascia might assist in the production of an extensor moment of the lumbar spine. It was suggested that the orientation of the fibres of the posterior layer of the thoracolumbar fascia could aid an extension moment by converting lateral tension into longitudinal tension. From the lateral raphe, superficial lamina fibres of the thoracolumbar fascia run caudomedially and deep fibres run craniomedially to the midline, forming a series of triangles that extend over two levels. It was proposed that contraction of transversus abdominis exerted tension on the posterior layer of the thoracolumbar fascia and the force exerted at the base of each triangle had a horizontal and vertical vector. Bilateral tension could produce a force approximating the spinous processes, thereby extending the lumbar spine and providing a mechanism by which transversus abdominis could contribute to spinal extension. Recent evidence suggests that the contribution of transversus abdominis and the thoracolumbar fascia to extension is negligible (Macintosh et al, 1987; Tesh et al, 1987; McGill and Norman, 1988).

Muscles which produce rotation of the trunk

- Obliquus internus abdominis (see pp. 123-124)
- Obliquus externus abdominis (see pp. 122-123)
- Multifidus (see pp. 132-134)
- Rotatores (see p. 141)
- Semispinalis

Semispinalis

Semispinalis is present in the thoracic and cervical regions only and consists of three parts:

Semispinalis thoracis arises from the transverse processes of the 6th–10th thoracic vertebrae and attaches to the spinous processes of the upper two thoracic and lower two cervical vertebrae.

Semispinalis cervicis arises from the transverse processes of the upper 5–6 thoracic vertebrae and attaches to the spinous processes of the 2nd–5th cervical vertebrae.

Semispinalis capitis arises from the tips of the transverse processes of the upper 6–7 thoracic and 7th cervical vertebrae and from the articular processes of the 4th–6th cervical vertebrae. It attaches between the superior and inferior nuchal lines of the occipital bone. The medial part of this muscle is named *spinalis capitis*.

Nerve supply. The dorsal rami of the adjacent cervical and thoracic spinal nerves.

Actions. Semispinalis thoracis and cervicis contract bilaterally to produce extension of the thoracic and cervical vertebral column. Unilateral contraction causes rotation of the trunk and neck towards the opposite side.

Spinalis capitis extends the head and turns the face slightly towards the opposite side.

Muscles which produce lateral flexion of the trunk

- Obliquus externus abdominis (see pp. 122-123)
- Obliquus internus abdominis (see pp. 123-124)
- Rectus abdominis (see p. 124)
- Erector spinae (see pp. 134-140)
- Multifidus (see pp. 132-134)
- Quadratus lumborum
- Intertransversarii (see pp. 141-142)

Quadratus lumborum

Quadratus lumborum is a wide, quadrilateral muscle running between the ilium and 12th rib, deep to erector spinae. It has medial and lateral fibres. The medial portion of the muscle attaches distally to the ilium and centrally to the anterior surface of the transverse processes of the lumbar vertebrae. The lateral fibres arise from the lateral ilium and attach onto the medial half of the lower anterior surface of the 12th rib.

The muscle is enveloped by the anterior and middle layers of the thoracolumbar fascia.

Nerve supply.   The ventral rami of the 12th thoracic and upper 3–4 lumbar spinal nerves.

Actions.   Quadratus lumborum acts as a muscle of inspiration by fixing the 12th rib, thereby stabilizing the origin of the diaphragm. It acts to move and stabilize the pelvis and lumbar spine in the frontal and horizontal planes. During lateral flexion of the trunk, the quadratus lumborum on the opposite side to the direction in which the trunk moves works eccentrically to help control the rate of descent. Return to the upright position is assisted by concentric contraction of the same muscle. Postural stability in the frontal plane is assisted by eccentric and concentric contraction of quadratus lumborum. The medial fibres of quadratus lumborum are thought to help provide segmental stability via the muscle's segmental attachments (McGill et al, 1996).

Muscles which produce extension of the trunk

- Quadratus lumborum (see above)
- Multifidus
- Semispinalis (see p. 131)
- Erector spinae
- Interspinales (see p. 141)

Multifidus (Fig. 3.15)

Multifidus consists of a number of tendinous fascicles which lie deep to semispinalis and erector spinae, filling in the groove at the sides of the spinous processes of the vertebrae from the sacrum to the axis. The muscle has five separate bands of fascicles, which arise from the spinous processes and laminae of the lumbar vertebrae. The deepest and shortest fascicles arise from the posteroinferior aspect of the laminae and apophyseal joint and insert onto the mamillary process of the vertebrae two levels caudad (Bogduk, 1997). The rest of the muscle arises medially from the spinous process and blends with the lamina fibres laterally to insert onto the mamillary processes of the vertebrae three, four or five segments below. The longest fascicles of L1, L2 and L3 have some attachment onto the posterior superior iliac spine. The fibres from L4 insert onto the lateral sacral crest, while those from L5 insert onto the intermediate sacral crest inferior to S3. Some of the deeper fibres attach to the capsules of the apophyseal joints next to the mamillary process. These attachments prevent the joint capsules from being trapped inside the joints during movements executed by multifidus.

Figure 3.15   Deep posterior muscles of the spine.

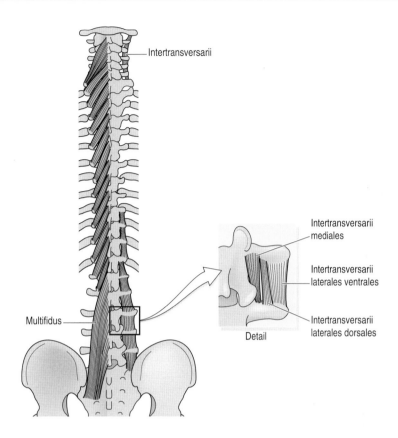

In the pelvis, multifidus has attachments to the sacrotuberous ligament, the aponeurosis of erector spinae and the posterior sacroiliac ligament (Porterfield and DeRosa, 1998). It also attaches to the deep lamina of the thoracolumbar fascia at a raphe which separates it from gluteus maximus.

In the thoracic spine, multifidus arises from the spinous processes and laminae and attaches to the transverse processes of the vertebra below. In the cervical spine the muscle is small and closely attached to the sides of the spinous processes and inserts onto the articular processes of the lower four or five vertebrae.

Nerve supply.   The fascicles arising from a spinous process of a particular vertebra are innervated by the medial branch of the dorsal ramus that comes from the vertebra below (Bogduk et al, 1982). Hence, the muscles that act on a particular segment are innervated by the nerve of that segment.

Actions.   The direction of the fibres is oblique, and therefore three actions may be possible:

1. When working bilaterally, multifidus may produce posterior sagittal rotation of its vertebra of origin, i.e. the 'rocking' component of extension, or control this component during flexion. Each fascicle of lumbar multifidus is ideally placed to create posterior rocking, but is unable to produce

the posterior translation which normally accompanies extension (Macintosh and Bogduk, 1986). While multifidus acts principally on individual spinous processes, some of its fascicles extend over several segments and have an indirect effect on the vertebrae interposed between attachments. In the lumbar spine it has a bowstring effect, which accentuates the lumbar lordosis.

2. Multifidus is active in contralateral and ipsilateral axial rotation of the trunk (Donisch and Basmajian, 1972). However, its role is not to produce rotation; the oblique abdominal muscles are better suited to do this, but when the obliques contract they also simultaneously produce flexion. Erector spinae and multifidus oppose this flexion effect, thereby maintaining pure axial rotation. Multifidus is therefore an important stabilizer during rotation.

3. Multifidus is also active in lateral flexion of the trunk to the same side.

Contraction of multifidus exerts a compressive force on the lumbar vertebrae and intervertebral discs, and by 'squeezing' the segments together the muscle may contribute to spinal stability.

Histological studies have shown that there is a greater percentage of type I than type II fibres in lumbar multifidus, suggesting that this muscle has an important stabilizing function (Sirca and Kostevc, 1985). Changes in the internal structure of multifidus have been demonstrated in patients with low back pain: atrophy of type II muscle fibres and internal structural changes in the type I fibres were demonstrated in a study of patients undergoing surgery for low back pain (Rantanen et al, 1993). Hides et al (1994) studied lumbar multifidus in patients with acute low back pain using real-time ultrasound imaging. They compared the multifidus of patients with a first episode of acute low back pain of approximately two weeks' duration with the multifidus of normal subjects. They found marked side-to-side asymmetry of the cross-sectional area of multifidus in the subjects with low back pain, but this was not apparent in the normal asymptomatic subjects. The smaller muscle was found on the same side as the symptoms and at the symptomatic segment. Further studies have shown that recovery of multifidus is not spontaneous after an episode of low back pain, even if pain has eased and the range of movement is restored (Hides et al, 1996). However, the cross-sectional area can be restored by a specific reconditioning programme for the muscle.

Patients with low back pain show a higher rate of fatigability of multifidus than asymptomatic controls (Roy et al, 1989; Biedermann et al, 1991). Fatigue of lumbar multifidus may lead to reduced control of segmental movement.

Contraction of multifidus causes the sacrum to nutate. Multifidus may act with levator ani as a force couple to control sacral nutation/counternutation (Snijders et al, 1997).

Erector spinae (Fig. 3.16)

Erector spinae is a large, powerful musculotendinous mass consisting of three columns: iliocostalis, longissimus and spinalis. It extends from the dorsal aspect of the skull to the sacrum, lying lateral to multifidus and forming the prominent contours on either side of the spine.

Erector spinae arises principally from a wide, flat aponeurosis which is attached to the 11th and 12th thoracic spinous processes, and the lumbar and sacral spinous processes, their supraspinous ligaments, the medial aspects of the iliac crests and the sacrum. The aponeurosis is mainly formed by tendons of muscles acting on *thoracic* levels – longissimus thoracis and iliocostalis thoracis – but also receives a few fibres of multifidus from the upper lumbar spine. The lumbar fibres of erector spinae do not themselves attach to the aponeurosis, and it can consequently move freely over them, which suggests that they are able to act independently from the rest of erector spinae.

From its extensive origin, erector spinae passes upwards deep to latissimus dorsi and in the *upper* lumbar spine splits into three columns:

Lateral – iliocostalis
Intermediate – longissimus
Medial – spinalis.

Figure 3.16   The erector spinae muscles.

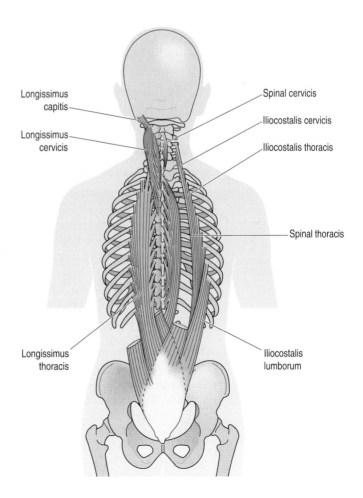

In the *low* lumbar spine, erector spinae consists of two muscles: iliocostalis lumborum and longissimus thoracis. These muscles are separated by the lumbar intermuscular aponeurosis, which is an anterior continuation of the erector spinae aponeurosis (Bogduk, 1980).

Each muscle column also receives fibres from the different spinal regions, and is itself divided into three parts.

1. Iliocostalis

a. *Iliocostalis lumborum* has been described as having both lumbar and thoracic components. The thoracic component inserts via flattened tendons into the angles of the lower 8–9 ribs. This part of the muscle spans the lumbar spine, but has no direct attachment to it. There is a lumbar component to the muscle called *iliocostalis lumborum pars lumborum*. These intrinsic lumbar fibres arise from the tips of the L1–4 transverse processes and the thoracolumbar fascia and insert independently of the erector spinae aponeurosis into the iliac crest and the posterior aspect of the posterior superior iliac spine (Macintosh and Bogduk, 1987). This muscle constitutes a substantial portion of the total muscle mass acting directly on the lumbar vertebrae.

b. *Iliocostalis thoracis* arises medial to iliocostalis lumborum from the upper borders of the angles of the 7th–12th ribs and inserts into the upper borders of the angles of the 1st–6th ribs and the posterior aspect of the transverse process of the 7th cervical vertebra.

c. *Iliocostalis cervicis* arises medial to iliocostalis thoracis from the angles of the 3rd–6th ribs and inserts into the posterior tubercles of the transverse processes of the 4th–6th cervical vertebrae.

Nerve supply. The dorsal rami of adjacent spinal nerves.

Actions. Iliocostalis contracts bilaterally to extend the spine. In the case of iliocostalis lumborum, bilateral contraction exerts an indirect 'bowstring' effect on the lumbar spine, causing an increase in its lordosis.

Unilateral contraction of iliocostalis laterally flexes the respective regions of the spine to the same side. Iliocostalis lumborum, in addition to laterally flexing the thoracic spine, also indirectly laterally flexes the lumbar spine.

Iliocostalis lumborum has little effect on ipsilateral rotation because the distance between the ribs does not shorten very much. However, in contralateral rotation, this distance is greatly increased and the muscle can serve to derotate the thoracic cage and, therefore, the lumbar spine (Bogduk and Twomey, 1987).

Iliocostalis lumborum pars lumborum acts with multifidus in opposing the flexion effect that occurs when the trunk is rotated by the abdominal muscles. As iliocostalis lumborum pars lumborum contracts to produce axial rotation, it simultaneously acts as an extensor.

2. Longissimus

a. *Longissimus thoracis.* This muscle is the largest of the erector spinae group. It is attached distally to the lumbar and sacral spinous processes and the sacrum between the spinous process of the 3rd sacral vertebra and the posterior superior iliac spine. Its tendons form the main part of the erector spinae aponeurosis. Proximally it is attached to the transverse processes of the 1st–12th thoracic vertebrae and between the tubercle and angle of the 2nd–12th ribs.

b. *Longissimus thoracis pars lumborum.* These are deep fibres of the lumbar erector spinae that arise from the accessory and transverse processes of all the lumbar vertebrae and insert into the ilium, posterior superior iliac spine and sacroiliac ligament. They are covered by the lumbar intermuscular aponeurosis, an anteroposterior continuation of the erector spinae aponeurosis. The muscle fibres are twisted so that the fibres from the lower lumbar transverse processes are inserted onto the superolateral aspect of the ilium while the fibres from the upper lumbar transverse processes insert onto the inferomedial part of the ilium.

c. *Longissimus cervicis.* This muscle runs from the transverse processes of the upper 4–5 thoracic vertebrae to the posterior tubercles of the transverse processes of the 2nd–6th cervical vertebrae, medial to longissimus thoracis.

d. *Longissimus capitis* lies between longissimus cervicis and semispinalis capitis. It arises from the transverse processes of the upper 4–5 thoracic vertebrae and the articular processes of the lower 3–4 cervical vertebrae and inserts into the posterior margin of the mastoid process.

Nerve supply.   The dorsal rami of the spinal nerves according to their position.

Actions.   Bilateral contraction of longissimus thoracis acts principally on the ribs and thoracic vertebrae, producing an extension moment over the lumbar spine. The muscle also works eccentrically to control movement of the trunk during forward bending (Ortengren and Andersson, 1977). It also acts indirectly on the lumbar spine, causing an increase in the lumbar lordosis. Unilateral contraction laterally flexes the thoracic spine and, thereby, indirectly the lumbar spine to the same side.
Longissimus thoracis pars lumborum is active in lumbar extension, but because its attachments are closer to the axes of sagittal rotation, it is less efficient in this action than multifidus. The orientation of the fibres of longissimus thoracis pars lumborum produces a posterior shear or translation of the lumbar vertebrae. At the low lumbar levels the muscle helps to resist the anterior translation of the vertebrae that occurs during flexion.
Unilateral contraction of the muscle produces lateral flexion of the lumbar spine.
Bilateral contraction of longissimus cervicis produces extension of the cervical spine. Unilaterally it initiates lateral flexion of the neck to the same side; the longissimus cervicis fibres on the opposite side to which the neck is laterally flexed contract eccentrically to control the lateral flexion.

Bilaterally, longissimus capitis contracts to extend the head on the neck. Unilaterally, it acts to turn the face towards the same side.

3. Spinalis

a. *Spinalis thoracis* is the most clearly demarcated of the spinales and is attached distally to the spinous processes of a varying number of upper thoracic vertebrae (4–8), and proximally to those of the 11th and 12th thoracic vertebrae and the 1st and 2nd lumbar vertebrae.

b. *Spinalis cervicis* is an inconstant muscle. When present, it is attached distally to the lower part of the ligamentum nuchae and the spinous process of the 7th cervical vertebrae. It is attached proximally to the spinous process of the axis and sometimes those of the 3rd and 4th cervical vertebrae.

c. *Spinalis capitis* is poorly developed and blends with semispinalis capitis.

Nerve supply.   The dorsal rami of the adjacent spinal nerves.

Actions.   The spinales extend the respective regions of the vertebral column.

Activity of erector spinae

During maintenance of posture.   Dysfunction in the erector spinae muscles, such as through spasm or tightness, is often present in patients with back problems, and an account of its static postural role and dynamic functions has a practical significance when considering the patient's activities of daily living, ergonomics, sport and exercise.

In the normal *standing* position, there is very little erector spinae activity, the mobile vertebral column being well balanced on the sacrum by joints and soft tissues. In approximately 75% of individuals, the line of gravity passes anterior to the 4th lumbar vertebra (Asmussen and Klausen, 1962) and consequently the erector spinae muscles show slight constant or intermittent activity as they counterbalance the tendency of the vertebral column to fall forwards (Floyd and Silver, 1951, 1955). Longissimus thoracis is more active than iliocostalis lumborum, suggesting that it has a greater postural role. The line of gravity may pass behind the lumbar spine in a significant number of individuals, and in these people abdominal muscle activity is recruited to prevent the vertebral column extending.

This low level of erector spinae activity is increased when either the head or the upper limbs are moved forwards. If a load is held, erector spinae activity is also increased in proportion to its weight and the further in front of the body the load is held (Kippers and Parker, 1985). Holding a low density, light object can still necessitate increased erector spinae activity if it is so large that, even when held close to the body, its centre of mass is a significant distance in front of it (Fig. 3.17).

When a load is being carried, the distribution of the stresses in the spine depends on the position of the load. If it is carried high on the back, e.g. a rucksack, the trunk compensates by leaning forwards, so there is more erector spinae activity than in normal standing. If the load is car-

Figure 3.17 Activity of the erector spinae muscles. A, A load (L) requires increased erector spinae tension (ES) when it is held further in front of the body. B, Objects of different size and weight which require the same response from erector spinae when held in front of the body. The length of arrow (ES) indicates the erector spinae tension relative to the weight of the object represented by the length of each arrow (W, W/2, W/3, W/4). (Modified from Tichauer 1971, 1978.)

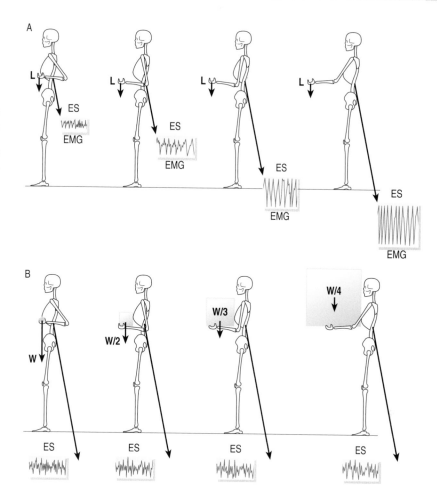

ried low on the back, erector spinae activity decreases to less than normal in standing, but there is increased activity in psoas major, indicating that the load is causing the vertebral column to extend (Klausen, 1965). Knowledge of muscular responses to the different positions in which a load can be carried will assist in devising strategies to recondition muscle groups that have become weak and fatigue early.

When the centre of gravity is displaced sideways, as when holding a weight in one hand, the contralateral erector spinae contracts to prevent undesired lateral flexion.

Erector spinae activity in *sitting* varies with the position. In an unsupported sitting position (without a backrest), activity in the lumbar erector spinae is at a constant low level, but there is an increase in the thoracic erector spinae activity. Muscle activity is greater in anterior sitting (leaning forward) than in posterior sitting. In supported sitting, erector spinae activity is reduced. The angle of the backrest has a significant influence; increasing its backward inclination reduces erector spinae activity (see pp. 335–336).

During trunk movements from the upright position. As the spine moves forward into flexion, there is an increase in erector spinae activity in proportion to the angle of flexion. If a load is carried, activity in erector spinae increases proportionately with the size of the load (Andersson et al, 1977).

Gravity produces the movement, but its rate is controlled by erector spinae and multifidus contracting eccentrically. Longissimus thoracis and iliocostalis lumborum control the movement of the thorax on the lumbar spine, anchoring them to the pelvis. In the lumbar region, multifidus, longissimus thoracis pars lumborum and iliocostalis lumborum pars lumborum also control anterior sagittal rotation and anterior translation of the lumbar vertebrae.

At approximately 90% of maximal flexion of the lumbar spine, a point is reached in most subjects where activity ceases in erector spinae. This is known as the *critical point* (Floyd and Silver, 1955). The vertebral column is then braced by the approximation of the apophyseal joints and tension in the posterior ligaments, but there is no active muscular protection of the spine or neuromuscular control of the movement. This implies, as is borne out clinically, that working in stooped postures is hazardous. As a general guide, when the fingertips are below knee height there is a high probability that the critical point has been reached (Watanabe, 1980). If a weight is carried, the critical point occurs later in the range of vertebral flexion.

Considerable erector spinae activity occurs in extension of the trunk from the flexed position. Iliocostalis and longissimus act around the thoracic kyphosis to bring the thorax back on the lumbar spine. Posterior sagittal rotation of the lumbar vertebrae is brought about by multifidus, causing the superior surface of the lumbar vertebrae to be progressively tilted upwards to support the thorax.

Further extension of the trunk from the upright position is initiated by erector spinae but, once the line of gravity has been displaced, the trunk moves under the effect of gravity and erector spinae activity ceases. If movement is forced or resisted, the muscles come into play again.

Lateral flexion from the upright position is initiated by the muscles on the ipsilateral side; once the centre of gravity is displaced, the movement occurs under the effects of gravity and is controlled by the muscles on the contralateral side.

Intradiscal pressure during erector spinae activity. When the erector spinae muscles contract, they exert longitudinal compression on the lumbar vertebral column which raises the intradiscal pressure. Increased muscular activity through certain activities is associated with an increase in intradiscal pressure (see pp. 71–73).

Muscle activity in individuals who are stressed and tense is higher than the normal resting muscle activity (Lundervold, 1951). It therefore follows that intradiscal pressure is also likely to be higher in these individuals.

Muscles which stabilize the spine

- Multifidus (see pp. 132–134)
- Rotatores
- Interspinales
- Intertransversarii

These deep, short muscles probably act principally as postural muscles, stabilizing adjacent vertebrae and controlling their movements, allowing the longer, more superficial muscles to act efficiently.

Rotatores

Rotatores are best developed in the thoracic region where there are 11 on each side. Here they are attached distally to the upper and posterior part of the transverse process of the vertebra. The fibres pass upwards and medially to attach to the lower border and lateral surface of the lamina of the next vertebra above as far as the root of its spinous process.

In the cervical and lumbar regions, the rotatores are represented by variable muscle bundles with attachments similar to those in the thoracic region.

Nerve supply.   The dorsal rami of adjacent spinal nerves.

Actions.   Historically, the rotatores have been considered to be rotators of the spine, particularly in the thoracic region, but their main function is probably stabilization of the vertebral column.

Interspinales

Interspinales are short muscles lying on either side of the interspinous ligament. They connect the spinous processes of adjacent vertebrae between the axis and the 1st or 2nd thoracic vertebra, and between the 11th or 12th thoracic vertebrae and the 5th lumbar vertebra.

Nerve supply.   The dorsal rami of adjacent spinal nerves.

Actions.   The interspinales produce posterior sagittal rotation of the vertebra above and are therefore active during extension. They also play a significant role in stabilizing the vertebrae during movement.

Intertransversarii (see Fig. 3.15, p. 133)

The intertransversarii are small slips of muscle between the transverse processes of adjacent vertebrae in the cervical, lower thoracic and lumbar regions.

In the *cervical region*, they consist of anterior and posterior slips which are separated by the ventral rami of the spinal nerves. The posterior muscles are divisible into medial and lateral parts. The anterior muscles and the lateral parts of the posterior muscles connect the costal processes of adjacent vertebrae, while the medial parts of the posterior muscles connect the transverse processes. There are seven pairs of muscles between the atlas and the 1st thoracic vertebra.

In the *thoracic region*, they consist of single muscles connecting the transverse processes of the 10th thoracic and 1st lumbar vertebrae.

In the *lumbar region*, the intertransversarii consist of two muscles – intertransversarii mediales and intertransversarii laterales.

The intertransversarii mediales connect the accessory process and mamillary process of one vertebra proximally to the mamillary process of the vertebra below.

The intertransversarii laterales are divisible into anterior and posterior parts. The anterior part connects the margins of adjacent transverse processes, and the posterior part connects the accessory process of one vertebra to the transverse process below.

Nerve supply. The medial parts of the posterior intertransversarii in the cervical region, the thoracic intertransversarii laterales and the intertransversarii mediales in the lumbar region are supplied by the dorsal rami of adjacent spinal nerves. The remainder are supplied by the ventral rami and are, therefore, not traditionally included among the back muscles, which are all innervated by the dorsal rami.

Actions. The intertransversarii are small muscles that lie lateral to the axis of lateral flexion and behind the axis of sagittal rotation. It is unclear whether they are capable of producing sufficient force to assist lateral flexion or posterior sagittal rotation. It is more likely that they function as stabilizing muscles.

The cervical intertransversarii contain a particularly high density of muscle spindles (Abrahams, 1977), and it has been suggested that they act as large proprioceptive transducers by monitoring spinal movements and providing feedback to the surrounding muscles, thereby influencing their action.

Muscles which control anteroposterior pelvic tilting (Fig. 3.18)

Forward tilting
- Erector spinae (see pp. 134-140)
- Psoas major (see pp. 120-121)

Backward tilting
- Rectus abdominis (see p. 124)
- Obliquus internus abdominis (see pp. 123-124)
- Obliquus externus abdominis (see pp. 122-123)
- Gluteus maximus
- The hamstrings:
  Semitendinosus
  Semimembranosus
  Biceps femoris

The action of tilting the pelvis on the femoral heads in an anteroposterior direction is often assessed in those with low back pain. Alteration in the length and activity of any of the muscles that help to control pelvic tilting will inevitably affect pelvic tilt in the standing posture and also normal physiological movements.

Movement of the anterior part of the pelvis proximally is referred to as *backward* tilting, and distally as *forward* tilting. In the standing position, backward tilting is produced anterosuperiorly by concentric con-

Figure 3.18   Pelvic tilting.

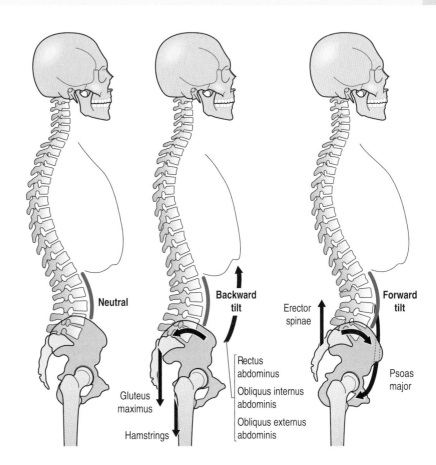

Neutral

Backward
tilt

Forward
tilt

Erector
spinae

Rectus
abdominus

Obliquus internus
abdominis

Obliquus externus
abdominis

Gluteus
maximus

Hamstrings

Psoas
major

traction of the recti and oblique abdominals, working posteroinferiorly with gluteus maximus and the hamstrings, which pull the posterior part of the pelvis downwards. At the same time, the lumbar spine is flexed and intradiscal pressure is increased. Forward tilting is produced principally by erector spinae raising the posterior part of the pelvis. The lumbar lordosis is then increased and the increased activity in the lumbar erector spinae increases intradiscal pressure.

The muscle work involved will, of course, vary depending on the starting position used.

Gluteus maximus   Gluteus maximus is a powerful, quadrilateral muscle forming the prominence of the buttock. Proximally, it is attached to the gluteal surface of the ilium behind the posterior gluteal line, the posterior border of the ilium and adjacent part of the iliac crest, the aponeurosis of erector spinae, the posterior aspect of the sacrum, including the upper part of the sacrotuberous ligament, and the side of the coccyx. Its muscle fibres pass downwards and laterally, the majority of the fibres (three quarters) forming a separate tendinous lamina which narrows down and attaches to the iliotibial tract of the fascia lata. The remaining quarter of the muscle fibres attach to the gluteal tuberosity of the femur.

Nerve supply.   The inferior gluteal nerve, L5, S1 and S2.

Actions.   When acting from the pelvis, gluteus maximus is a powerful extensor of the flexed thigh, laterally rotating it at the same time, and plays a major role in activities such as climbing the stairs and running, when it is intermittently active. In ordinary walking, the muscle shows some intermittent activity. During running, gluteus maximus works eccentrically to slow down the leg as it moves into hip flexion. Its upper fibres are active in powerful abduction of the thigh.

When acting from its distal attachments, gluteus maximus working with the hamstrings helps to raise the trunk from a flexed position by rotating the pelvis backwards on the head of the femoral heads. Weakness of gluteus maximus combined with increased activity in erector spinae promotes forward tilting of the pelvis and can adversely affect both the static posture and dynamic function of this region.

Through its attachments to the iliotibial tract, gluteus maximus provides a powerful support on the lateral side of the knee. In standing, the ability of the muscle to rotate the femur laterally assists in raising the medial longitudinal arch of the foot.

Contraction of the contralateral gluteus maximus and latissimus dorsi increases the tension in the thoracolumbar fascia and helps to stabilize the sacroiliac joint (Vleeming et al, 1995). The pull of gluteus maximus also increases tension in the sacrotuberous ligament, so that motion between the sacrum and ilium is minimized and stability of the sacroiliac joint is enhanced (Vleeming et al, 1989).

The hamstrings   The hamstrings are the posterior femoral muscles: semitendinosus and semimembranosus (the medial hamstring) and biceps femoris (the lateral hamstring).

Semitendinosus. The proximal attachment of this muscle is to the ischial tuberosity from a tendon shared with the long head of biceps femoris, and from an aponeurosis connecting the two muscles. The muscle fibres soon end in a long tendon which attaches to the upper part of the medial condyle of the tibia.

Nerve supply.   The sciatic nerve through its tibial division, L5, S1 and S2.

Semimembranosus. This muscle lies deep to semitendinosus. It is attached proximally to the ischial tuberosity by a tendon that spreads into an aponeurosis from which muscular fibres arise. It is attached distally mainly to the posterior aspect of the medial tibial condyle, but also sends slips in different directions, particularly upwards and laterally forming the oblique popliteal ligament.

Nerve supply.   The sciatic nerve through its tibial division, L5, S1 and S2.

Biceps femoris. This muscle is situated on the posterolateral aspect of the thigh. Proximally it arises by two heads: a *long head* from the ischial tuberosity from a tendon shared with semitendinosus and the lower part of the sacrotuberous ligament; and a *short head* from the linea aspera on the femur and from the lateral supracondylar line. The fibres of the long head cross the sciatic nerve and receive those of the short head on its deep surface. The muscle gradually narrows down into a short tendon which is attached to the head of the fibula, the fibular collateral ligament and the lateral condyle of the tibia.

Nerve supply.   The sciatic nerve – the long head through the tibial part and the short head through the common peroneal part L5, S1 and S2.

Actions of the hamstrings

The hamstrings act upon both the hip and knee joints. Acting from above, they flex the knee joint. Acting from below, the muscles, in particular biceps femoris, help to raise the trunk from a flexed position by extending the hip. They also play an important role in balancing the pelvis on the femoral heads. Working with the abdominal muscles anterosuperiorly and gluteus maximus posteroinferiorly, they can tilt the pelvis backwards, which consequently flexes the lumbar spine.

When the knee is flexed or the hip extended, biceps femoris can produce lateral rotation of the hip, and semitendinosus and semimembranosus can produce medial rotation.

The length of the hamstrings varies markedly in different individuals. In symptom-free subjects, straight-leg raising in the lying position can vary from 45° to 120°. An increase in hamstring stiffness can constrain the rotation of the pelvis during forward bending and lead to a compensatory increase in lumbar and thoracic flexion.

Contraction of biceps femoris increases tension in the sacrotuberous ligament, pulling the sacrum against the ilium and contributing to stability of the sacroiliac joint.

Other muscles which are relevant in spinal disorders

- Latissimus dorsi
- Piriformis
- Rectus femoris
- Pelvic floor muscles

Latissimus dorsi (Fig. 3.19)

Latissimus dorsi is a large, flat, triangular sheet of muscle extending from the trunk to the upper arm. Although it is principally a muscle acting on the shoulder joint it also affects the lumbar spine and sacroiliac joints.

It is attached distally by tendinous fibres to the spinous processes of the 7th–12th thoracic vertebrae anterior to trapezius, and from the posterior layer of the thoracolumbar fascia which is attached to the spinous processes of all the lumbar and sacral vertebrae, supraspinous ligaments and iliac crest. It also has muscular fibres arising from the iliac crest, and is attached to the lowest 3–4 ribs, interdigitating with obliquus externus abdominis.

The muscular fibres of latissimus dorsi pass laterally and the lower ones almost vertically upwards to converge into a thick fasciculus. This crosses and attaches to the inferior angle of the scapula and then wraps

Figure 3.19   Latissimus dorsi.

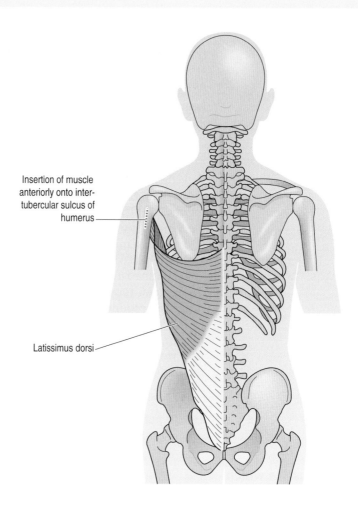

Insertion of muscle anteriorly onto intertubercular sulcus of humerus

Latissimus dorsi

round teres major, forming with it the posterior fold of the axilla. It ends in a long tendon which is attached to the lower end of the intertubercular sulcus of the humerus.

Nerve supply.   The thoracodorsal nerve, C6–8.

Actions.   Latissimus dorsi is a strong adductor, extensor and medial rotator of the arm. It acts with pectoralis major and teres minor to depress the elevated arm against resistance as, for instance, when these muscles pull the trunk upwards and forwards. It is particularly active in the downstroke in swimming. Through its attachment to the ribs, it also takes part in all sudden expiratory movements such as coughing and sneezing.

There is an important mechanical link between the contralateral latissimus dorsi, gluteus maximus and the thoracolumbar fascia (see pp. 126–131). Contraction of contralateral gluteus maximus and latissimus dorsi increases tension in the thoracolumbar fascia that lies perpendicular to the sacroiliac joint; the forces produced enhance lumbosacral stability.

Bilateral contraction of latissimus dorsi pulls on the thoracolumbar fascia that has its insertion into the lumbar spinous and transverse processes; by increasing fascial tension it assists in checking rotation and flexion of the lumbar spine.

Piriformis

Piriformis is a triangular muscle lying deep inside the buttock, with its base within the pelvis and its apex posterior to the hip joint. Medially, its base is attached to the front of the sacrum between and lateral to the 1st and 4th sacral foramina, the gluteal surface of the ilium near the posterior superior iliac spine, the capsule of the sacroiliac joint and the pelvic surface of the sacrotuberous ligament. Its fibres pass downwards, laterally and forwards, through the greater sciatic foramen, narrowing into a tendon which is attached to the upper border of the greater trochanter of the femur. As the muscle passes out of the greater sciatic foramen, it lies just above the sciatic nerve and is often pierced by its common peroneal portion.

Nerve supply.   The ventral rami of L5, S1 and S2.

Actions.   Piriformis laterally rotates the extended thigh and helps to stabilize the pelvis in the standing position by compressing the sacroiliac joint. If the hip joint is flexed as in the sitting position, the muscle can abduct the thigh, for instance when getting out of a car.

Spasm or an alteration in the length of the muscle – either lengthened or shortened – is sometimes a feature of sacroiliac joint dysfunction. Piriformis trigger points are commonly found in sacroiliac dysfunction and may be palpated lateral to the sacrum and distally, proximal to its insertion into the greater trochanter (Bachrach, 1997). A lengthened or shortened piriformis can increase loading on the sciatic nerve and result in distal symptoms within the distribution of the sciatic nerve.

Rectus femoris

Rectus femoris is the part of the quadriceps femoris group which has an attachment to the pelvis. Its proximal attachment is by two tendons from the anterior inferior iliac spines and above the acetabulum and capsule of the hip joint. The two heads spread into an aponeurosis from which muscular fibres arise. Approximately two thirds of the way down the thigh, the muscle starts to narrow down into a thick tendon which is attached to the base of the patella.

Nerve supply.   The femoral nerve, L2–4.

Actions.   Quadriceps femoris is the main extensor of the knee joint. Rectus femoris can also assist in flexing the hip joint or, if the thigh is fixed, help to flex the pelvis. Tightness in the muscle can affect the mechanics of the pelvis and is sometimes associated with disorders of the sacroiliac joint. In the standing position, if rectus femoris is shortened bilaterally it results in an anterior rotatory moment of the pelvis so that there is an increase in the lumbosacral angle and lumbar lordosis.

Pelvic floor muscles   The pelvic floor muscles are the only transverse load-bearing muscle group in the body (Sapsford, 2004) and they provide antigravity support.

There are three layers of pelvic floor muscles:

Superficial: bulbospongiosus, ischiocavernosus and superficial transverse perineal muscles and the external anal sphincter.

Intermediate: intrinsic urethral sphincter, deep transverse perinei. In females only: compressor urethrae and the urethrovaginal sphincter (DeLancey, 1990).

Deep: levator ani can be divided into four parts: puborectalis, pubococcygeus, iliococcygeus and ischiococcygeus. Anteriorly, puborectalis and pubococcygeus attach to the body of the pubis and the anterior part of the obturator fascia. Puborectalis does not have a posterior bony attachment but it passes posteriorly and laterally to join puborectalis on the opposite side to form a muscular sling at the anorectal flexure. Pubococcygeus passes posterior and inferiorly to puborectalis to attach to a midline raphe posterior to the rectum. Fibres from this raphe pass posteriorly and attach to the anterior aspect of the two most inferior coccygeal segments.

Iliococcygeus and ischiococcygeus arise from the medial aspect of the ischial spine, the posterior part of the obturator fascia and the medial aspect of the sacrospinous ligament. They attach to the anterior aspect of the apex of the sacrum at S5.

During functional activities such as coughing and sneezing, the pelvic floor and abdominal muscles are recruited to increase the intra-abdominal pressure, create an expiratory force and maintain continence. Activation of the abdominal muscles is a normal response to activation of the pelvic floor muscles (Sapsford et al, 2001).

Contraction of iliococcygeus and ischiococcygeus may counternutate the sacrum and act as part of a force couple with multifidus which nutates the sacrum (Lee, 1999).

References

Abrahams VC (1977) The physiology of neck muscles; their role in head movement and maintenance of posture. *Canadian Journal of Physiology and Pharmacology* 55: 332.

Andersson GBJ, Ortengren R, Nachemson A (1977) Intradiscal pressure, intra-abdominal pressure and myoelectric back muscle activity related to posture and loading. *Clinical Orthopaedics and Related Research* 129: 156.

Asmussen E, Klausen K (1962) Form and function of the erect human spine. *Clinical Orthopaedics and Related Research* 25: 55.

Bachrach RM (1997) Psoas dysfunction/insufficiency, sacroiliac dysfunction and low back pain. In: Vleeming A, Mooney V, Dorman T, Snijders C, Stoeckart R (eds) *Movement, Stability and Low Back Pain*. Churchill Livingstone, Edinburgh, Ch. 25, pp. 309–318.

Bannister R (1985) *Brian's Clinical Neurology*, 64th edn. Oxford University Press, London.

Bearn JG (1961) An electromyographic study of trapezius, deltoid, pectoralis major, biceps and triceps muscles, during static loading of the upper limb. *Anatomical Record* 140: 103.

Beeton K, Jull GA (1994) The effectiveness of manipulative physiotherapy in the management of cervicogenic headache: A single case study. *Physiotherapy* 80: 417–423.

Bergmark A (1989) Stability of the lumbar spine. A study in mechanical engineering. *Acta Orthopaedica Scandinavica* 230(suppl.): 20–24.

Biedermann HJ, Shanks GL, Forrest WJ, Inglis J (1991) Power spectrum analyses of electromyographic activity: discriminators in the differential assessment of patients with chronic low-back pain. *Spine* 10: 179–184.

Bogduk N (1980) A reappraisal of the anatomy of the human lumbar erector spinae. *Journal of Anatomy* 131: 525–540.

Bogduk N, Macintosh JE (1984) The applied anatomy of the thoracolumbar fascia. *Spine* 9: 164–170.

Bogduk N, Twomey LT (1987) *Clinical Anatomy of the Lumbar Spine*. Churchill Livingstone, Edinburgh.

Bogduk N, Wilson AS, Tynan W (1982) The human lumbar dorsal rami. *Journal of Anatomy* 134: 383–397.

Bogduk NLT (1997) *Clinical Anatomy of the Lumbar Spine and Sacrum*, 3rd edn. Churchill Livingstone, New York.

Booth FW, Gollnick PD (1983) Effects of disuse on the structure and function of skeletal muscle. *Medicine and Science in Sports and Exercise* 15: 415–420.

Brooke MH, Kaiser KK (1970) Muscle fiber types: how many and what kind? *Archives of Neurology* 23: 369–379.

Campbell EJM, Green JH (1955) The behaviour of the abdominal muscles and the intra-abdominal pressure during quiet breathing and increased pulmonary ventilation. *Journal of Physiology* 127: 423–426.

Carman DJ, Blanton PL, Biggs NL (1972) Electromyographic study of the antero-lateral abdominal musculature using indwelling electrodes. *American Journal of Physical Medicine* 15: 113–129.

Comerford M, Mottram S (2001) Movement and stability dysfunction – contemporary developments. *Manual Therapy* 6: 15–26.

Conley M.S., Meyer R.A., Bloomnerg J.J., Feeback D.L., Dudley G.A. (1995). Noninvasive analysis of human neck muscle function. Spine 20, 2505–2512.

Cooper RG, St Clair Forbes W, Jayson MIV (1992) Radiographic demonstration of paraspinal muscle wasting in patients with chronic low back pain. *Journal of Rheumatology* 31: 389–394.

Cresswell AG, Grundstrom H, Thorstensson A (1992) Observations on intra-abdominal pressure and patterns of abdominal intra-muscular activity in man. *Acta Physiologica Scandinavica* 144: 409–418.

Dangaria TR, Naesh O (1998) Changes in cross-sectional area of psoas major muscle in unilateral sciatica caused by disc herniation. *Spine* 23: 928–931.

DeLancey JOL (1990) Anatomy and physiology of continence. *Clinical Obstetrics and Gynaecology* 33: 298–307.

DeTroyer A, Estenns M, Ninane V, VanGansbeke D, Gorini M (1990) Transversus abdominis function in humans. *Journal of Applied Physiology* 68: 1010–1016.

Dolan P, Earley M, Adams MA (1994) Bending and compressive stresses acting on the lumbar spine during lifting activities. *Journal of Biomechanics* 27: 1237.

Donisch EW, Basmajian JV (1972) Electromyography of deep back muscles in man. *American Journal of Anatomy* 133: 25.

Editorial (1979) Stay young by good posture. *New Scientist* 82: 544.

Elder GC, Bradbury K, Roberts R (1982) Variability of fiber type distributions within human muscles. *Journal of Applied Physiology: Respiratory Environmental and Exercise Physiology* 53: 1473–1480.

Fairbank JCT, O'Brien JP, Davis PR (1980) Intra-abdominal pressure rise during weight lifting as an objective measure of low-back pain. *Spine* 5: 179–184.

Feinstein B (1977) Referred pain from the paravertebral structures. In: Buerger AA, Tobis JF (eds) *Approaches to the Validation of Manipulative Therapy*. Thomas, Springfield, Illinois, p. 139.

Fielding JW, Hawkins RJ (1978) Atlanto-axial rotatory deformities. *Orthopedic Clinics of North America* 9: 995.

Floyd WF, Silver PHS (1950) Electromyographic study of patterns of the anterior abdominal wall muscles in man. *Journal of Anatomy* 84: 132–145.

Floyd WF, Silver PHS (1951) Function of the erectores spinae in flexion of the trunk. *Lancet* 20: 133–134.

Floyd WF, Silver PHS (1955) The function of the erectores spinae muscles in certain movements and postures in man. *Journal of Physiology* 129: 184.

Goff B (1972) The application of recent advances in neurophysiology to Miss Roods' concept of neuromuscular facilitation. *Physiotherapy* 58: 409–415.

Gossman MR, Sahrmann SA, Rose SJ (1982) Review of length-associated changes in muscle. *Physical Therapy* 62: 1799–1808.

Grandjean E (1971) *Fitting the Task to the Man. An Ergonomic Approach*. Taylor and Francis, London.

Hallgren RC, Greenman P, Rechtein J (1994) Atrophy of suboccipital muscles in patients with chronic pain: a pilot study. *Journal of the American Osteopathic Association* 94: 1032–1038.

Hides JA, Stokes MJ, Saide M, Jull GA, Cooper DH (1994) Evidence of multifidus wasting ipsilateral to symptoms in patients with acute/subacute low back pain. *Spine* 19: 165–177.

Hides JA, Richardson CA, Jull GA (1996) Multifidus recovery is not automatic after resolution of acute, first-episode low back pain. *Spine* 21: 2763–2769.

Hodges PW, Richardson C (1997) Feedforward contraction of transversus abdominis is not influenced by the direction of arm movement. *Experimental Brain Research* 114: 62–370.

Hukins DWL, Kirby MC, Sikoryn TA, Aspden RM, Cox AJ (1990) Comparison of structure, mechanical properties, and function of lumbar spinal ligaments. *Spine* 15: 787–795.

Janda V (1976) The muscular factor in the pathogenesis of back pain syndrome. Physiotherapy Symposium, Oslo.

Janda V (1983) On the concept of postural muscles and posture in man. *Australian Journal of Physiotherapy* 29: 83–84.

Janda V (1996) Evaluation of muscle imbalance. In: Liebenson C (ed.) *Rehabilitation of the Spine*. Williams and Wilkins, Baltimore.

Janda VL (1985) Pain in the locomotor system – A broad approach. In: Glasgow EF (ed.) *Aspects of Manipulative Therapy*. Churchill Livingstone, Melbourne, pp. 148–151.

Janda VL (1994) Muscles and motor control in cervicogenic disorders: assessment and management. In: Grant R (ed.) *Physical Therapy of the Cervical and Thoracic Spine*, 2nd edn. Churchill Livingstone, Edinburgh, Ch. 10, pp. 195–216.

Johnson G, Bogduk N, Nowitzke A, House D (1994) Anatomy and actions of the trapezius muscle. *Clinical Biomechanics* 9: 44–50.

Jowett RL, Fidler MW (1975) Histochemical changes in multifidus in mechanical derangements of the spine. *Orthopedic Clinics of North America* 6: 45.

Jull G (1997) Management of cervical headache. *Manual Therapy* 2: 182–190.

Jull G, Barrett C, Magee R, Ho P (1999) Further clinical clarification of the muscle dysfunction in cervical headache. *Cephalalgia* 19: 179–185.

Jull GA (2000) Deep cervical flexor muscle dysfunction in whiplash. *Journal of Musculoskeletal Pain* 8: 143–154.

Kader DF, Wardlow D, Smith FW (2000) Correlation between the MRI changes in multifidus muscles and leg pain. *Clinical Radiology* 55: 145–149.

Keagy RD, Brumlik J, Bergan JL (1966) Direct electromyography of the psoas major muscle in man. *Journal of Bone and Joint Surgery (Am.)* 48: 1377.

Kendall FP, McCreary EK, Provance PG (1993) *Muscle Testing and Function*, 4th edn. Williams and Wilkins, Baltimore.

Kippers V, Parker AW (1985) Electromyographic studies of erectores spinae: symmetrical postures and sagittal trunk motion. *Australian Journal of Physiotherapy* 3: 95.

Kirkaldy Willis WH, Hill RJ (1979) A more precise diagnosis for low back pain. *Spine* 4: 102.

Klausen K (1965) The form and function of the loaded human spine. *Acta Physiologica Scandinavica* 65: 176–190.

Lee D (1999) *The Pelvic Girdle. An Approach to the Examination and Treatment of the Lumbo-pelvi-hip Region.* Churchill Livingstone, Edinburgh, p. 59.

Lieber R (1992) *Skeletal Muscle Structure and Function. Implications for Rehabilitation and Sports Medicine.* Lippincott Williams and Wilkins, Baltimore, pp. 1–48.

Lundervold AJS (1951) *Electromyographic Investigations of Position and Manner of Working in Typewriting.* W. Brøggers Boktrykkeri, Oslo.

Macintosh JE, Bogduk N (1986) The biomechanics of the lumbar multifidus. *Clinical Biomechanics* 1: 205.

Macintosh JE, Bogduk N (1987) The morphology of the lumbar erector spinae. *Spine* 12: 658.

Macintosh JE, Bogduk N, Gracovetsky S (1987) The biomechanics of the thoracolumbar fascia. *Clinical Biomechanics* 2: 78–83.

McArdle WD, Katch FI, Katch VL (1986). Skeletal muscle: Structure and function. In: McArdle WD, Katch FI, Katch VL (eds) *Exercise Physiology: Energy, Nutrition and Human Performance.* Lea & Febiger, Philadelphia, p. 289.

McGill SM, Norman RW (1986) Partitioning of the L4-L5 dynamic movement into disc, ligamentous and muscular components during lifting. *Spine* 11: 566.

McGill SM, Norman RW (1988) Potential of the lumbodorsal fascia forces to generate back extension moments in squat lifts. *Journal of Biomedical Engineering* 10: 312–318.

McGill SM, Juker D, Kropf P (1996) Quantitative intramuscular myoelectric activity of quadratus lumborum during a wide variety of tasks. *Clinical Biomechanics* 11: 170–172.

McPartland J, Brodeur R, Hallgren R (1997) Chronic neck pain, standing balance and suboccipital muscle atrophy – a pilot study. *Journal of Manipulative and Physiological Therapeutics* 20: 24–29.

Nachemson A (1966) Electromyographic studies of the vertebral portion of the psoas muscle. *Acta Orthopaedica Scandinavica* 37: 177.

Nolan JP, Sherk HH (1988) Biomechanical evaluation of the extensor musculature of the cervical spine. *Spine* 13: 9–11.

Ortengren R, Andersson GBJ (1977) Electromyographic studies of trunk muscles with special reference to functional anatomy of the spine. *Spine* 2: 44.

Palastanga N, Field D, Soames R (1989) *Anatomy and Human Movement.* Heinemann Medical Books, Oxford.

Peachy LD, Eisenberg BR (1978) Helicoids in the T system and striations of frog skeletal muscle fibres seen by high voltage electron microscopy. *Biophysical Journal* 22: 145–154.

Peter JB, Barnard RJ, Edgerton VR, et al (1972) Metabolic profiles of three fiber types of skeletal muscle. *Biochemistry* 11: 2627–2633.

Porterfield J, DeRosa C (1997) *Mechanical Low Back Pain. Perspectives in Functional Anatomy.* 2nd edn. Saunders, Philadelphia, pp. 53–119.

Porterfield JA, DeRosa C (1994) *Mechanical Neck Pain. Perspectives in Functional Anatomy.* Saunders, Philadelphia, pp. 47–81.

Rantanen J, Hurme M, Falck B, et al (1993) The lumbar multifidus muscle five years after surgery for a lumbar intervertebral disc herniation. *Spine* 18: 568–574.

Richardson C, Jull G, Hodges P, Hides JA (1999) *Therapeutic Exercise for Spinal Segmental Stabilization in Low Back Pain: Scientific Basis and Clinical Approach.* Churchill Livingstone, Edinburgh.

Richardson CA, Sims K (1991) An inner range holding contraction. An objective measure of stabilizing function of an antigravity muscle. In: *Proceedings of XI International Congress of World Confederation for Physical Therapy,* London, pp. 829–831.

Rose SJ, Rothstein JM (1982) Muscle mutability. *Physical Therapy* 62: 1773–1787.

Roy SH, Deluca CJ, Casavant DA (1989) Lumbar muscle fatigue and chronic low back pain. *Spine* 14: 992–1001.

Sahrmann SA (2000) *Diagnosis and Treatment of Movement Impairment Syndromes.* London. Course manual.

Sapsford R (2004) Rehabilitation of pelvic floor muscles utilizing trunk stabilization. *Manual Therapy* 9: 3–12.

Sapsford RR, Hodges PW, Richardson CA, Cooper DH, Markwell SJ, Jull GA (2001) Co-activation of the abdominal and pelvic floor muscles during voluntary exercises. *Neurology and Urodynamics* 20: 31–42.

Sirca A, Kostevc V (1985) The fibre type composition of thoracic and lumbar paravertebral muscles in man. *Journal of Anatomy* 141: 131–137.

Snijders CJ, Vleeming A, Stoekart R, Mens JMA, Kleinrensink GJ (1995) Biomechanical modelling of sacroiliac joint stability in different postures. *Spine, State of the Art Reviews.* Hanley & Belfus, Philadephia.

Snijders CJ, Vleeming A, Stoeckart R, Mens JMA, Kleinrensink GJ (1997) Biomechanics of the interface between spine and pelvis in different postures. In:

Vleeming A, Mooney V, Dorman T, Snijders C, Stoeckart R (eds) *Movement, Stability and Low Back Pain*. Churchill Livingstone, Edinburgh, Ch. 6, p. 103.

Stokes MA, Cooper R, Morris G, Jayson MIV (1992) Selective changes in multifidus dimensions in patients with chronic low back pain. *European Spine Journal*, 1: 38–42.

Suzuki N, Endo S (1983) A quantitative study of trunk muscle strength and fatigability in the low back pain syndrome. *Spine* 8: 69.

Tesh KM, ShawDunn J, Evans JH (1987) The abdominal muscles and vertebral stability. *Spine* 12: 501–508.

Vleeming A, Stoeckart R, Snidjers CJ (1989) The sacrotuberous ligament: A conceptual approach to its dynamic role in stabilizing the sacroiliac joint. *Clinical Biomechanics* 4: 201.

Vleeming A, Pool-Goudzwaard AL, Stoeckart R, van Windergarden JP, Snijders CJ (1995) The posterior layer of the thoracolumbar fascia: Its function in load transfer from spine to legs. *Spine* 20: 753.

Voss D, Ionta M, Myers B (1985) *Proprioceptive Neuromuscular Facilitation*, 3rd edn. Harper and Row, Philadelphia.

Watanabe K (1980) Biomechanical implications of EMG activity of erector spinae and gluteus maximus muscles in postural changes of the trunk. In: Morecki A, Fidelus K, Kedzior K, et al (eds) *Biomechanics VII-B*. University Park Press, Baltimore, pp. 23–30.

Watson DH, Trott PH (1993) Cervical headache. An investigation of natural head posture and upper cervical flexor muscle performance. *Cephalalgia* 13: 272–284.

Wheeler SD (1982) Pathology of muscle and motor units. *Physical Therapy* 62: 1809–1822.

Wiemann K, Klee A, Stratmann M (1998) Fibrillar sources of the muscle resting tension and therapy of muscular imbalances. *Deutsche Zeitschrift für Sportmedizin* 49: 111–118.

Willard FH (1997) The muscular, ligamentous and neural structure of the low back and its relation to back pain. In: Vleeming A, Mooney V, Dorman T, Snijders C, Stoeckart R (eds) *Movement, Stability and Low Back Pain. The Essential Role of the Pelvis*. Churchill Livingstone, Edinburgh, pp. 3–35.

Winters JM, Peles JD (1990) Neck activity and 3-D head kinematics during quasi-static and dynamic tracking movements. In: Winters JM, Woo SLY (eds) *Multiple Muscle Systems: Biomechanics and Movement Organization*. Springer-Verlag, New York, pp. 461–480.

Chapter 4

Blood supply of the spinal cord and the vertebral column

BLOOD SUPPLY OF THE SPINAL CORD

The spinal cord has been described as a solitary integrated organ that extends nearly the whole length of the spine (Schmorl and Junghanns, 1959). The metabolic demands of the brain and spinal cord are high, and together they consume approximately 20% of the available oxygen in the circulating blood. The spinal grey matter has a higher metabolic demand than the white matter; consequently, blood flow within the grey matter is 15.4 times greater than in the white matter. The blood flow to the spinal cord is provided via the aorta, medullary feeder arteries, longitudinal arterial trunks of the cord, small arteries, arterioles, precapillaries and capillaries (Dommisse, 1986).

LONGITUDINAL ARTERIAL TRUNKS (Fig. 4.1)

The arterial supply of the cord is derived from one anterior and two posterolateral longitudinal arterial trunks (anterior spinal artery and posterior spinal arteries). The anterior longitudinal trunk lies over the anterior median sulcus. In its upper part, it communicates with the small

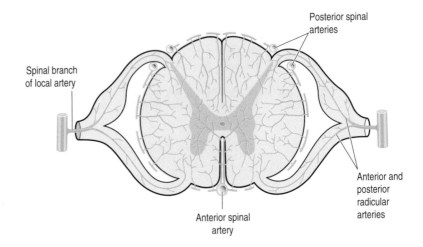

Figure 4.1   Intrinsic arteries of the spinal cord – transverse section. (Adapted from Williams PL, Warwick R 1980 *Gray's Anatomy*, 36th edn. Churchill Livingstone, Edinburgh, p. 896.)

anterior spinal arteries and branches of both vertebral arteries. The posterior longitudinal trunks are paired vessels extending the length of the cord. They pass around and between the posterior nerve rootlets. In the upper part, they communicate with the posterior inferior cerebellar branches of both vertebral arteries by means of two posterior spinal arteries.

The anterior and posterior longitudinal trunks form an anastomosis distally around the conus medullaris.

MEDULLARY FEEDER ARTERIES

The longitudinal trunks are supplied and maintained by medullary feeder arteries. The site, number and source of origin of the medullary feeders vary in each individual. A cadaveric study (Dommisse, 1994) found an average of 7.5 anterior feeders per cadaver, the numbers varying from 2 to 17. The average number of posterior feeders was 12.5 per cadaver, with a range of 6 to 25. The medullary feeders are particularly numerous in the region of the brachial and lumbosacral plexuses. There are relatively fewer medullary feeders in the thoracic region and, as it has the narrowest spinal canal lumen, it is a critical vascular zone. Medullary feeders arise from the segmental arteries and enter the intervertebral foramen to join the longitudinal arterial trunks on the cord surface.

PERFORATING ARTERIES

Three sets of perforating arteries penetrate the spinal cord:

1. Anterior perforating arteries arise from the anterior longitudinal arterial trunk and penetrate the median sulcus to supply the major portion of the cord substance. The anterior perforators are largest and most numerous in the region of the brachial and lumbosacral plexuses. The anterior perforators and anterior longitudinal trunk are vital for normal function. Occlusion of these vessels results in 'anterior spinal artery syndrome' with motor paralysis and impairment of thermal and pain sensations, although tactile and pressure senses are preserved.

2. Small posterior perforating arteries enter the cord substance with the posterior rootlets and are distributed in the posterior one third of the cord. They anastomose with the capillary plexus.

3. Small perforating arteries provide surface communications between the anterior and posterior perforating arteries. They also anastomose with the capillary plexus.

CAPILLARIES OF THE SPINAL CORD

An uninterrupted plexus of capillaries extends from the medulla oblongata to the conus medullaris. The capillary density is greatest in the grey matter where the nerves have a high metabolic demand. The dorsal root ganglia, spinal nerve rootlets and spinal nerves have an abundant blood supply. The supply to the dorsal root ganglia is particularly rich, being commensurate with that of the spinal cord grey matter.

ARTERIAL SUPPLY OF THE VERTEBRAL COLUMN

The arterial supply of the vertebral column is derived from branches of the segmental arteries. The cervical region receives branches from the vertebral and ascending cervical arteries; the thoracic column branches arise from the costocervical and posterior intercostal arteries; the branches to the lumbar region arise from the lumbar and iliolumbar arteries; while the pelvis takes its supply from the lateral sacral arteries.

LUMBAR SPINE

Each lumbar artery passes laterally and back around the vertebral body until it reaches the intervertebral foramen. Branches of the lumbar arteries supply the vertebral bodies (see pp. 155–158).

Branches of the lumbar arteries

Just outside the intervertebral foramina each lumbar artery divides into several branches.

1. Anterior branches supply the abdominal wall.

2. Posterior branches supply the paravertebral muscles, the apophyseal joints and the bony arch of the vertebral bodies.

3. Three spinal canal branches arise from the lumbar arteries opposite the intervertebral foramen:
   a) The *anterior spinal canal branch* enters the canal and bifurcates to form ascending and descending branches. The ascending branch crosses the outer third of the intervertebral disc and joins the descending branch from the artery above. These branches form an arcade system on the anterior wall of the spinal canal.

   b) The *posterior spinal canal branches* are also disposed in an arcuate pattern, forming a closely woven network over the anterior surface of the lamina and ligamenta flava. Branches also pass to the laminae, spinous processes, extradural fat and the anterior plexus on the dura mater.

c) The *radicular branches* supply the lumbar nerve roots.

Blood supply of the spinal nerve roots

The lumbar nerve roots are supplied, proximally, by the vessels from the conus medullaris of the spinal cord and, distally, in the intervertebral foramina from the radicular branches of the lumbar arteries.

At their attachment to the conus medullaris, the ventral and dorsal rootlets are supplied by five branches from the conus medullaris for a few centimetres. The remainder of the root is supplied by the proximal and distal radicular arteries.

The proximal radicular arteries arise from the anterior and posterior spinal arteries. Each proximal radicular artery passes with its root embedded in its own pial sheath. The artery enters the root several centimetres from the spinal cord and follows one of the main nerve bundles along its length.

The radicular artery is a branch of the lumbar artery. It enters the spinal nerve, dividing into branches that enter the ventral and dorsal roots, becoming the distal radicular artery. The distal radicular artery forms a plexus around the dorsal root ganglion. The distal radicular artery passes proximally along the root until it meets and anastomoses with the proximal radicular artery.

Branches of the distal and proximal artery communicate with one another. These communicating branches are coiled (Parke and Watanabe, 1985). The arteries themselves are also coiled proximal and distal to the origin of these branches. These coils accommodate the movement of the nerve root that occurs during spinal movements.

The nerve roots have proximal and distal radicular veins. The proximal veins tend to drain towards the spinal cord, while the distal veins tend to drain towards the intervertebral foramina, where they anastomose with the lumbar veins. The radicular veins lie deep in the nerve and take a wavy course.

Blood supply of the vertebral bodies
(Fig. 4.2)

The segmental arteries (lumbar arteries, intercostal arteries and deep cervical arteries) pass around the vertebral bodies, giving rise to ascending and descending branches called the *primary periosteal arteries*. These branches supply the periosteum of the vertebral bodies. Periosteal branches also arise from the anterior spinal canal arteries to supply the posterior wall of the vertebral bodies.

At the superior and inferior borders of each vertebra, the primary periosteal arteries form an anastomotic ring called the *metaphysial anastomosis*. Branches of this anastomosis, the *metaphysial arteries*, supply the superior and inferior borders of the vertebral body.

The centre of the vertebral body derives its blood supply from the branches of the segmental arteries and the anterior spinal canal arteries.

Branches of the anterior spinal canal arteries are named *nutrient arteries*; they pierce the middle of the posterior surface of the vertebral body.

Figure 4.2   Blood supply of the vertebral bodies. A, Transverse section of superior or inferior end of vertebral body. B, Frontal section through the middle of vertebral body (after Ratcliffe JF 1980 The arterial anatomy of the adult human vertebral body: a micrarteriographic study. *Journal of Anatomy* 131: 57–79). C, Sagittal section through a lumbar vertebra (adapted from Crock HV, Yoshizawa H 1976 The blood supply of the lumbar vertebral column. *Clinical Orthopaedics and Related Research* 6–21).

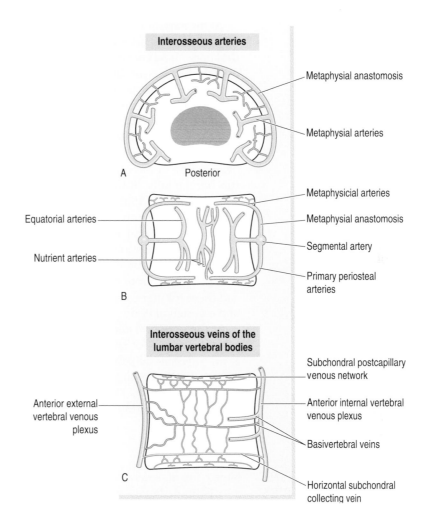

Branches of the segmental arteries are named *equatorial arteries*; they pierce the anterior and lateral aspect of the vertebral body.

Branches of the nutrient and equatorial arteries form an arterial grid in the centre of the vertebral body. These branches form pathways towards the respective vertebral end plates.

During ageing, atherosclerosis of the arteries occurs, so that the lumen of the blood vessels is reduced or obliterated, resulting in a reduction or cessation of blood flow. Arteries which follow a tortuous course are particularly affected, and the nutrient and metaphysial arteries of the vertebral bodies are among the first to undergo these changes. As ageing occurs, the periphery of the vertebral body therefore receives a better blood flow than the central region (Palastanga et al, 1989). Reduction in the blood supply to the centre of the vertebral body affects the nutrition of the centre of the intervertebral disc.

At the vertebral end plate, terminal branches of the metaphysial arteries and nutrient arteries form a dense capillary network in the subchondral bone. It has been noted from studies in dogs that the capillary ends over the nucleus are large and globular, while the capillary terminals over the annulus fibrosus are smaller, less numerous and simpler in appearance (Crock and Goldwasser, 1984). Consequently, the blood supply to the nucleus is probably greater, ensuring that the nutrition of the centre of the disc is adequate.

The principal veins of the vertebral body are *basivertebral veins*, which are situated in the centre of the vertebral body. The basivertebral veins run horizontally in the middle of the vertebral body forming a large-scale venous grid into which the vertebral veins of the vertebral body flow from above and below.

The basivertebral veins drain primarily posteriorly into the anterior internal vertebral venous plexus. They also drain anteriorly into the anterior external vertebral venous plexus. The basivertebral veins receive vertical tributaries from the upper and lower halves of the vertebral body, and these tributaries receive oblique tributaries from the peripheral parts of the vertebral body.

At the vertebral end plate, small vertical capillaries drain into a horizontal network of small veins that lie parallel to the end plate. This is the *subchondral postcapillary venous network*. Short veins drain from this plexus into a larger venous channel, the *horizontal subarticular collecting vein system*. This system of veins also lies parallel to the end plate. Veins from this network pass vertically towards the centre of the vertebral body.

THORACIC SPINE AND RIBS

Nine pairs of *posterior intercostal arteries* arise from the thoracic aorta and are distributed in the nine lower intercostal spaces. The 1st and 2nd intercostal spaces are supplied by the *superior intercostal artery*.

Branches of the posterior intercostal arteries

Muscular branches pass to the intercostal and pectoral muscles and to serratus anterior.

Lateral cutaneous branches pass with the lateral cutaneous branches of the thoracic nerves.

The *collateral intercostal branch* arises from the posterior intercostal artery near the angle of the rib. It crosses to the upper border of the rib below to anastomose with an intercostal branch of the thoracic artery.

Mammary branches arise from the arteries at the 2nd, 3rd and 4th spaces.

The *dorsal branch* passes back between the necks of the ribs superiorly and inferiorly, lateral to the vertebral body and medial to the costotransverse ligaments. Opposite the intervertebral canal, it gives rise to spinal canal branches. These branches (anterior spinal canal branch, posterior spinal canal branch, radicular branch) follow a similar course to those of the lumbar spine (see *p.* 155) to supply the vertebra, spinal cord and nerve roots. The dorsal branch also supplies the paravertebral back muscles.

CERVICAL COLUMN

Vertebral artery
(Figs 4.3, 4.4)

The vertebral artery has four parts:

Part 1.   It arises from the upper and posterior area of the first part of the subclavian artery and runs backwards between longus colli and scalenus anterior. The vertebral vein and common carotid artery lie in front of it, and behind it lie the inferior cervical ganglion and the ventral rami of the 7th and 8th cervical nerves.

Part 2.   It enters the foramen transversarium of the 6th cervical vertebra and passes through each cervical vertebra to the foramen transversarium of the axis, where it passes upwards and laterally to the foramen transversarium of the atlas. The vertebral artery is relatively fixed at the foramina of C1 and C2 so that it is particularly vulnerable to stretch at this motion segment.

   As it ascends, it is accompanied by a branch of the inferior cervical ganglion and a plexus of veins which eventually form the vertebral vein. It lies in front of the ventral rami of the 2nd–6th cervical nerve roots and lateral to the uncovertebral joints.

Part 3.   The artery emerges from the foramen of the atlas, medial to rectus capitis lateralis, and curves backwards behind the lateral mass of the atlas with the ventral rami of C1 medial to it. The artery then lies on a groove in the posterior arch of the atlas and passes below the arched border of the posterior atlanto-occipital membrane to enter the spinal canal. The dorsal ramus of C1 lies between the artery and the posterior arch of the atlas.

Figure 4.3   Course of the right vertebral and carotid arteries. (Adapted from Williams PL, Warwick R 1980 *Gray's Anatomy*, 36th edn. Churchill Livingstone, Edinburgh, p. 896.)

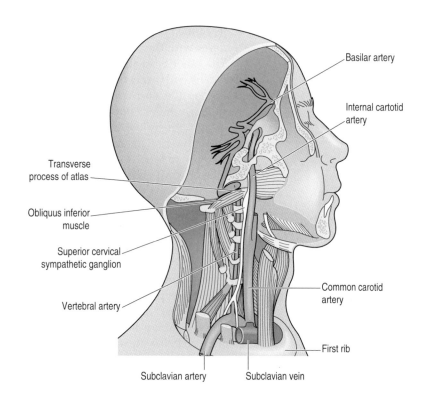

Basilar artery

Internal cartotid artery

Transverse process of atlas

Obliquus inferior muscle

Superior cervical sympathetic ganglion

Vertebral artery

Common carotid artery

First rib

Subclavian artery   Subclavian vein

Part 4. After entering the spinal canal, the artery pierces the dura and arachnoid mater and inclines medially to the front of the medulla oblongata where, at the lower border of the pons, it unites with the opposite artery to form the basilar artery.

Variations of the vertebral artery

The origin of the artery may vary depending on side. On the left, it can originate from the arch of the aorta, between the left common carotid and subclavian arteries. Occasionally, it may arise from the descending aorta.

The artery normally enters the 6th cervical foramen transversarium but not infrequently it may enter via the 7th or 5th cervical vertebra, and it has even been reported entering the foramen as high as the 3rd cervical vertebra (Taitz et al, 1978). This variation may be unilateral or bilateral.

In a study of 150 cadavers, Stopford (1916) found that the vertebral arteries were of unequal size in 92% of instances. In 22 cadavers, the vessel on one side was at least twice the size of the vessel on the opposite side. In the presence of a marked difference in the calibres of the vertebral arteries, the supply to the basilar artery is virtually entirely through the dominant artery.

There are variations in the elastic and muscular tissues in different parts of the vertebral artery. The first and third parts are adapted for greater elasticity, mobility and lack of support in these regions.

Spinal branches of the vertebral artery

The spinal branches enter the vertebral canal through the intervertebral foramina and divide into two branches. One branch passes along the roots of the nerve to supply the spinal cord and its membranes. It anastomoses with the other arteries of the spinal cord.

The other branch divides into an ascending and descending branch that joins with branches from above and below to form two anastomotic chains on the posterolateral surfaces of the vertebral bodies. Branches from these chains supply the periosteum and vertebral bodies, communicating with similar branches from the opposite side. These communications give rise to small branches, which join similar branches above and below to form a central anastomotic chain on the posterior surfaces of the vertebral bodies.

Muscular branches of the vertebral artery

As the vertebral artery passes around the lateral mass of the atlas, muscular branches are given off and supply the deep muscles of the region.

Cranial branches of the vertebral artery

In the cranium, the main branches form the anterior and posterior spinal arteries. The posterior inferior cerebellar artery is the largest branch of the vertebral artery in the cranium and supplies the lateral aspect of the medulla, choroid plexus of the 4th ventricle and the lower surface of the cerebellar hemisphere. Meningeal branches and the medullary artery also arise from the vertebral artery.

The two vertebral arteries unite at the lower border of the pons to form the basilar artery, and branches supply the medulla, pons, brainstem and cerebellum.

Circle of Willis
(Fig. 4.4)

The vertebral arteries and the circle of Willis (circulus arteriosus) supply a large area of the brain.

The circle is situated at the base of the brain. It is formed in front by two anterior cerebral arteries that are joined together by the anterior communicating artery. Behind, the basilar artery divides into two posterior cerebral arteries, each of which is joined to the internal carotid artery of the same side by the posterior communicating artery.

The arteries forming the circle vary enormously and some are often absent: 60% of individuals have anomalies of the circle of Willis.

The direction of blood flow within the circle varies. Physical and chemical factors are thought to determine the direction of flow.

Figure 4.4 Schematic view of principal arteries at the base of the brain. (Adapted from Williams PL, Warwick R 1980 *Gray's Anatomy*, 36th edn. Churchill Livingstone, Edinburgh, p. 896.)

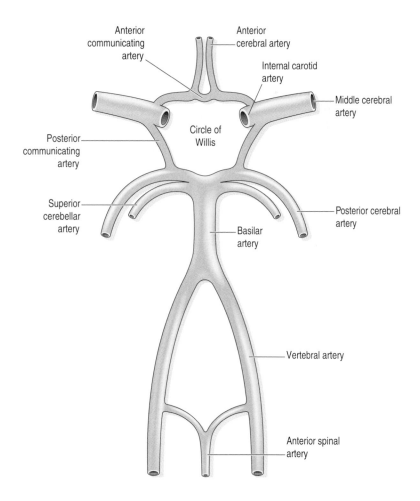

Anterior communicating artery

Anterior cerebral artery

Internal carotid artery

Middle cerebral artery

Circle of Willis

Posterior communicating artery

Superior cerebellar artery

Basilar artery

Posterior cerebral artery

Vertebral artery

Anterior spinal artery

THE VERTEBROBASILAR SYSTEM

Symptomology

The vestibular nuclei receive their blood supply entirely from branches of the vertebral and basilar arteries (Fisher, 1967). If the blood flow to these nuclei is reduced, vestibular function is impaired. Dizziness is usually the most common and predominant symptom of vertebrobasilar disease.

Other symptoms are also associated with vertebrobasilar insufficiency. As the vertebrobasilar arteries supply areas other than the vestibular nuclei, any accompanying symptoms vary according to the area of the brainstem affected by ischaemia. Symptoms associated with vertebrobasilar vascular disease include visual disturbances, diplopia, 'drop attacks', dysarthria, dysphagia, nausea, ataxia, impairment of trigeminal sensation, sympathoplegia, hemianaesthesia and hemiplegia (Bogduk, 1986).

Pathology

It has been suggested that irritation of the sympathetic plexus accompanying the vertebral artery can produce symptoms of vertebrobasilar insufficiency (Neuworth, 1954; Stewart, 1962; Lewit, 1969). It was hypothesized that irritation of the sympathetic plexus by osteophytic encroachment or prolapsed intervertebral disc could lead to spasm of the distal part of the vertebrobasilar complex, which may result in brainstem ischaemia. However, in experiments on monkeys (Bogduk et al, 1981), the vertebral blood flow was completely unresponsive to stimulation of any part of the cervical sympathetic system, and it was concluded that there was no evidence to support this theory.

Mechanical factors affecting the vertebrobasilar system

Pathological changes in the cervical spine or within the vertebral artery may influence blood flow within the artery and hence the blood supply to the brain. These mechanical disorders may be classified as either intrinsic or extrinsic.

Extrinsic disorders

Extrinsic disorders are those which compress the external wall of the vertebral artery, thereby narrowing the lumen of the vessel and compromising the blood flow within it. Soft tissue thickening, lipping of the vertebral body and osteophytic impingement are examples of mechanical factors which may impinge the vertebral artery or displace it. Displacement of the artery can be slight or so marked that the course of the artery is altered considerably and, consequently, the blood flow within it may be affected.

In the first part of the vertebral artery, three types of anomaly may compromise the vessel (Bogduk, 1986):

1. An anomalous origin of the vertebral artery from the subclavian artery so that during rotation of the neck the artery becomes distorted and occluded (Power et al, 1961)
2. Bands of cervical fascia crossing the vertebral artery which constrict the vessel during rotation of the neck (Hardin and Poser, 1963)
3. An anomalous course of the artery between the fascicles of longus colli or scalenus anterior at their attachment to the C6 transverse

process; during neck rotation the artery may be squeezed by the muscle bundles (Husni and Storer, 1967a and b).

Osteophytic compression can occur as the vertebral artery ascends through the foramina transversaria. The vertebral artery may be subject to compression or angulation by osteophytes projecting laterally from the uncinate processes. Compression of the vertebral artery is seen most commonly at the C5/6 level with a lesser incidence at the C4/5 and C6/7 levels (Bogduk, 1986). When the neck is in the neutral position, osteophytic encroachment may or may not distort the vertebral artery but, as the neck is rotated, distortion of the artery is either increased or produced. The vertebral artery on the side to which the head is rotated is most likely to be affected by uncinate osteophytes. Dizziness is the most common symptom of osteophytic impingement within the foramina transversaria. At operation, in addition to bony outgrowths, adhesions surrounding the vertebral artery have frequently been observed. Resection of the osteophytes is not always sufficient to restore adequate blood flow, and the patency of the vessel may only be achieved by removal of the adventitial adhesions as well.

At the atlanto-axial joint the vertebral artery may be compromised if the atlas subluxes on the axis (e.g. in rheumatoid arthritis, aplasia of the odontoid and os odontoideum). In these cases, post mortem studies have shown thrombus of the atlanto-axial section of the vertebral artery. The thrombus formation is probably initiated by the distortion of the vessel (Webb et al, 1968).

Intrinsic disorders   Atherosclerosis is the major intrinsic disorder to affect the vertebrobasilar system. Atheromatous changes have been noted in all the arteries of the body, and are commonly found in the vertebral and basilar arteries. In the vertebral artery, narrowing may occur focally due to formation of isolated plaques or it may be more widespread so that considerable parts of the length are affected. These changes within the artery increase the likelihood of obstruction or stenosis occurring. If the vertebral artery is narrowed internally due to arteriosclerosis, and it also becomes compromised by an extrinsic factor such as osteophytic encroachment, blood flow will be particularly at risk.

Thrombosis of the vertebral and basilar arteries is a complication of atherosclerosis, and emboli tend to lodge in the distal branches of the vertebrobasilar system, particularly the posterior cerebral artery (Fisher and Karnes, 1965).

Clinical biomechanics

A number of studies have investigated the effect of head and neck position on blood flow within the vertebral arteries. Many of these studies have been performed on cadavers (Tatlow and Bammer, 1957; Toole and Tucker, 1960; Brown and Tatlow, 1963) and it is possible that they do not accurately reflect what happens in vivo.

Brown and Tatlow (1963) carried out angiographic studies on 41 cadavers to observe the effect of head position on the vertebral arteries. They found that extension alone did not affect the vertebral arteries, but that rotation and extension together occluded the vessels in 5 specimens. When traction was applied with the head rotated and extended, occlusion was noted in 17 out of 21 specimens. In 24 out of 41 specimens, occlusion did not occur on rotation and extension. When occlusion did occur, in each case the artery on the contralateral side was occluded, and it was always at or above C2.

The addition of a traction force causes a narrowing of the vertebral arteries and places the arteries on a stretch. This may make the vertebral artery more susceptible to trauma, particularly if a high-velocity thrust is used in a position of rotation with the addition of strong axial traction. The use of traction in combination with a manipulative thrust is potentially dangerous and must be avoided (Grant, 1988).

The effect of head position on the flow of perfused water within the carotid and vertebral arteries of cadavers was studied in an attempt to quantify any reduction of blood flow during neck rotation (Toole and Tucker, 1960). In most specimens, flexion, extension and rotation all affected the arterial flow, but rotation to less than 45° was the principal compromising manoeuvre. Whenever decreased flow was noted, a further 5–10° of movement occluded the vessel completely. Decreased flow was observed at points well within the normal physiological range of neck movement. It was found that flow within the vertebral artery could be reduced to 10% of the initial rate by neck rotation.

In contrast, an in vivo study (Hardesty et al, 1963) measured vertebral blood flow during rotation of the neck in two patients and recorded a reduction in blood flow of 23% and 9% respectively.

In a Doppler study of 280 vertebral arteries, Haynes (1996) found that 5% lost Doppler sounds during rotation to end range, but none developed any signs of vertebrobasilar insufficiency. Lateral flexion had no effect on Doppler signs.

Blood flow within the vertebral arteries fluctuates during normal everyday activities (Bakay and Sweet, 1953). Partial or complete occlusion of the vertebral artery, while compromising blood flow, will not be symptomatic unless there is a critical reduction in the blood supply to the brainstem. Angiographic studies on two patients who complained of dizziness and brainstem symptoms revealed that the contralateral vertebral artery was narrowed when the head was rotated, but this position failed to reproduce the patients' symptoms of brainstem ischaemia (Barton and Margolis, 1975).

Reduction of blood flow itself may not be critical in an individual with a normal healthy vertebrobasilar system, where adequate collateral flow is available. Occlusion of one vertebral artery in the neck may be compensated for by collateral blood flow from the opposite vertebral artery, the ascending and deep cervical arteries, the occipital artery, and blood flow via the circle of Willis. Symptoms of vertebrobasilar insufficiency (VBI) are more likely to occur when these compensating mechanisms are not available due to congenital anomalies or concurrent disease (Bogduk, 1986).

It has been shown that the vertebral arteries are of unequal size in 92% of individuals. Damage to or compression of the dominant artery may lead to brainstem ischaemia if the contralateral artery is unable to maintain an adequate blood supply. Studies have shown that when blood flow within one vertebral artery is occluded, symptoms of brainstem ischaemia have been produced when the contralateral artery is rudimentary or poorly filling (Husni et al, 1966; Pasztor, 1978). These mechanical lesions might not have been symptomatic if the opposite artery had provided an adequate blood flow.

Sites of injury

The vertebral arteries can be subjected to crushing, stretching or shearing at any point along their length. The most common site of injury following manipulative therapy is the atlanto-axial joint, where the vertebral artery is relatively fixed at the C1 and C2 transverse foramina and therefore vulnerable to stretching.

As the vertebral artery ascends through the foramina transversaria it is susceptible to compression or angulation from osteophytic outgrowths that originate at the uncinate processes.

Clinical implications

Incidents of trauma to the vertebral artery following manipulative treatment have been widely reported (Kanshepolsky et al, 1972; Parkin et al, 1978; Fast et al, 1987; Dvorak and Orelli, 1985; Terrett, 1987). Complications following cervical manipulation may vary from a transient light-headedness to dizziness or fainting. There have also been serious incidents reported of stroke and even death subsequent to cervical manipulation. The incidence of complications following cervical manipulation is unknown but it must be noted that the estimated incidence increases as the subject is better investigated (Terrett, 1998).

Although complications following cervical manipulation might be expected to be more prevalent in the elderly due to spondylitic and atherosclerotic changes, literature reviews have revealed that complications following manipulation can occur at any age (Kreuger and Okazaki, 1980; Grant, 1988; Terrett and Kleynhans, 1992). In these reviews, the reported age range of patients suffering severe complications was 7–68 years with a mean of 37.8 years. The increased number of incidents seen in the 30–45-year age group may reflect the fact that this age group is most likely to seek treatment from a practitioner specializing in manipulation (Terrett and Kleynhans, 1992).

Most individuals in the 30–45-year age group are unlikely to have significant spondylitic and atherosclerotic changes, and the presence or absence of these changes may not therefore be sufficient to assess the patient's risk of manipulative iatrogenesis (Terrett and Kleynhans, 1992). Risk factors associated with vertebrobasilar insufficiency and manipulation have been identified by many authors and were summarized by Barker et al (2000). These risk factors are as follows:

Continues

Continued

- Dizziness or vertigo, particularly associated with head positioning
- Drop attacks, fainting, blackouts
- Visual disturbances (e.g. decreased or blurred vision, diplopia, nystagmus)
- Nausea, vomiting, general feeling of being unwell
- Ataxia and unsteadiness of gait
- Tingling or numbness of the lips or face, particularly if it is hemianaesthesia
- Difficulty in speaking or swallowing
- Hearing disturbances (e.g. tinnitus)
- Headaches and acute neck pain
- Past history of trauma
- Cardiac disease, altered blood pressure, previous cerebrovascular accident or transient ischaemic attacks
- Blood clotting disorders
- Anticoagulant therapy
- Oral contraceptives
- Long-term oral steroids
- History of smoking
- Immediately post partum

There have been a number of incidents following ordinary daily activities where sustained or repetitive positioning of the head has caused brainstem ischaemic accidents. These activities include extending the neck over a hairdresser's basin, yoga (Hanus et al, 1977) and driving (Yang et al, 1985).

A review of 185 cases of accidents following cervical manipulation (Terrett, 1998) showed that the onset of symptoms relative to the time of the manipulation was cited in 138 cases as follows:

- 69% during the manipulation
- 3% within minutes of the manipulation
- 8.5% within 1 hour of manipulation
- 8.5% 1–6 hours after manipulation
- 5% 7–24 hours after manipulation
- 6% 24 hours or more after manipulation.

Mechanisms of injury

Evidence from post mortem examination, surgery, angiograms and Doppler sonography has shown that the mechanism of injury following cervical manipulation is either spasm or damage to the artery wall. This is probably a result of trauma to the artery from the manipulative technique.

In some cases, serious complications have followed cervical manipulation but investigations have demonstrated no evidence of vascular injury. Arterial spasm may be the cause of the post-manipulation symptoms in these individuals (Terrett, 1998). The patient may make a complete recovery providing there is no further trauma to the artery. Arterial spasm may be transient; however, if there is hypoplasia or atherosclerosis of the contralateral vertebral artery, it can have devastating effects and cause permanent neurological deficit.

Angiographic and autopsy findings have shown that post-manipulation damage to the arterial wall includes lacerations, intramural hemorrhages, dissections, aneurysms, thrombus and embolus formation. These injuries will all result in permanent neurological deficit.

Clinicians use a number of tests to test the patency of the vertebral artery prior to cervical manipulation (Kleynhans & Terrett, 1985; Grant, 1988). These tests usually involve holding the patient's head in a variety of positions for a sustained period of time (10 seconds to 30 seconds). The therapist observes the patient for any signs of vertebrobasilar insufficiency such as dizziness or nystagmus. If these tests are positive, it indicates that the symptoms may *possibly* be due to brainstem ischaemia from compression of one vertebral artery and inadequacy of the contralateral vertebral artery. In these cases cervical manipulation is contraindicated. The tests themselves involve a certain risk: there have been documented cases of stroke from merely placing the head in a rotated position (Gatterman, 1982).

There is no evidence to show that these tests can exclude any underlying arteriopathy or anatomical anomaly, indeed Bolton et al (1989) used angiography to demonstrate occlusion of one vertebral artery when pre-manipulative testing had been clear. The problem with the testing procedures is that they differ from manipulative thrusts in two respects: force and speed. It seems probable that these two factors increase the likelihood of damage to the vertebral artery. It must be understood that a passive neck rotation test is unlikely to give any indication as to the susceptibility of the vertebral artery to vascular injury on a forceful rotation.

Treatment techniques for the cervical spine should only be used in the full knowledge of contraindications to their use and after comprehensive examination and testing procedures have been employed.

Risk reduction

The following points should be taken into consideration when using cervical manipulation:

1. There is always an element of unpredictability. Complications have arisen even in patients in whom pre-manipulative testing was negative or previous manipulative treatment was uneventful. Using clinical tests alone, it is not possible to screen all patients for pre-existing arteriopathy. The absence of vertebrobasilar insufficiency symptoms does not mean that the patient does not have arterial disease.

2. A review of 185 cases of stroke following cervical manipulation showed that in 94.8% of cases a rotation movement (with or without other movements) was used (Terrett, 1998).

3. The flow of blood within the vertebral arteries is unaffected by lateral flexion (Toole and Tucker, 1960; Haynes, 1996) and a lateral flexion movement should be considered when the treatment rationale indicates that cervical manipulation is appropriate (Terrett and Kleynhans, 1992).

4. The addition of traction to a cervical manipulation is considered dangerous; it should not be used.

5. Repeated manipulations are unnecessary and more likely to traumatize the vertebral artery. An early sign of vertebral artery damage is head and neck pain. This can occur immediately after the manipulation and is often unlike pains the patient has experienced before. The pain may be accompanied by signs of ischaemia such as fainting, nausea and dizziness. If the patient is unfortunate enough to develop head and neck pain after a cervical manipulation, the practitioner must not re-manipulate the neck but observe the patient carefully for a short time. If the symptoms do not subside, the patient should quickly be referred to hospital.

6. Dizziness testing should be fully recorded.

7. The pre-manipulative test procedures themselves hold certain risks.

VEINS OF THE VERTEBRAL COLUMN

The venous drainage of the vertebral column is derived from an intricate plexus that lies both inside and outside the vertebral canal. The veins of the plexus do not have valves; hence the blood may flow in both directions. There are many anastomoses within the plexus. Variations in gross anatomy are common.

The vertebral venous plexus has been described as a pool for receiving backflow from adjacent veins (Herlihy, 1947). As there is no direction of flow, blood is able to ebb and flow, and any unequal pressure in the adjacent veins is quickly equalized.

EXTERNAL VERTEBRAL VENOUS PLEXUS

The external vertebral plexuses are most developed in the cervical region. The *anterior* external vertebral venous plexus lies in front of the vertebral bodies and anastomoses with the basivertebral veins, intervertebral veins and tributaries from the vertebral bodies. The *posterior* external vertebral venous plexus lies over the posterior surfaces of the laminae, the spinous processes, the transverse processes and the articular processes. It anastomoses with the internal vertebral venous plexus and ends in the vertebral, posterior intercostal and lumbar veins.

INTERNAL VERTEBRAL VENOUS PLEXUS

The internal vertebral plexus is also known as Batson's plexus (Batson, 1940). The plexus lies within the spinal canal and extends from the basiocciput to the coccyx. It subserves the venous drainage of the brain and spinal cord. The plexus is orientated around the anterior and posterior walls of the spinal canal and is arranged as four longitudinal veins: two anterior and two posterior.

The *anterior* internal vertebral plexus lies on the posterior surface of the vertebral bodies and intervertebral disc on each side of the posterior longitudinal ligament. The veins are disposed in an arcuate system on either side, joining in the midline. The veins are thin-walled, but have a large calibre when distended. They anastomose with the basivertebral veins.

The two *posterior* internal vertebral plexuses lie posterolaterally within the spinal canal and join in the midline.

The internal and external vertebral venous plexuses anastomose around the emerging nerve root at the intervertebral foramen.

These plexuses provide a place for storage of blood, but also allow outflow of blood under all conditions. A large proportion of the cardiac output is directed at the brain and spinal cord: inflow must be matched by outflow to maintain an effective circulation.

The plexuses act as pressure absorbers and equalize unequal pressure in adjacent veins. The plexus itself has no pressure, thereby ensuring that cerebral flow is not interrupted during normal conditions, such as breathing, coughing and sneezing.

These thin-walled sinuses can be a source of serious bleeding and are potential contributors to postoperative arachnoiditis and radiculopathy (Dommisse and Grobler, 1976).

The *basivertebral veins* emerge from the intervertebral foramina on the posterior surfaces of the vertebral bodies (see 'Blood supply of the vertebral bodies', p. 156). The veins enlarge in old age.

The *intervertebral veins* accompany the spinal nerves through the intervertebral foramina, draining the veins from the spinal cord and the internal and external vertebral venous plexuses. These veins end in the vertebral, posterior intercostal, lumbar and lateral sacral veins.

It is not known whether the intervertebral veins have effective valves, but experimental studies suggest that blood flow in them may be reversed (Batson, 1957). This may explain how neoplasms may produce metastases in the vertebral bodies and spread from pelvis and lungs to the brain.

VEINS OF THE SPINAL CORD

The veins are situated in the pia mater. There are two *median longitudinal* veins: one in front of the anterior median fissure and the other behind the posterior median septum of the spinal cord.

Two anterolateral and two posterolateral longitudinal channels run behind the ventral and dorsal roots respectively. This plexus drains into the internal vertebral venous plexus.

FACTORS INFLUENCING BLOOD FLOW TO NERVOUS TISSUE

The spinal cord, dorsal root ganglia and spinal nerve roots are critical zones of vascular supply. Blood flow to these structures may be affected by congenital, traumatic, inflammatory, neoplastic, metabolic, degenerative or iatrogenic factors.

Spinal stenosis has been defined as narrowing of the spinal canal, nerve root canals or intervertebral foramina. It may be local, segmental or generalized, and can be caused by bony or soft tissue narrowing (Arnoldi et al, 1976). The spinal cord, dorsal root ganglia and spinal nerve roots may be compromised by spinal stenosis.

Lumen of the spinal canal (Fig. 4.5)

The cross-sectional area of the spinal canal varies in shape and dimensions in the different regions of the spine. The canal is largest in the cervical spine and at the thoraco-lumbar junction. It becomes narrow between the 4th and 9th thoracic vertebrae, the narrowest point being at the 6th thoracic vertebra. The spinal column in this region is a critical vascular zone. Minimal reduction in the space will result in compression and ischaemia.

In the lumbar spine, the vertebral canal is flattened in the anteroposterior direction and wider laterally to accommodate the cauda equina.

The neural canals

The spinal nerves and dorsal root ganglia are vulnerable within the neural canal. The length of the canal varies in the different spinal regions.

Figure 4.5 The lumen of the spinal cord. (Adapted from Dommisse GF 1986 The blood supply of the spinal cord. In: Grieve GP, ed. *Modern Manual Therapy.* Churchill Livingstone, Edinburgh, pp. 37–52.)

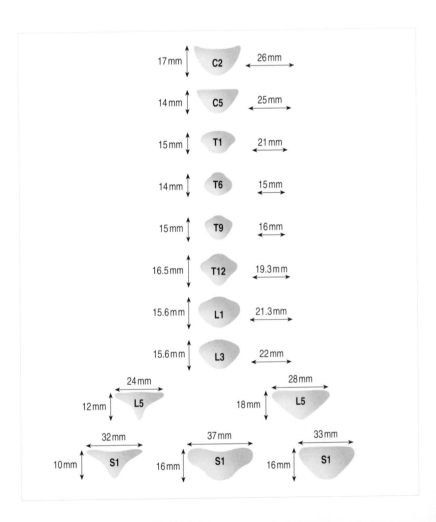

In the cervical spine the neural canals are 10–15 mm in length, in the thoracic region the canals are just small openings, and in the lumbar region the canals are 20–35 mm in length.

In the lumbar spine, the neural canals contain many veins and arteries, the dorsal root ganglia and the spinal nerves. The contents of the canal may be compressed by soft tissue (e.g. herniating disc) or bone (e.g. osteophytes). Compression of the neural structures will give rise to ischaemic pain, and permanent fibrotic changes will occur if the pressure is not relieved.

Arachnoiditis

The dura mater is a highly vascular structure. If it is damaged following an invasive procedure (e.g. surgery or myelogram), an inflammatory reaction takes place which results in permanent fibrotic changes. The spinal nerve sheaths are no longer patent; these changes are irreversible (Dommisse, 1986).

References

Arnoldi CC, Brodsky AE, Cauchoix J, et al (1976) Lumbar spinal stenosis. *Clinical Orthopaedics and Related Research* 115: 4.

Bakay L, Sweet WH (1953) Intra-arterial pressures in the neck and brain. *Journal of Neurosurgery* 10: 353–359.

Barker S, Kesson M, Ashmore J, et al (2000) Guidance for pre-manipulative testing of the cervical spine. *Manual Therapy* 5: 37–41.

Barton JW, Margolis MT (1975) Rotational obstruction of the vertebral artery at the atlanto-axial joint. *Neuroradiology* 9: 117.

Batson OV (1940) The function of the vertebral veins and their role in the spread of metastases. *Annals of Surgery* 112: 138.

Batson OV (1957) The vertebral vein system. Caldwell Lecture, 1956. *American Journal of Roentgenology* 78: 195.

Bogduk N (1986) Cervical causes of headaches and dizziness. In: Grieve GP (ed.) *Modern Manual Therapy*. Churchill Livingstone, Edinburgh, Ch. 27, pp. 289–302.

Bogduk N, Lambert G, Duckworth JW (1981) The anatomy and physiology of the vertebral nerve in relation to cervical migraine. *Cephalalgia* 1: 1.

Bolton PS, Stick PE, Lord RSA (1989) Failure of clinical tests to predict ischemia before neck manipulation. *Journal of Manipulative and Physiological Therapeutics* 12: 304–307.

Brown B St. J, Tatlow WFT (1963) Radiographic studies of the vertebral arteries in cadavers: effects of head position and traction of the head. *Radiology* 81: 80–88.

Crock HV, Goldwasser M (1984) Anatomic studies of the circulation in the region of the vertebral end plate in adult grey-hound dogs. *Spine* 9: 702.

Dommisse GF (1986) The blood supply of the spinal cord. In: Grieve GP (ed.) *Modern Manual Therapy*. Churchill Livingstone, Edinburgh, Ch 4, pp. 37–52.

Dommisse GF (1994) The blood supply of the spinal cord and the consequences of failure. In: Boyling JD,

Palastanga N (eds) *Grieve's Modern Manual Therapy,* 2nd edn. Churchill Livingstone, Edinburgh, pp. 3–20.

Dommisse GF, Grobler L (1976) Arteries and veins of the lumbar nerve roots and cauda equina. *Clinical Orthopaedics and Related Research* 115: 22.

Dvorak J, Orelli F (1985) How dangerous is manipulation of the cervical spine? *Manual Medicine* 2: 1–4.

Fast A, Zinicola DF, Marin EL (1987) Vertebral artery damage complicating cervical manipulation. *Spine* 12: 840.

Fisher CM (1967) Vertigo in cerebrovascular disease. *Archives of Otolaryngology* 85: 529.

Fisher CM, Karnes WE (1965) Local embolism. *Journal of Neuropathology and Experimental Neurology* 24: 174.

Gatterman MI (1982) Extreme caution advised. *Journal of Chiropractic* 19: 14.

Grant R (1988) Dizziness testing and manipulation of the cervical spine. In: Grant R (ed.) *Physical Therapy of the Cervical and Thoracic Spine*. Churchill Livingstone, Edinburgh, Ch. 7, pp. 111–124.

Hanus SH, Homer TD, Harter DH (1977) Vertebral artery occlusion complicating yoga exercises. *Archives of Neurology* 34: 574–575.

Hardesty WH, Whiteacre WB, Toole JF, et al (1963) Studies on vertebral blood flow in man. *Surgery, Gynaecology Obstetrics.* 116: 662.

Hardin CA, Poser CM (1963) Rotational obstruction of the vertebral artery due to redundancy and extraluminal cervical fascial bands. *Annals of Surgery* 158: 133.

Haynes MJ (1996) Doppler studies comparing the effects of cervical rotation and lateral flexion on vertebral artery flow. *Journal of Manipulative and Physiological Therapeutics* 19: 378–384.

Herlihy WF (1947) Revision if the venous system: the role of the vertebral veins. *Medical Journal of Australia* 22: 661–672.

Husni EA, Storer J (1967a) The syndrome of mechanical occlusion of the vertebral artery. *Journal of the American Medical Association* 196: 475.

Husni EA, Storer J (1967b) The syndrome of mechanical occlusion of the vertebral artery: further observations. *Angiology* 18: 106.

Husni EA, Bell HS, Storer J (1966) Mechanical occlusion of the vertebral artery: a new clinical concept. *Journal of the American Medical Association* 196: 475.

Kanshepolsky J, Danielson H, Flynn RE (1972) Vertebral artery insufficiency and cerebellar infarct due to manipulation of the neck. *Bulletin of the Los Angeles Neurological Society* 37: 62–66.

Kleynhans AM, Terrett AGJ (1985) The prevention of complications from spinal manipulative therapy. In: Glasgow EF, et al (eds) *Aspects of Manipulative Therapy*, 2nd edn. Churchill Livingstone, London, pp. 161–175.

Kreuger BR, Okazaki H (1980) Vertebral-basilar distribution infarction following chiropractic cervical manipulation. *Proceedings of the Staff Meetings of the Mayo Clinic* 55: 322.

Lewit K (1969) Vertebral artery insufficiency and the cervical spine. *British Journal of Geriatric Practice* 6: 37.

Neuworth E (1954) Neurologic complications of osteoarthritis of the cervical spine. *New York State Journal of Medicine* 54: 2583.

Palastanga N, Field D, Soames R (1989) *Anatomy and Human Movement: Structure and Function*. Heinemann Medical, Oxford.

Parke WW, Watanabe R (1985) The intrinsic vasculature of the lumbosacral spinal nerve roots. *Spine* 10: 508.

Parkin PJ, Wallis WE, Wilson JL (1978) Vertebral artery occlusion following manipulation of the neck. *New Zealand Medical Journal* 88: 441–443.

Pasztor E (1978) Decompression of the vertebral artery in cases of cervical spondylosis. *Surgical Neurology* 9: 371.

Power SR, Drislane TM, Nevin S (1961) Intermittent vertebral artery compression; a new syndrome. *Surgery* 49: 257.

Schmorl G, Junghanns H (1959) *The Human Spine in Health and Disease*. Grune and Stratton, New York.

Stewart DY (1962) Current concepts of 'Barre syndrome' or the 'posterior cervical sympathetic syndrome'. *Clinical Orthopaedics and Related Research* 24: 40.

Stopford JSB (1916) The arteries of the pons and medulla oblongata: part 1. *Journal of Anatomy* 50: 131.

Taitz C, Nathan H, Arensburg B (1978) Anatomical observations of the foramina transversaria. *Journal of Neurology, Neurosurgery and Psychiatry* 41: 170.

Tatlow WFT, Bammer HG (1957) Syndrome of vertebral artery compression. *Neurology* 7: 331–340.

Terrett AGJ (1987) Vascular accidents from cervical spine manipulation; report on 107 cases. *Journal of Australian Chiropractic Association* 17: 15–24.

Terrett AGJ (1998) Contraindications to cervical manipulation. In: Giles LGF, Singer KP (eds) *Clinical Anatomy and Management of Cervical Spine Pain*, Vol. 3. Butterworth Heinemann, Oxford, Ch. 12.

Terrett AGJ, Kleynhans AM (1992) Cerebrovascular complications of manipulation. In: Haldeman S (ed.) Principles and Practice of Chiropractic, 2nd edn. Appleton & Lange, Norwalk, CT, pp. 579–598.

Toole JF, Tucker SH (1960) Influence of head position on cerebral circulation. *Archives of Neurology* 2: 616 – 623.

Webb FWS, Hickman JA, Brew D St. J (1968) Death from vertebral artery thrombosis in rheumatoid arthritis. *British Medical Journal* 2: 537.

Yang PJ, Latack JT, Gabrielson TO, et al (1985) Rotational vertebral artery occlusion at C1-2. *American Journal of Neuroradiology* 6: 98–100.

Chapter 5

Normal movement

Normal movements between two adjacent vertebrae are relatively small, but the cumulative effect of these movements gives a considerable range to the vertebral column as a whole.

Numerous studies have attempted to measure intersegmental and regional spinal movement, but large variations in 'normal' movement have been recorded. Figures 5.1 and 5.2 show the estimated range and representative degrees of rotation around three axes based on a review of literature and the authors' analysis (White and Panjabi, 1978a). Many factors influence movement, and variations in range recorded reflect differences in the age, race, sex, numbers of subjects and also differences in experimental design such as various methods of measurement, lack of reliability and validity, and errors in measurement.

Studies of cadavers have provided valuable insight into intersegmental motion, but it is not known how closely these movements reflect in vivo movement at the motion segment. Functional interdependence of

Figure 5.1 Average ranges of segmental movement. These are *average* values. Wide variations occur according to age, body structure, pathology, etc. (see text).

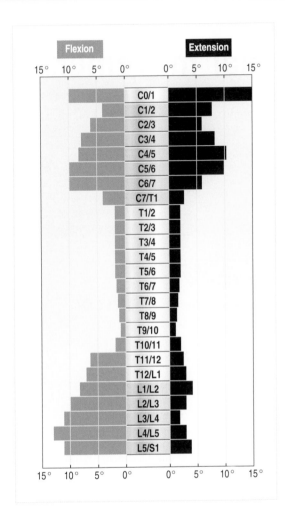

the bony and muscular elements of the spine was highlighted by Campbell and Parsons (1944). Inevitably, normal muscle tone and muscles acting in their functional capacity as prime movers, antagonists and fixators will affect spinal movement. Recent developments in non-invasive measurement techniques, the use of functional MRI scans and three-dimensional analysis are improving our understanding of normal movement.

Although it is useful clinically to have a working knowledge of relative spinal ranges, there is such disparity in mean ranges recorded that too much emphasis should not be placed on these values. The essence of a good spinal examination is to be able to observe movement abnormalities and relate these to the patient's signs and symptoms. A skilled clinician is able to relate the range and quality of movement to what might be expected from that subject when age, sex, race and body type are taken into account.

Figure 5.2   Average ranges of segmental movement (values given are to *one* side). These are *average* values. Wide variations occur according to age, body structure, pathology, etc. (see text).

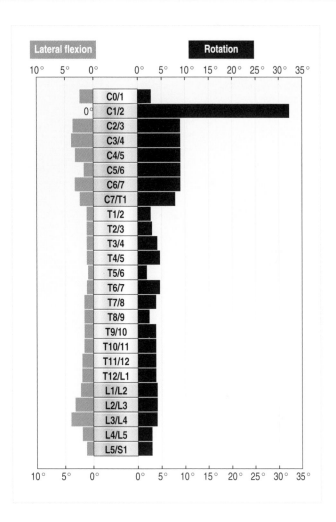

PLANES OF THE BODY AND AXES OF MOVEMENT (Fig. 5.3)

A three-dimensional coordinate system allows analysis and definition of any position or movement in space. There are three principal planes of the body. Each plane is perpendicular to the other two planes.

PLANES

- The *sagittal* or *median* plane is a vertical plane passing through the body, dividing it into right and left halves.
- The *frontal* or *coronal* plane is a vertical plane, which divides the body into anterior and posterior halves.
- The *horizontal* or *transverse* plane divides the body into upper and lower halves.

Figure 5.3 Planes of the body and axes of movement. AB, frontal plane; CD, sagittal plane; the circle represents the horizontal plane. X–X', vertical axis; Y–Y', frontal axis; Z–Z', sagittal axis.

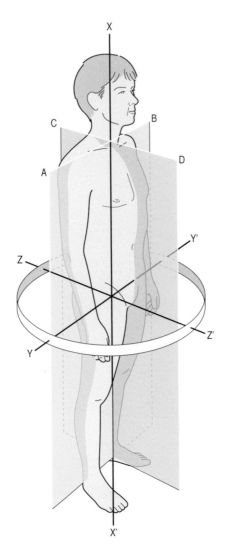

An external force acting on the spine can be resolved into component forces and movements acting along or about three axes. Each axis is perpendicular to the plane in which movement occurs.

AXES

- The *vertical* axis is perpendicular to the ground (X axis).
- The *frontal* axis passes horizontally from side to side (Y axis).
- The *sagittal* axis passes horizontally from front to back (Z axis).

The movement of a mass around an axis is described as *rotation*. The axis may be inside or outside the rotating body. A body is in rotation when all particles along some straight line within the body (or hypothetical extension of it) have a zero velocity to a fixed reference point. A body is in *translation* when all particles in the body at a given time have the same velocity relevant to some reference.

A *degree of freedom* is motion in which a rigid body has the possibility of translating forwards and backwards along a straight line or rotating back and forward in a clockwise and counterclockwise direction about a perpendicular axis (White and Panjabi, 1978a).

At a segmental level, the vertebral body can move in the sagittal, vertical and frontal planes, and it also rotates around the three same axes. Each vertebral body, therefore, has six degrees of movement and can move in six different ways:

1. Glide forwards and backwards in the sagittal plane (i.e. anterior and posterior translation)
2. Tilt forwards and backwards around a frontal axis (i.e. anterior and posterior sagittal rotation)
3. Glide laterally in the frontal plane (lateral translation)
4. Tilt laterally in the frontal plane around a sagittal axis, e.g. during lateral flexion
5. Distract and compress in the horizontal axis of the spine
6. Rotate in a horizontal plane around a vertical axis (axial rotation).

When a vertebral body moves, the axis or 'centre of rotation' of the body is different from one instant to the next. The point around which movement occurs is termed the *instantaneous axis of rotation*. It represents a mean axis around which coupled accessory movements occur during motion in a cardinal plane.

At one instant, motion of a rigid body in three-dimensional space can be analysed as a simple screw motion. This motion is a combination of rotation and translation about and along the same axis. The axis has the same direction as the resultant of the three rotations given sequentially about the X, Y and Z axes (Fig. 5.4). It describes movements among the three planes and is known as the *helical axis of motion*.

MOTION SEGMENTS (Fig. 5.5)

Between the skull and the sacrum there are 25 levels at which movement may occur. The terms *motion segment*, *mobile segment* or *articular triad* are used to describe an intervertebral disc and its articulations with the adjacent vertebral bodies above and below. The motion segment is the traditional unit of study in spinal kinematics.

A typical motion segment consists of:

- Symphyses between the intervertebral disc and the adjacent vertebral bodies, i.e. the interbody joints
- Articular processes of the apophyseal joints
- Uncovertebral joints (cervical spine only)
- Articulations of the ribs (thoracic spine only)

Figure 5.4 Degrees of motion of a vertebra. A motion segment has six degrees of freedom, producing three translations and three rotations. (From Giles LGF, Singer KP 2000 *Clinical Anatomy and Management of Thoracic Spine Pain*. Butterworth Heinemann, Oxford. Vol. 2, Fig. 4.1, p. 47.)

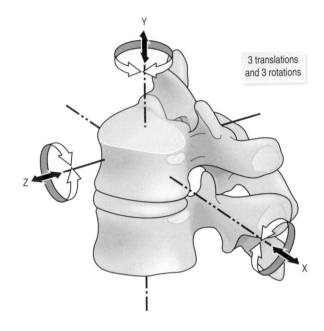

3 translations and 3 rotations

Figure 5.5 The motion segment – lumbar region.

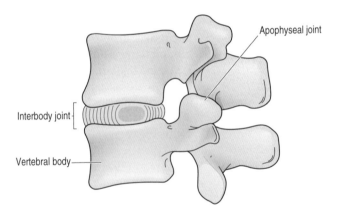

The factors that influence movement at a motion segment include the thickness of the intervertebral disc, the compliance of its fibrocartilage and the dimensions and shape of the adjacent vertebral end plates. A large range of movement occurs when the disc height is relatively great and the vertebral end plate horizontal dimensions relatively short (Taylor and Twomey, 1984; Fig. 5.6). Adolescent and young females have shorter vertebral end plates than males, while the disc height and stiffness is the same (see page 182). Hence, young women are likely to have a greater range of movement than males of a comparable age (Twomey and Taylor, 1987).

The shape and orientation of the articular facets, the ligaments and the muscles determine the direction of movement, guide the type of

Figure 5.6 The anterior vertebral elements (mobile segment). A, Vertebral end plate; b, Disc thickness. (From Twomey LL, Taylor JR 1986 Factors influencing ranges of movement in the lumbar spine. In: Grieve GP, ed. *Modern Manual Therapy of the Vertebral Column*. Churchill Livingstone, Edinburgh, Fig. 11.1, p. 139.)

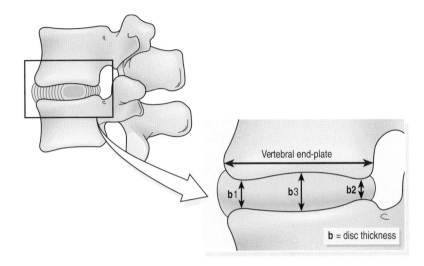

movement and govern the amount of movement possible at a motion segment. Movement ranges are restricted by ligament and muscle tension or bony apposition, and the structures limiting movement vary at different motion segments.

The orientation of the apophyseal joints varies in the different spinal regions. (For the direction of apophyseal joints, see Ch. 1.) The orientation of these joints does not exactly coincide with the plane of movement, and commonly two or more types of movement occur at the same time. Rotation or translation of a vertebral body about one axis is consistently associated with rotation or translation of the same vertebral body about another axis – this is known as *coupling*. For example, rotation of the spine is always accompanied by some degree of lateral flexion. Likewise, lateral flexion of the spine is accompanied by some degree of vertebral rotation (Stoddard, 1962).

Assessment of normal spinal movement must take into account the combination of movements that normally occur. It is inadequate and inaccurate to observe in isolation the physiological movements of flexion, extension, lateral flexion and rotation. Spinal physiological movements exhibit either coupled or 'tripled' movement, so in order to understand normal and abnormal movement patterns in relation to pathology, it is important that combinations of movement patterns are observed. It may be desirable to use a combination of movement patterns for treatment purposes.

Movement of an individual joint of a particular motion segment cannot occur in isolation. Treatment aimed at creating movement at a specific joint will inevitably affect the other joints in the articular triad.

During movement, subchondral bone and articular cartilage deform equally under pressure (Radin et al, 1970) and bone deformation contributes in a small proportion to vertebral movement. If the bony posterior elements are fused, there is still enough plasticity in the bone anterior to the pedicles to allow movement between the vertebral body and disc on vertical loading. A posterior spinal fusion will, therefore, stabilize an unstable segment, but it will not completely immobilize the segment.

REGIONAL CHARACTERISTICS OF NORMAL MOVEMENT

Movement in one direction may restrict or allow movement in another direction.

CERVICAL SPINE

Between C2 and C7, in neutral, in flexion or in extension, lateral flexion to one side makes rotation to the same side easier, e.g. lateral flexion of the neck to the right is accompanied by rotation to the right.

THORACIC SPINE

The thoracic spine has been less extensively investigated than the cervical and thoracic spine and some of the movement studies are based on three-dimensional mathematical models (Saumarez, 1986; Ben-Haim and Saidel, 1990). It is not known whether these studies give an accurate reflection of in vivo movement. Stoddard (1962) states that, below the 3rd thoracic vertebra, if the spine is in neutral or extension, lateral flexion to one side is accompanied by rotation to the same side. In a series of experiments on cadavers, White (1969) demonstrated that in the upper thoracic spine, during lateral flexion, the vertebral body rotated axially into the concavity of the lateral curve. In the middle and lower thoracic spine the same pattern predominated but was not as marked as in the upper thoracic spine. It was noted that in some cases the reverse coupling occurred as axial rotation of the vertebra was towards the convexity of the lateral curve.

Panjabi et al (1976) investigated the mechanical properties of the thoracic spine through an in vitro study. They found that rotation around the Y axis (axial rotation) was coupled with contralateral rotation around the Z axis (lateral bending) and contralateral translation along the X axis (see Fig. 5.4). This is inconsistent with clinical observation, as in the mid thoracic spine rotation around the Y axis has been found to be coupled with ipsilateral rotation around the Z axis and contralateral translation along the X axis (Lee, 1994). In the study by Panjabi et al (1976), the ribs and anterior elements of the thorax were removed 3 cm lateral to the costotransverse joints, so the effects of an intact functional costal unit on thoracic spine movements were not demonstrated and this may have influenced the coupled movements observed.

LUMBAR SPINE

In the upper four segments, axial rotation of the vertebra is normally accompanied by lateral flexion to the opposite side, and lateral flexion is accompanied by rotation to the opposite side.

Conversely, at the joints between the 5th lumbar vertebra and the sacrum, axial rotation of the vertebra is accompanied by lateral flexion to the same side, and lateral flexion of the joint is accompanied by rotation to the same side (Bogduk and Twomey, 1987).

If there is any degree of articular tropism (see pp. 55–56) at the lumbosacral junction, the coupling of movements will be affected accordingly.

GENERAL CHARACTERISTICS OF NORMAL MOVEMENT

When one physiological movement has occurred, it has the effect of reducing other additional movements, for instance:

1. In flexion, the amount of lateral flexion and rotation possible is reduced.

2. Extension reduces the amount of lateral flexion and rotation possible.

3. Lateral flexion restricts normal flexion and extension.

4. Rotation restricts normal flexion and extension.

These characteristics of normal movement are of particular relevance in patients presenting with a spinal deformity. For example, lateral flexion and rotation to the opposite side is reduced in a subject with a kyphoscoliosis. Similarly, flexion and extension is reduced in a patient who has a lateral deviation of the lumbar spine.

If treatment is aimed at gaining physiological range, it is essential that the patient be placed in a position that allows optimal gain in range. For example, if posteroanterior vertebral pressures are applied to the lumbar spinous processes with the aim of increasing lumbar extension, the treatment is less likely to be effective if the patient has been carelessly positioned so that the pelvis is shifted to one side and the spine is not straight.

Normal mobility of the spinal column varies considerably. It may be influenced by one or more of the following factors: age, sex, ligamentous laxity, congenital factors, and pathology.

AGE   There is a decline in spinal mobility of all ranges with increasing age. As hormonal differences reduce with increasing age, the sexual differentiations in vertebral shape, posture and spinal range of movement disappear, so that in old age lumbar movement in men and women is almost identical (Twomey and Taylor, 1987).

A large disc height is associated with increased movement, and the principal reason for decreased range of movement is increased disc stiffness. In old age, most discs increase in volume (Taylor and Twomey, 1981), becoming thicker centrally and convex at the disc–vertebra interface: so that the frequently given reason that thinning of the discs decreases movement is incorrect. Histological and biochemical changes within the disc increase disc stiffness by as much as 40%, and this is associated with a decrease in physiological range. Changes that affect disc stiffness include an increase in the number of collagen fibres and in the ratio of Type I to Type II collagen, a change in the proteoglycan ratios and a subsequent decrease in water content. 'Fatigue failure' of the collagen in older cartilage may also occur, but it is unclear whether the individual collagen fibres fatigue or the bonds between adjacent fibres break down (Stockwell, 1979). The ageing disc is less able to dissipate force and transmits loads along the vertebral column.

Thoracic and lumbar mobility increases between the ages of 15 and 24 (Moll and Wright, 1971). After 25, there is a general decrease in movement and it may eventually decline by as much as 50%. In a study performed on cadavers and living subjects, Twomey and Taylor (1987) found decreasing mobility in both the lumbar sagittal and horizontal planes after the age of 25.

SEX

There are conflicting views as to whether males or females have greater spinal mobility. Studies of a normal population of males and females showed that up to the age of 65 men had a greater total sagittal mobility, but after 65 years women had greater total sagittal mobility (Sturrock et al, 1973).

A greater range of movement occurs when there is a combination of relatively greater disc height and relatively shorter vertebral end plate horizontal dimensions. Disc heights are the same in young males and females, but in females the vertebral end plates are shorter. Therefore young females are more likely to have greater range of movement than young males.

In a study on cadavers, Twomey and Taylor (1987) found that adolescent and young females had between 13% and 26% more sagittal mobility than males of the same age. Both sexes had substantially the same sagittal movement in middle-aged and elderly groups. However, young adults measured in a live study did not show the sex differential in the total sagittal range that was demonstrated with the cadavers, suggesting that muscles play an important role in limiting the amount of movement possible.

LIGAMENTOUS LAXITY

A hypermobile joint is one whose range of movement exceeds that which is considered to be normal in an individual when age, sex and ethnic background are taken into consideration (Grahame, 1999). Ligamentous laxity causing hypermobility of a joint may be present as a single joint entity, it may affect just peripheral joints or just spinal joints, or it may be generalized. The true incidence of joint hypermobility in the adult population is not known, but it has been estimated to occur in up to 10% of individuals in Western populations, and the figure may be as high as 25% in certain ethnic groups.

Joint laxity is usually greatest at birth, decreases during childhood and continues to reduce during adolescence and adult life. The tightness or relative laxity of a ligament is an important element in governing the available joint range of an individual. Laxity of ligaments is determined by an individual's genetic make-up, and the genes that encode collagen, elastin and fibrillin are important in influencing joint flexibility.

Hypermobility may be inherited or acquired; joint mobility can be increased with training. Some groups such as ballet dancers and gymnasts with 'normal tissues' can increase range of movement through stretching and training programmes. It is probable that individuals who have joints of average flexibility have better protection from injury by their 'normal tissues', and those who have developed a hypermobile range from specific training enhance stability of their joints through good muscle strength and control. Although an increase in joint laxity is considered an advantage for some sports and activities, the generally weaker tissue of a hypermobile individual means that they are more susceptible to injury and instability (Grahame and Jenkins 1972). Hypermobile tissues are less resilient so that muscle tears and tendon–bone attachment lesions occur more readily.

The increased ligamentous laxity in hypermobility may result in the annular fibres of the intervertebral disc being subjected to greater torsional stress in rotation. In the cervical spine the increased flexibility can be such that the neural structures of the brachial plexus are placed on a considerable stretch at the end of range of the physiological movements of rotation and lateral flexion. Structures that help to restrain spinal movements include the facet joints, the interspinous ligaments and the discs themselves. In those with hypermobility the spine does not have the protection of 'normal tight tissues' and the discs are more vulnerable to the strains of daily life.

When treating an individual with generalized hypermobility, it is essential not to use forceful or sustained manipulative techniques at the end of the individual's physiological range of movement. This will help to ensure that the fragile hypermobile tissue is not subjected to trauma. Cervical manipulation is contraindicated in an individual with generalized hypermobility.

CONGENITAL FACTORS

Congenital anomalies, e.g. sacralization of the 5th lumbar vertebra or congenital fusion of adjacent vertebrae, will affect the range of motion available at the segment involved.

PATHOLOGY

Degenerative changes of the spine do not necessarily affect range of movement. However, pathology that alters the normal alignment of the apophyseal joints will inevitably affect the range and type of motion possible at the affected segment.

OTHER FACTORS

Other factors that influence spinal mobility include height, obesity, race and the level of general fitness of an individual. Spinal mobility can also vary with the time of day, and may be temporarily reduced after adopting a sustained posture such as working at a visual display unit. Individuals with degenerative joint changes in the spine frequently experience joint stiffness in the early morning that eases during the day.

SEGMENTAL MOVEMENT

Kinematics is the study of measuring and observing motion without taking into account the influences of force and mass. Kinetics is a study of the effects of mass and force on movements.

Radiographic studies have analysed normal motion of the cervical spine (Penning, 1978, 1992). Movements of the head and neck are described and observed clinically in the three main planes: flexion and extension in the sagittal plane; lateral bending to the left and right in the frontal plane; and rotation to the right and left in the transverse plane. Translatory motion also occurs, mainly in the sagittal plane. Movements of the head and neck result in movement occurring between the cervical vertebrae in a combination of rotations and translations about one or more axes simultaneously. Movements of the head bear no relation to the actual range of head and neck movement, and the total range of movement is the sum of neck and head movements. (Adams and Logue, 1971).

The upper and lower parts of the cervical spine can move independently of each other, so that in the sagittal plane independent sagittal rotation of the upper or lower cervical spine is possible.

The upper and lower sections of the cervical spine may also move in opposite directions, e.g. the upper cervical spine may be extended and the lower cervical spine flexed simultaneously. This particular combination of segmental postures is often seen clinically in those with poor posture and also those with degenerate necks.

The degree of upper cervical flexion that can be achieved is greater if the lower cervical spine is held in a relatively neutral position than when the whole of the cervical spine is flexed. There are several possible explanations for this difference in upper cervical range. In some individuals, when the neck is fully flexed, the chin approximates the sternum so that the occiput may be deflected into extension at the end of range (Dirheimer, 1977). It has been suggested that passive insufficiency of sternocleidomastoid is more likely to cause the upper cervical deflexion during neck flexion (Kapandji, 1974). *Passive insufficiency* of a muscle occurs when full range of movement at a joint is limited by the length of the muscle that crosses it. During upper and lower cervical flexion, the length of sternocleidomastoid may be insufficient to allow full cervical flexion, so that the upper cervical spine moves into slight extension. Insufficient length of the cervical ligaments may have a similar effect by passive coordination of the joints. *Passive coordination* occurs when at least one of the participating bones is not acted on directly by muscles or there is a physical link across two or more joints (Barnett et al, 1961). If there is insufficient length of the ligamentum nuchae to allow maximum separation of all the spinous processes, as well as separation of the occiput from the posterior tubercle of the atlas, then, in full flexion, the gap between the basiocciput and the posterior atlantal arch will appear less than in the neutral position (Worth, 1988).

Structures within the spinal canal may also affect cervical flexion. The spinal cord and meninges extend throughout the length of the cervical spine and are attached to the bodies of the 2nd and 3rd cervical vertebrae. Insufficient length or restricted movement of the spinal cord and meninges may prevent full flexion of both upper and lower cervical spine. The upper cervical spine may extend at the end of movement to relieve this stretch and it does so by the mechanism of passive coordination (Worth, 1988).

During movement of the cervical spine as a whole, individual segments may temporarily move in the opposite direction. This is termed *paradox motion* and Gutmann (1960) described an extension motion occurring at the atlanto-occipital joint at the end of full cervical flexion. Paradox motion does not occur during physiological nodding movements of the head, but only when the cervical spine is fully flexed. Paradox motion has also been shown to occur at C1/2, C6/7 and occasionally C5/6 (van Mameren et al, 1990).

The upper and lower cervical spines move in opposite directions during the chin-in/chin-out manoeuvre. In the chin-in position, the upper cervical spine translates posteriorly so that the upper cervical spine is in flexion and the lower part of the cervical spine is extended. In the chin-out position, the upper cervical spine translates anteriorly and is extended, while the lower part is flexed. The reversal of the direction of movement takes place anywhere between C2 and C5 and the range of motion available is reduced in the region of the reversal of movement (Penning, 1992).

Movements in the upper and lower cervical spines are described separately: the upper segment from C0 to C2, and the lower segment from the inferior facets of C2 to the superior facets of C7. Movements at the cervico-thoracic junction are also considered. Movements at C0/1 and C1/2 are described first, followed by the resulting combined movements at the upper cervical segment.

MOVEMENTS OF THE CRANIOVERTEBRAL JOINTS

Motion at the craniovertebral joints is complex because of the uniqueness of the joints involved. Asymmetry of the bony and ligamentous structures of this region is common, e.g. joint surfaces on the superior surface of the atlas may not lie in the same plane (Van Roy et al, 1997), or one of the occipital condyles may be smaller than the other (Dalseth, 1974). Asymmetry or anomalies are likely to affect the range of direction of movement possible.

There is marked variability in the reported ranges of movement at the craniovertebral joints. This may be in part due to differences in experimental method and measurement techniques, lack of reliability and validity studies, and errors of measurement (Worth and Selvik, 1986). Even with the use of modern imaging techniques and sophisticated technology, it is difficult to obtain accurate and reproducible measurements of motion at the craniovertebral joints (Porterfield and De Rosa, 1995).

Attempts by the physiotherapist to measure in vivo movements of the craniovertebral joints with any degree of accuracy are fraught with difficulty. Placing a goniometer on a subject's head will only measure head movement and not demonstrate three-dimensional vertebral movement. Orthodox radiographic views of the cervical spine are only two-dimensional, and the complexity of movement in this region can only be truly revealed by methods that allow three-dimensional analysis of movement. Three-dimensional techniques that have been used to measure cervical movement include photogrammetry, where three cameras record motion simultaneously (Snyder et al, 1975), and positioning five electrogoniometers that measure motion simultaneously in the three planes (Alund and Larsson, 1990). Many of the methods used in studies measure gross movements of the head and neck and do not reflect the intersegmental motion.

Movement at the occipito-atlantal and atlanto-axial joints occurs as rotation about any of the three axes at these joints with concomitant rotations about, and translations along, the other axes at these joints (Worth and Selvik, 1986).

CO/1: The two atlanto-occipital joints

Maximum movement at these joints occurs in the sagittal plane, i.e. flexion and extension, or nodding of the head. Penning (1978) gave the average range for this movement as 30°, Fielding (1957) reported 10° of flexion and 25° of extension, while Panjabi et al (1988) recorded 24° of motion.

During normal physiological flexion of the head and neck, there is a rocking or angular movement and a gliding movement of the occiput. The glide of the occiput is in the opposite direction to the angular movement so that, during flexion, the occipital condyles roll forwards and glide backwards on the superior facets of the atlas (Bogduk, 1988). Flexion is limited by the bony contact between the anterior rim of the foramen magnum and the superior surface of the dens (Fig. 5.7; Porterfield and DeRosa, 1995). On extension of the head and neck, the occiput rolls backwards and glides forwards on the facets of the atlas. Extension is limited by tension of the tectorial membrane and the anterior atlanto-occipital membranes (White and Panjabi, 1990).

Quantitative values for the amount of forward and backward translation accompanying flexion and extension vary. Worth and Selvik (1986) measured a mean of 5.46 mm ± 0.20 mm of translation, whereas Weisel and Rothman (1979) state that sagittal plane translation rarely exceeds 1 mm.

Some authors believe that rotation at the atlanto-occipital joints cannot occur because of the configuration of the bony surfaces (Last, 1972; White and Panjabi, 1978a), but some studies have shown that a very small

Figure 5.7 Flexion at CO/1. The rim of the foramen magnum checks flexion as the occiput impacts on the dens. (From Porterfield JA, De Rosa C 1995 *Mechanical Neck Pain. Perspectives in Functional Anatomy*. Saunders, Philadelphia, p. 99, Fig. 4.23.)

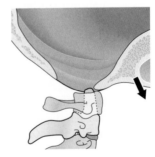

amount of rotation can occur. Values for atlanto-occipital rotation are given in Table 5.1. The shape of the articular surfaces and the alar ligaments restrict rotation.

A small amount of lateral displacement accompanies rotation at the atlanto-occipital joint (Penning and Wilmink, 1987). There is a lateral displacement of approximately 4 mm of the atlas relative to the foramen magnum in a direction contralateral to the direction of rotation of the head.

C1/2: The two lateral atlanto-axial joints and the median atlanto-axial joint

The greatest amount of spinal rotation occurs at C1/2 and movement occurs simultaneously at all three joints of the motion segment. Values for rotation to one side vary from 30° to 47° (Table 5.2).

Median atlanto–axial joint.   The dens is the centre of rotation at the C1/2 joint. The transverse ligament and atlas form an osseoligamentous ring which pivots around the odontoid during rotation.

Lateral atlanto–axial joints.   The surfaces of the articular facets are relatively flat to convex and this allows a large amount of rotary movement to occur. During rotation to the left, the right lateral mass of the atlas moves forwards on the superior facet of the axis and the left lateral mass moves backwards. Rotation to the left is limited by tension of those fibres of the left alar ligament which are attached to the dens in front of the axis of movement and those of the right alar ligament which attach to the dens behind the axis of movement.

It has been noted that rotary movement and returning to the neutral position alternately decrease and increase the vertical height of the atlas on the axis by 2–3 mm (Hohl and Baker, 1964). However, experiments by Worth and Selvik (1986) showed that there was no significant vertical approximation during axial rotation at C1/2.

Table 5.1   Range of movement at the atlanto-occipital joint

Source	Axial rotation
Worth and Selvik (1986)	3.43° ± 0.39°
Penning and Wilmink (1987)	2°
Dvorak et al (1987)	4.3°
White and Panjabi (1990)	0°

Table 5.2   Range of axial rotation in one direction at the atlanto-axial joints

Source	Axial rotation
Werne (1957)	47°
Dvorak et al (1987)	39°
Panjabi et al (1988)	39°
White and Panjabi (1990)	47°

Flexion/extension   The total range of flexion/extension is approximately 15°. The transverse ligament of the atlas maintains the dens in apposition to the anterior arch of the atlas. During flexion of the atlas on the axis, the joint surfaces make tilting movements and the dens is pushed posteriorly against the thick transverse ligament, limiting sagittal rotation. The osseoligamentous ring also limits anterior translation. The posterior arch of the atlas and spinous process of the axis separate during flexion and approximate on extension.

Lateral flexion   The downward oblique orientation of the lateral atlanto-axial joints restricts movement in the frontal plane. Kapandji (1974) and Werne (1957) state that lateral flexion does not occur at C1/2. Worth and Selvik (1986) measured a mean of 4.07° ± 2.01° of lateral flexion at the atlanto-axial joint and Fielding (1957) observed a small amount of lateral shift between the atlas and axis.

C0/1/2 combined movements   During rotation of the head, the occiput and atlas move as one unit on the axis, pivoting around the dens. As rotation of C1/2 reaches its limit, a small amount of rotation then occurs at C0/1; in addition the axis starts to rotate on C3 and the spinous process of C2 can be felt to move in the opposite direction to which the head is rotated. During normal movement, when the head is rotated to the left, the spinous process of C2 moves to the right. Sliding movements of 20 mm or more occur at the atlanto-axial joints during rotation (Lewit et al, 1964).

Rotation of the head to the left is accompanied by occiput to C2 rotation to the left; by occiput to C2 lateral bending to the right; and by lateral sliding of the head upon the atlas to the left (Giles and Singer, 1998). During rotation the head slides in the direction of the rotation.

On *lateral bending*, the head always slides laterally upon the atlas to the opposite side of the lateral bending, so that on lateral bending to the left, the occipital condyles glide a small amount to the right. Lateral bending is also accompanied by occiput to C2 rotation to the opposite direction. Therefore, when the head bends laterally to the left, it is accompanied by lateral bending of occiput to C2 to the left, rotation of occiput to C2 rotation to the right, and gliding of the head to the right.

The relationship between the atlas and axis alters during lateral bending. Lateral bending of the head and neck up to 15° produces rotation of the axis (but not head rotation). Beyond 15° of lateral bending, more rotation occurs at the atlanto-axial joints and there is greater lateral displacement of the articular margin of the inferior facet on the lateral mass of the atlas as compared with the corresponding articular margin of the superior facet of the axis (Hohl and Baker, 1964).

C2–6   In the lower cervical spine, movement at a motion segment occurs simultaneously in the two lateral apophyseal joints, the interbody joints and the uncovertebral joints. C4/5 and C5/6 are the most mobile and, therefore, particularly susceptible to functional stress. Consequently, degenerative changes at these levels are common.

The apophyseal joints of C2–6 lack inner stability due to their parallel orientation and they rely on the intervertebral disc and ligamentum flavum for stability. The apophyseal joints perform sliding movements. The location of the centre of motion from C2 to T1 bears no relationship to the slope of the articular facets; instead the location of the centre of motion is related to differences in the height of the articular processes (Penning, 1968a; Nowitzke et al, 1994). The type of movement pattern occurring at the intervertebral disc can vary and it is influenced by the location of the centre of motion. At the C2/3 intervertebral disc a sliding type of motion occurs, whereas at the C7/T1 disc it is a more tilting type of motion (Penning, 1988).

Flexion and *extension* occur in the sagittal plane. During flexion at a motion segment, the upper vertebral body tilts and simultaneously slides anteriorly on the one beneath. The centre of rotation around which the movement occurs lies within the subjacent vertebral body (Penning, 1968b). The total amount of translation in the sagittal plane is approximately 3.5 mm. There is slightly more anterior translation (1.9 mm) than posterior translation (1.6 mm) (Panjabi et al, 1986). The plane of the facets is a primary restraint to the anterior shear that occurs in cervical flexion. The shearing effect is particularly pronounced in a child's neck.

On flexion, the inferior articular facet of the superior facet slides upwards and anteriorly on the vertebra below and the interspace is opened posteriorly. The uncinate processes that extend upwards from the superior vertebral body margin assist in guiding motion in the sagittal plane. The intervertebral space is compressed anteriorly and a tensile stress is imparted to the posterior annular fibres as they are stretched. Flexion is limited by tension in the posterior ligamentous structures.

Cervical discs undergo more distortion during movements in the sagittal plane than discs in other spinal regions (Grieve, 1988). A lateral radiographic view of a normal cervical spine in full flexion shows that the line of the anterior vertebral body margins is broken in a series of steps. This is reversed when the neck is viewed in extension. If the interspinous spaces are palpated during sagittal movement, it can be felt that the spinous processes move apart in flexion and come closer in extension.

During extension, the upper vertebral body tilts and slides posteriorly. The intervertebral space is compressed posteriorly and the anterior annular fibres are stretched. The inferior facet of the superior vertebra slides downwards and posteriorly on the superior facet and tilts posteriorly, opening the interspace of the joints anteriorly. Extension causes a slight reduction in the sagittal diameter of the vertebral canal (Rauschning, 1991) and normally a minor retrolisthesis occurs due to the posterior translation.

Extension is limited by tension in the anterior longitudinal ligament, by the bony impact of the superior articular process of the lower vertebra on the lamina of the upper vertebra, and by ligamentous bulk from the posterior arches.

Rotation and *lateral flexion* are coupled motions and this is probably due to the combined mechanics of both the apophyseal joints and the uncovertebral joints. The uncinate processes that project from the superior vertebral body have a rounded concave shape. The inner aspect of the uncinate process resembles an arc of a circle around which the superior vertebra of a motion segment can pivot (Penning and Wilmink, 1987). In a study of C2–T1 in 28 autopsy specimens, Lysell (1969) found that in average full rotation of 45° there was a coupled motion of 24° lateral bending to the same side. Full lateral bending C2–T1 of 49° was coupled with 28° rotation to the same side. The amount of lateral flexion that is combined with rotation at each level is not uniform. The plane of the facets changes, and caudally the cervical facets have a more horizontal inclination which allows more rotation. When the facets lie more in the frontal plane, rotation becomes more limited. The facets of C7 have a more frontal plane orientation, which reduces the amount of rotation possible (Fig. 5.8).

Rotation to the right is coupled with lateral flexion to the same side and sometimes slight extension. The right inferior articular facet of the vertebra above glides inferiorly, posteriorly and translates medially on the superior articular facet of the vertebra below, falling inside its margins; the left inferior facet of the vertebra above glides superiorly, anteriorly and translates laterally outside the margin of the opposing facet of the vertebra below (Fig. 5.9). The axis of rotation lies in the midline at the anterior part of the vertebral body. When the neck is rotated to the right, the right side of the spine is approximated while the left side becomes longer.

During lateral flexion, the facets on the concave side glide backwards, thereby inducing rotation to the same side. Therefore, lateral flexion is normally accompanied by rotation to the same side (Fig. 5.10). During this movement, the dimensions of the intervertebral foramina on the ipsilateral side are reduced (Fig. 5.11), potentially compromising the foraminal contents.

Figure 5.8   Plane of cervical apophyseal joints. Note how a more horizontal plane of the facet is conducive to rotation and a more frontal orientation precludes rotation. (From Porterfield JA, De Rosa C 1995 *Mechanical Neck Pain. Perspectives in Functional Anatomy.* Saunders, Philadelphia, p. 93, Fig. 4.14.)

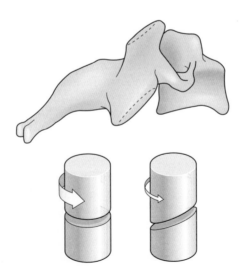

Figure 5.9   Rotation to the right coupled with lateral flexion in mid and lower cervical region.

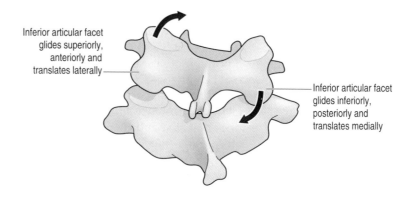

Inferior articular facet glides superiorly, anteriorly and translates laterally

Inferior articular facet glides inferiorly, posteriorly and translates medially

Figure 5.10   Combined movement in the lower cervical spine. A, Neutral. B, Lateral flexion to the right combined with rotation of vertebral bodies to the right (and spinous processes to the left).

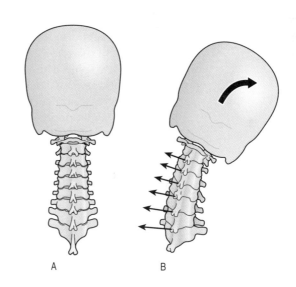

A

B

Figure 5.11   Reduction in dimensions of intervertebral foramen with movement. A, Neutral. B, Lateral flexion to the left and rotation to the left.

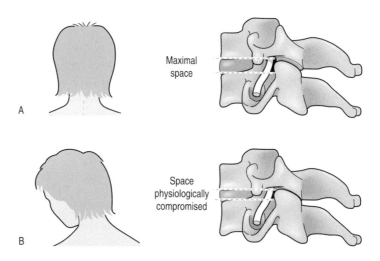

A

Maximal space

B

Space physiologically compromised

Compensatory movements in the cervical spine

Pure rotation of the head can only be achieved by intricate compensatory movements which eliminate the coupled movements that normally occur. Jirout (1971) examined 768 radiographic films taken of the neck in a position of lateral bending. He observed that in 237 examples the lateral bending was accompanied by flexion, in 118 it was combined with extension, and in 413 there was no added forward or backward tilt. The lack of consistency in these findings suggests that a normal stereotype does not exist and it follows that any manipulation philosophy based on 'normal' movement patterns derived 'logically' from the plane of the facets may be fallacious (Grieve, 1988). It is therefore essential that clinical assessment of individual movements takes precedence over biomechanical theories and theories of treatment techniques.

CERVICO-THORACIC JUNCTION C6–T2

There has been little evaluation of normal movement at the cervico-thoracic junction. There is a gradual change from the obliquely orientated facets in the cervical spine to the more vertically orientated facets in the thoracic spine. The end plates of C6 and C7 are significantly larger than those of the more superior cervical vertebra and there is an increase in the transverse dimensions of the cervical vertebral bodies and the superior articular facets from C3 to T1 (Milne, 1991). The uncinate processes are well developed between C3 and C6 and are less developed, but still evident, down to T2 or T3. It is therefore considered that the upper boundary of the cervico-thoracic junction is probably C6. The upper thoracic vertebrae (T1–4) have a narrow spinal canal and the dimensions of the end plates are smaller: Panjabi et al (1991) state that the lower boundary of this transitional area is T4. These changes in shape and dimensions affect the range and direction of motion.

Motion at each segment at the cervico-thoracic junction reduces caudally, but not in a graduated manner. The amount of flexion and extension decreases, although it is not as restricted as in the lower thoracic spine.

At the cervico-thoracic junction, the mobile cervical spine is adjacent to the relatively stiff thoracic spine, and this area is a common source of symptoms. A motion segment adjacent to a stiff segment is particularly susceptible to the stresses of movement of the cervical spine; these stresses are accentuated by the transmission of the weight of the head (the approximate weight of the head is 5 kg).

When degenerative changes occur at the cervico-thoracic junction, the spinous processes of C7 and T1 often become very prominent and they are termed a 'bison's hump'. The paravertebral soft tissues become tight and thickened and may be particularly tender to palpation. Movement abnormalities occur with these changes and all ranges quickly diminish. In addition, the lower cervical spine can become fixed in a flexed position, so consequently the upper cervical spine is extended to compensate and allow a normal visual field.

T3–10

The thoracic spine is the least mobile area of the spine. Protection of the viscera and internal organs is of prime importance and the thoracic spine and rib cage provide the necessary protection and stability at the expense of mobility. Reduced mobility is attributed to several factors: thin discs, facet planes, ligamentum flavum, attachments of the rib cage and sternum, configuration and proximity of the spinous processes, and an increased moment of inertia which stiffens the spine when rotatory forces are sustained. All movements are decreased in the thoracic spine, although rotation the least so.

Panjabi et al (1976) investigated the motions that occur in the thoracic spine with an in vitro study using specimens in the age range from 19 to 59 years. The ribs were removed 3 cm from the costotransverse joint so that although the functional spinal unit remained intact, the anterior chest was removed. The removal of the functional chest unit may have influenced the motion recorded at the motion segment. The joints studied at the motion segment included the anterior interbody joint, the posterior zygapophyseal joints, and the costotransverse and costovertebral joints. Panjabi et al (1976) showed that coupling patterns occur in all six degrees of freedom in the thoracic segments (see Fig. 5.4). In addition to the physiological movements of flexion, extension, lateral bending and axial rotation, the ribs are constantly moving simultaneously during inspiration and expiration.

In an experimental model, Panjabi et al (1976) found that during flexion there was anterior sagittal rotation around the X axis coupled with slight anterior translation along the Z axis and very slight distraction. When anterior translation was induced, anterior sagittal rotation around the X axis and slight compression occurred (see Fig. 5.4). During flexion, the interspace between two vertebrae opens out posteriorly. The inferior facets of the apophyseal joints of the superior vertebra slide superiorly. This movement is accompanied by only a small amount of forward translation of the superior vertebra, as the almost vertical disposition of the superior articular facets prohibits forward translation in the thoracic spine. The heads of the ribs are closely connected to the vertebral bodies by the radiate and interarticular ligaments. The effect of spinal movements on the ribs has not been studied, but Lee (1994) proposes that three movement patterns of the ribs can be observed clinically and are dependent on the relative flexibility between the spinal column and rib cage.

Before puberty, the superior costovertebral joint has not completely developed and the thoracic spine and chest is therefore more mobile. Based on clinical observations, Lee (1994) proposes that, during flexion in the young mobile thorax, the anterior translation of the vertebral body pulls the superior aspect of the head of the rib forward at the costovertebral joint, inducing an anterior rotation of the rib. As the rib rotates along a paraconal axis along the line of the neck of the rib, the anterior end of the rib moves inferiorly and the posterior aspect of the rib travels superiorly (Fig. 5.12). The anterior rotation of the neck of the rib results in a superior glide of the tubercle at the costotransverse joint. The facet on the transverse process is concave and that of the rib is convex so that the superior glide of the tubercle results in anterior rotation of the neck of the rib (Lee, 1993).

Figure 5.12 Flexion. (From Lee D 1994 Biomechanics of the thorax. In: Grant R, ed. *Physical Therapy of the Cervical and Thoracic Spine*, 2nd edn. Churchill Livingstone, Edinburgh, p. 51, Fig. 3.3, with permission.)

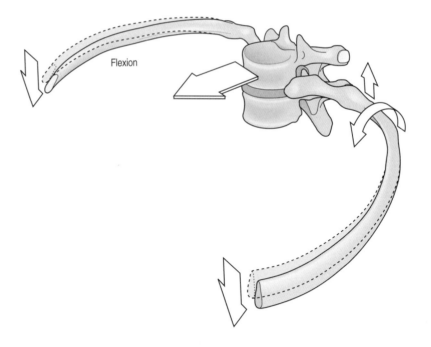

Flexion

In the skeletally mature, there is less flexibility of the spinal unit and the rib cage. During trunk flexion, Lee (1993) suggests that in the skeletally mature the same movement pattern of the ribs occurs initially until the amount of rib movement is exhausted. Once movement of the rib cage has ceased, the thoracic vertebrae continue to move on the stationary ribs. At the costotransverse joint, the concave facet on the transverse process travels superiorly relative to the tubercle of the rib so that there is a relative *inferior* glide of the tubercle of the rib at the costotransverse joint. When relative flexibility of the spinal column and rib cage is the same there is no apparent movement between the thoracic vertebrae and the ribs.

Flexion is limited by the posterior ligamentous structures and the posterior half of the intervertebral disc. In some individuals, anterior rib overcrowding is an important limiting factor (Grieve, 1986). The costovertebral joints are essential in maintaining stability during anterior translation of the thoracic vertebrae (Panjabi et al, 1981).

The location of the instantaneous axis of rotation is difficult to measure and in the thoracic spine there is a large scatter in its reported position. This may be partly due to errors in measurement, but it may also reflect that the location of the instantaneous axis of rotation is variable (Giles and Singer, 2000). White and Panjabi (1978a) described the location of the instantaneous axis of rotation during flexion as being just anterior to and a little above the centre of the subjacent vertebral body.

The total sagittal range of movement in the thoracic spine is relatively small. The thoracic spine contributes 25% of total spinal flexion and extension (Loebl, 1967). Between T3 and T6 there is the least amount of sagittal movement. Measurement of movement in the sagittal plane has shown that the median flexion/extension range between T1 and T6 is 4°, between T7 and T10 it is 6° and between T11 and L1 it is 9–12° (White and Panjabi, 1978b). There is greater flexion than extension in the sagittal plane and extension accounts for 30–42% of total sagittal movement.

In the experimental model, Panjabi et al (1976) found that during extension, posterior sagittal rotation occurred around the X axis and was coupled with posterior translation along the Z axis and slight distraction. When backward translation was induced along the Z axis it was accompanied by posterior sagittal rotation around the X axis and slight compression (see Fig. 5.4).

During extension, the inferior facets of the superior vertebra descend on the superior facets of the vertebra below. The thoracic vertebra tilts posteriorly and there is a small amount of posterior translation. These movements are accompanied by slight distraction (Panjabi et al, 1976). Posteriorly, the vertebrae are approximated and the posterior annulus and posterior longitudinal ligament are compressed. If the interspinous space is palpated, the spinous processes can be felt to move closer together during extension. A tensile stress is placed on the anterior part of the disc and the anterior longitudinal ligament. During extension, the instantaneous axis of rotation is just anterior to and a little below the centre of the vertebra above (White and Panjabi, 1978b).

Movement of the ribs probably accompanies extension at a motion segment. Lee (1994) proposes that the pattern of movement of the ribs during extension may depend upon whether the individual is skeletally mature. In the young mobile thorax it is suggested that the backward rotation and posterior translation of the vertebra pushes the superior aspect of the head of the rib backwards at the costotransverse joint. This induces rotation of the rib about a paraconal axis, resulting in the anterior end of the rib moving superiorly and the posterior end travelling inferiorly. As the rib rotates posteriorly it creates an inferior glide of the rib tubercle at the costotransverse joint (Fig. 5.13).

Lee (1994) suggests that in the skeletally mature, the same pattern of movement is initiated and the rib travels inferiorly until rib cage movement has been exhausted. At that point, the vertebrae continue to move on stationary ribs so that the facet on the transverse process travels inferiorly relative to the ribs. This causes a relative superior glide of the tubercle of the rib at the costotransverse joint.

Extension is limited by the ligaments anterior to and including the posterior longitudinal ligament. Bony impact of the inferior articular processes on the lamina below may also limit movement. As the bony points approximate further, backward rotation is limited by the articular capsule and the anterior structures (Valencia, 1988). In some individuals extension may be restricted, particularly in the upper thoracic spine, by soft tissue contracture of the intercostals, pectoral musculature and clavipectoral fascia (Grieve, 1988).

As in other regions of the spine, axial rotation is coupled with lateral bending and vice versa. Analysis of the kinematic behaviour of autopsy specimens of the thoracic spine suggests that the upper and lower parts behave differently from the middle (White, 1969).

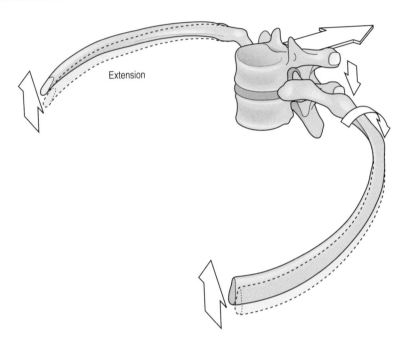

Figure 5.13 Extension. (From Lee D 1994 Biomechanics of the thorax. In: Grant R, ed. *Physical Therapy of the Cervical and Thoracic Spine*, 2nd edn. Churchill Livingstone, Edinburgh, p. 54, Fig. 3.6, with permission.)

Extension

In the upper thoracic spine the direction of coupling is such that the axial rotation of the vertebral body is into the concavity of the lateral curve, i.e. lateral bending to one side is coupled with axial rotation to the same side. White noted that this pattern existed in the middle and lower thoracic spine, but it was not as marked or consistent. In some cases, the middle region showed the reverse behaviour, so that lateral bending was coupled with axial rotation to the opposite side. These experiments were carried out with the ribs and muscle mass dissected away and it is, therefore, unclear as to how accurately these findings truly represent in vivo motion. Panjabi et al (1976) found that axial rotation was coupled with lateral bending to the opposite side and contralateral translation. Lee (1994) states that this is not consistent with clinical observation and that axial rotation in the mid-thoracic spine is linked with lateral bending to the same side and that it may be that the thorax must be intact and stable to reproduce in vivo coupling of motion.

Panjabi et al (1976) found that during side bending (lateral flexion of the trunk), rotation around the Z axis was coupled with contralateral rotation around the Y axis and ipsilateral translation along the X axis (see Fig. 5.4). Translation along the X axis was coupled with ipsilateral rotation (side bending) around the Z axis and contralateral rotation around the Y axis.

During lateral bending to the left, the inferior facets of the superior vertebra on the right slide superiorly and translate fractionally forward, while those on the left slide inferiorly and translate backwards, thereby creating a small amount of rotation. In addition, a small amount of lateral translation occurs. Lee (1994) proposes that in lateral bending, the transverse processes of the thoracic vertebrae move relative to the tubercle of the ribs. In right lateral bending, the ribs on the right approximate and those on the left separate. In both the young and skeletally mature, when laterally bending the trunk, the ribs stop moving before the thoracic vertebra, which continues to glide on stationary ribs. In right lateral bending the transverse process on the right glides inferiorly in relation to the right rib so that the tubercle on the right rib is in a relative superior position (Fig. 5.14). The tubercle of the left rib glides in an inferior position relative to the transverse process. The superior glide of the right rib causes an anterior rotation of the rib and the inferior glide of the left rib causes a posterior rotation of the rib (Lee, 1994). Lateral bending is limited by the impact of the articular processes on the side of the movement, the opposite ligamenta flava, outer annular fibres, intertransverse ligaments and antagonistic muscles. Rib overcrowding on the concave side is also a limiting factor. On the convex side, the intercostal spaces widen when the thorax is elevated, and the thoracic cage is enlarged; on the concave side, the opposite occurs.

At each level, the median range of lateral bending is 6° at the segments between T1 and 10, while in the lower two segments the median range is 7–9°.

Rotation is the greatest movement found in this region. Panjabi et al (1976) found that in the experimental model with the anterior chest unit removed, rotation around the Y axis was coupled with contralateral rotation around the Z axis and contralateral translation along the X axis (see Fig. 5.4). Lee (1993) proposes that rotation of the thoracic vertebral body induces movement of the ribs at the motion segment. During rotation to the right, the superior vertebra rotates to the right and translates to the left (Fig. 5.15). As the vertebra rotates to the right, the head of the right rib is pushed posteriorly, inducing posterior rotation of the neck of the right rib. The head of the left rib is brought forward at the costotransverse joint, inducing anterior rotation of the neck of the left rib. The vertebra translates laterally to the left, pushing the left rib posterolaterally along the line of the neck of the rib and causes posterolateral translation of the rib at the

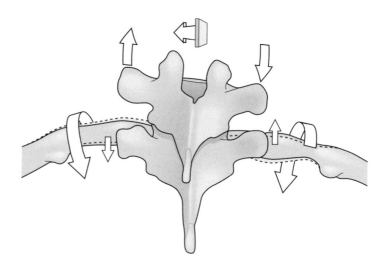

Figure 5.14   Lateral flexion of a thoracic motion segment to the right. Superior glide of the right rib induces anterior rotation of the same. (From Lee D 1994 Biomechanics of the thorax. In: Grant R, ed. *Physical Therapy of the Cervical and Thoracic Spine*, 2nd edn. Churchill Livingstone, Edinburgh, p. 57, Fig. 3.9, with permission.)

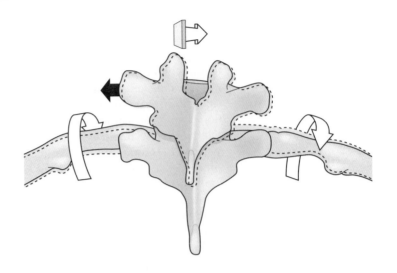

Figure 5.15   Rotation of a thoracic motion segment to the right. Translation of the superior thoracic vertebra to the left. (From Lee D 1994 Biomechanics of the thorax. In: Grant R, ed. *Physical Therapy of the Cervical and Thoracic Spine*, 2nd edn. Churchill Livingstone, Edinburgh, p. 61, Fig. 3.14, with permission.)

left costotransverse joint. The right rib is pulled anteromedially along the line of the neck of the rib and causes anteromedial translation of the rib at the right costotransverse joint (Lee, 1993).

When the vertebra has exhausted horizontal translation, the costotransverse and costovertebral ligaments are taut and the superior vertebra tilts to the same side to which the vertebral body is rotated, so that lateral bending occurs with rotation. Hence, in the mid-thoracic spine, rotation to the right can occur with side bending to the right.

The articular facets of the apophyseal joints slide relative to each other and the disc is twisted; only minimal shearing occurs here. Further rotation is prevented by the attachment of the ribs, which, in turn, are limited by their attachments to the sternum. The ribs, especially the cartilages, are distorted. The mean range of axial rotation at each segment is 8–9° in the upper segments and it reduces to 2° in the lowest three segments.

MOVEMENTS OF THE RIB CAGE IN RESPIRATION

The diaphragm is the main muscle of inspiration. It forms a musculotendinous dome, concave towards the abdomen, the central part being tendinous and the peripheral part muscular.

During inspiration, the lowest ribs are fixed and, as the muscular fibres contract, the central tendon is at first drawn downwards, pressing on the abdominal viscera and increasing the vertical diameter of the thorax. The extensibility of the abdominal wall allows this descent to a small extent, but the abdominal organs quickly limit this movement. The central tendon then becomes the fixed point for the action of the diaphragm, which then elevates the lower ribs. Elevation of the vertebrochondral ribs results in an outward and backward movement to produce an increase in the transverse diameter only. The anterior ends of the vertebrosternal ribs are pushed forwards and upwards, elevating the sternum and upper ribs, and increasing the anteroposterior dimension of the thorax. At the same time, these ribs are everted, thus increasing the transverse diameter.

Movements of the ribs at the costovertebral, costotransverse and sternocostal joints

Each rib has its own range and variety of movements. It can be seen as a lever, its fulcrum being just outside the costotransverse joint. Hence, if the shaft of the rib is elevated, the neck is depressed, and vice versa. The lever arm of the shaft of the rib is much longer than that at the vertebral end, so small movements of the latter result in much greater movements at the anterior end. In general, the individual rib shafts are highly flexible, but together they contribute to the stiffness of the thorax (Schultz et al, 1974).

When a rib moves, it does so at the costovertebral, costotransverse and sternocostal joints. The costovertebral and costotransverse joints form a joint couple mechanically linked. The axis of movement, running through the centre of each joint, acts as a swivel for the rib. The direction of the axis varies in the upper and lower ribs, thus affecting the direction of movement of the ribs (Fig. 5.16). For the lower ribs, the axis lies more or less anteroposteriorly, whereas in the upper ribs it is more in a medial/lateral direction. Therefore, elevation of the lower ribs increases

Figure 5.16   Axes of movement (X–X' and Y–Y') of the ribs: A, Vertebrosternal ribs. B, Vertebrochondral ribs.

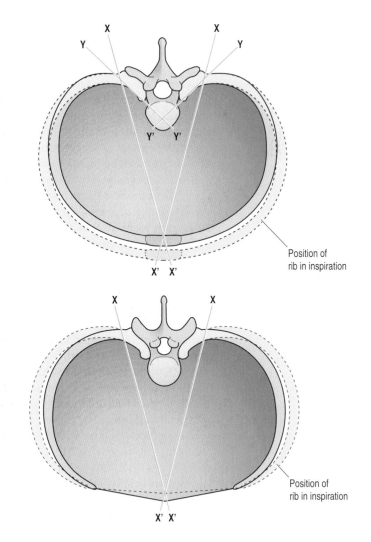

Position of rib in inspiration

Position of rib in inspiration

the transverse diameter of the lower thorax, and elevation of the upper ribs the anteroposterior diameter of the upper thorax. In the mid thorax, the axis lies between the above two axes at an angle of 45° to the sagittal plane. Therefore, on elevation of these ribs, both diameters are increased. The shortest, higher ribs are stiffer than the longer, lower ribs. The orientation and shape of the articular surfaces varies at every rib and thus influences direction of movement.

The 1st and 2nd ribs take little part in quiet respiration, but are more involved in forced respiration. Although only relatively small amplitudes of motion occur at these levels, they are often affected by degenerative changes at the cervicothoracic junction and are frequently a source of symptoms, in particular, unilateral suprascapular pain which may radiate to the shoulder.

As the articulating surfaces on the tubercles of the upper six ribs are convex from above downwards and the corresponding surfaces on the transverse processes are concave, elevation and depression of the ribs results in rotation of the rib neck about this axis. Elevation of the rib results in rotation upwards of the front of the neck of the rib, and depression results in rotation downwards. There is only very slight upward and downward movement of the neck of the rib itself.

The articulating surfaces of the 7th–10th tubercles of the ribs are flattened and face downwards, medially and backwards. Corresponding articular surfaces are on the upper aspects of the transverse processes of the vertebrae. Movement of these ribs involves upward, backward and medial gliding of the rib tubercle during inspiration and downward, forward and lateral movement on expiration. The whole neck of the rib undergoes the same movement, and it is accompanied by a small degree of rotation.

Movement occurs simultaneously at the sternocostal joints. The anterior ends of the ribs lie on a lower plane than the posterior, so that when the rib shaft is elevated, the anterior extremity is thrust forwards, taking the sternum with it. A gliding movement occurs at the sternocostal joints.

The 11th and 12th ribs are free at their anterior ends and do not have demifacets, intra-articular ligaments and costotransverse joints. Small movements can occur in all directions, but during respiration these ribs are depressed and fixed by quadratus lumborum, providing a fixed base for the action of the diaphragm.

The manubriosternal joint becomes ankylosed in 10% of people in the fourth decade and, later in life, the joints of the costal cartilages also ankylose, inevitably affecting the range of movement available for respiration (Grieve, 1986). It has been shown that although selective restriction of rib movement decreases the tidal volume of the restricted portion, it is associated with increased expansion of the non-restricted areas (Di Marco and Kelsen, 1981). Therefore, respiratory exchange may not be affected by localized rib lesions or corsets.

THORACO–LUMBAR JUNCTION

Movements in the sagittal plane progressively begin to increase in range caudally as the discs increase in height and the movements become less restricted by the ribs. The thoraco-lumbar junction is a transitional zone between T10 and L1. At this level the zygapophyseal joint orientation changes from the coronal plane in the thoracic spine to the sagittal plane in the lumbar spine. In an evaluation of 600 CT scans and 75 cadaveric specimens, Singer (1989) found that in 70% there was a progressive change in the orientation of the facets from T10/11 to T12/L1. Zygapophyseal joint tropism occurs frequently at the thoraco-lumbar joint (Singer, 1989). A 'mortice' effect has been described at the thoraco-lumbar junction (Davis, 1955). This is apparent when the spine is in full extension: there is a bone-to-bone block and no movement other than flexion is possible. It is important to remember when mobilizing or manipulating the spine at this level that, when it is in extension, there is no rotation or lateral flexion.

LUMBAR SPINE

The lumbar spine has its greatest range of movement in forward bending. In forward flexion, the motion segment of a healthy individual will be flexed approximately 8° at L1/2 and 11° at L4/5 and L5/S1 (Adams and Hutton, 1982; Pearcy et al, 1984). Flexion usually results in a partial or general eradication of the lumbar lordosis. When the lumbar spine is in a fully flexed position, the bony alignment is straight, although in hypermobile subjects or those under the age of 30 (Allbrook, 1957) the lumbar spine might have a slight anterior concavity. Reversal of the curve occurs mainly above the L3 vertebra. There may be some reversal at the L4/5 segment, but not at the L5/S1 level (Pearcy et al, 1984).

The largest amount of intersegmental flexion occurs at the L4/5 level, and the L5/S1 level has the greatest amount of individual variability (Adams, 1994).

Flexion of the lumbar spine is a combination of anterior sagittal rotation and anterior translation of the lumbar vertebrae (Fig. 5.17). These two components are resisted and stabilized by different structures and in different ways by the zygapophyseal joints. On flexion, the superior

Figure 5.17 Flexion and extension of a lumbar motion segment showing the two components of sagittal rotation and translation.

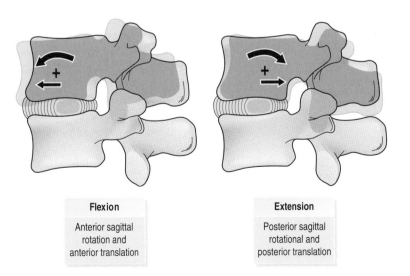

Flexion	Extension
Anterior sagittal rotation and anterior translation	Posterior sagittal rotational and posterior translation

vertebra rotates forward so that the inferior articular facets glide upwards and slightly backwards on the superior facets of the vertebra below. Thus, as anterior sagittal rotation occurs, there will be a small amount of gapping between the superior and inferior facets. As the body leans forwards, the effect of gravity or muscle contraction causes concomitant anterior translation of the superior vertebra, so that the gap between the superior and inferior facet closes. Forward translation is resisted by impaction of the inferior articular facets of one vertebra with the superior articular facets of the vertebra below. The facets play a major role in maintaining stability of the lumbar spine and preventing forward shear. The load is borne evenly across the entire articular surface of joints with flat articular surfaces (see p. 53) but, in joints with curved articular surfaces, most of the load is borne by the anteromedial portion of the superior and inferior articular facets (Bogduk and Twomey, 1987). Experiments have shown that, on flexion, the highest pressures are recorded at the medial portion of the lumbar apophyseal joints (Dunlop et al, 1984). These areas of stress are particularly vulnerable to degenerative changes.

The anterior sagittal rotation component of lumbar flexion is limited mainly by the joint capsules. In full flexion, the apophyseal joint capsules contribute approximately 39% to resisting the bending moment (Adams et al, 1980); the intervertebral disc contributes 29%, the interspinous and supraspinous ligaments 19% and the ligamentum flavum 13%. The interspinous and supraspinous ligaments realign at low angles of flexion, but are the first structures to be damaged when the elastic limit is reached. The articular surfaces probably play only a minor role in resisting the anterior sagittal rotation, but they are the major stabilizing structure in resisting anterior translation. Flexion is progressively slowed by the supraspinous ligaments, interspinous ligaments, ligamenta flava and the apophyseal joint capsules, but it ceases because of apposition of the superior and inferior articular facets (Twomey and Taylor, 1983). Experiments that investigate the effect of sequential severing of various structures on the joint movement will not demonstrate the relative and simultaneous contributions of the different elements at different phases of movement and the effects of muscle control on movement.

As the lumbar spine flexes, the intervertebral disc is compressed anteriorly, the posterior annular fibres are stretched (see pp. 76–78) and the spinous processes can be felt to separate. Intradiscal pressure increases by up to 80% in full flexion (Adams, 1994). Clinically, when flexion is examined, it should be considered that with increasing flexion, stress is placed not only on the soft tissue structures, but also on the bony elements as the apophyseal joints appose.

Lumbar spine extension is a combination of posterior sagittal rotation and a small amount of posterior translation of the vertebral bodies (see Fig. 5.17). The inferior articular facets glide downwards on the superior articular facets until the movement is limited by bony impaction of the tip of the inferior facets on the lamina of the vertebra below. The fat pads and loose areolar tissue of the inferior recesses of the apophyseal joints (Lewin, 1968; Bogduk and Engel, 1984) form a buffer between the hard, sharp inferior facets and the solid laminae, and help to attenuate the sudden jarring force of rapid full-range extension. This loading in extension is concentrated in a localized area of each inferior recess, and the load borne by the lamina at this point (the pars interarticularis) is attested by the sclerosis and thickening of compact bone observed in young adult spines (Twomey and Taylor, 1986).

Once the inferior facet has impacted on the lamina below, a continued increase in loading will cause axial rotation of the superior vertebra (Yang and King, 1984). The superior vertebra pivots on the impacted inferior articular process so that the opposite inferior articular process swings backwards. Its joint capsule becomes tense, and severe forces may cause the capsule to rupture (Yang and King, 1984). Symptoms arising from an extension injury may, therefore, arise from strain or damage to the backwardly rotating apophyseal joint, trapping of the joint capsule between the inferior articular process and the lamina, or erosion of the periosteum of the lamina at the site of impaction of the articular process.

Extension causes stretching of the anterior annular fibres while the posterior annulus bulges outwards and can decrease the size of the vertebral canal by approximately 2 mm (Schonstrom et al, 1989). Extension increases the stress distribution inside the disc: McNally and Adams (1992) report that just 2° of extension creates high peaks of compressive stress in the posterior annulus. In some circumstances, extension can reduce the stresses on the posterior annulus, while increasing the stresses on both the anterior annulus and apophyseal joints (Adams, 1994). This may explain why, in some individuals, central back pain can be relieved by extension exercises (Donelson et al, 1991). The intervertebral disc resists approximately 30–40% of the bending moment in extension (Adams et al, 1988).

Mechanical tests have shown that the anterior longitudinal ligament is much too weak to resist and limit extension of the spine. In rare cases of 'kissing spines', approximation of the spinous processes may limit movement; more typically they resist movement by trapping the interspinous ligament between them. If the spinous processes are particularly widely spaced, the apophyseal joints are vulnerable to injury in hyperextension. On palpation, the gap between the spinous processes is reduced or obliterated as the processes move closer together.

Rotation in the lumbar spine is approximately 3° to each side, although up to 8° of rotation has been noted in specimens with degenerative changes (Adams and Hutton, 1981). This greater range is probably the result of an increase in available motion caused by loss of articular cartilage from the articular surfaces of the apophyseal joints. The centre of axial rotation is not clearly defined and probably moves during the action of twisting. Experimental studies of a motion segment have shown that the centre of axial rotation lies in the posterior annulus fibrosus (Cossette et al, 1971; Adams and Hutton, 1981).

On axial rotation of a lumbar motion segment to the right, the spinous process will swing to the left and the supraspinous and infraspinous ligaments are placed under tension. The movement is limited by the impaction of one of the inferior articular facets of the upper vertebra with the opposing superior articular facet of the vertebra below. Hence, on rotation to the right, the left inferior facet of the upper vertebra impacts against the superior facet of the vertebra below and there is a slight gapping at the apophyseal joint on the right. Once impaction of the apophyseal joint occurs, any further rotation will take place about an axis located in the impacted joint.

The lumbar intervertebral discs also resist torsion. Annular fibres orientated in the direction of rotation are strained, while those in the opposite direction are relaxed. Collagen fibres can withstand 3–4% elongation, but sustain damage if stretched by more than 4% (Bogduk and Twomey, 1987). It has been calculated that the collagen fibres of the disc will allow 3° of movement, but if greater movement occurs the fibres will undergo micro-injury (Hickey and Hukins, 1980). Complete failure of the disc occurs at 12° of rotation (Farfan et al, 1970).

There is very little joint space at the lumbar apophyseal joints, so that the 3° of rotation that occur are principally due to compression of the articular cartilages of the facets, which are able to sustain compression because their major constituents are proteoglycans and water. Water is squeezed out of the cartilages under compression and it is gradually reabsorbed when the load is released (Bogduk and Twomey, 1987).

Rotation is primarily resisted by the apophyseal joints, so that rotatory movement in excess of 3° places the annulus under considerable torsional stress. Once 3° of rotation have occurred at a motion segment, the impacted joint becomes the axis of movement so that the vertebral body swings laterally and backwards and the opposite inferior articular process swings backwards and medially. As the vertebral body shifts laterally, it exerts a lateral shear on the subjacent disc that is in addition to any torsional stress of the disc that occurs on rotation. Backward movement of the opposite inferior articular process places the capsule of its apophyseal joint under greater stress.

A very strong rotatory force may cause failure of (1) the impacted apophyseal joint, (2) the disc which is strained by torsion and shear, or (3) the tensed capsule of the opposite apophyseal joint. The posterior elements contribute 65% to resisting torsion, while the disc contributes 35% (Farfan et al, 1970). Axial rotation is always accompanied by a degree of lateral flexion. Axial rotation between L1 and L4 is accompanied by lateral flexion to the contralateral side, while at L5/S1 axial rotation is coupled with lateral flexion to the same side.

Lateral flexion in the lumbar spine is a complex movement that is coupled with rotatory movements of the interbody joints and the apophyseal joints. Pure lateral flexion is not commonly performed during daily living, and in most instances lateral flexion is combined with another movement. There is approximately 10° of lateral bending from side to side in the upper lumbar spine, but this is reduced to 3° at L5/S1 where the iliolumbar ligaments restrict lateral bending. On the side to which lateral flexion occurs, the inferior articular facet of the upper vertebra slides inferiorly on the superior articular facet of the vertebra below. The cross-sectional area of the intervertebral foramen is reduced on the side of the lateral flexion. Consequently, the inferior facet on the opposite side slides upwards on the superior facet of the vertebra below and the vertical diameter of the intervertebral foramen on that side is increased.

Between L1 and L4, lateral flexion to one side is accompanied by axial rotation to the opposite side. At the L5/S1 segment, lateral flexion to one side is accompanied by rotation to the same side.

Axial distraction of the lumbar spine occurs during therapeutic traction. If the traction is applied with the intervertebral joints in mid-position between flexion and extension, the facets of the apophyseal joints glide relative to each other and the annular fibres are tensed equally. Twomey (1985) observed that 40% of the lengthening of the spine occurred as a result of flattening of the lumbar spine, while 60% was due to separation of the vertebral bodies, and it was calculated that only approximately 0.9 mm of distraction occurred at each joint. The increase in length retained when traction is released is only 0.1 mm per intervertebral joint and this is obliterated as soon as the patient weight-bears through the spine. Therefore, therapeutic traction does not have its effect by creating a permanent increase in length of the spine. The forces and movement created by therapeutic traction are also unable to draw or 'suck back' a herniated disc. The beneficial effects of traction must occur through some other mechanism.

References

Adams CBT, Logue V (1971) Studies in spondylotic myelopathy 2. The movement and contour of the spine in relation to the neural complications of cervical spondylosis. *Brain* 94: 569–586.

Adams M (1994) Biomechanics of the lumbar motion segment. In: Boyling JD, Palastanga N (eds) *Grieve's Modern Manual Therapy*, 2nd edn. Churchill Livingstone, Edinburgh, pp. 109–129.

Adams MA, Hutton WC (1981) The relevance of torsion to the mechanical derangement of the lumbar spine. *Spine* 6: 241–248.

Adams MA, Hutton WC (1982) Prolapsed intervertebral disc. A hyperflexion injury. *Spine* 7: 184–191.

Adams MA, Hutton WC, Stott JRR (1980) The resistance to flexion of the lumbar intervertebral joint. *Spine* 5: 245–253.

Adams MA, Dolan P, Hutton WC (1988) The lumbar spine in backward bending. *Spine* 13: 1019–1026.

Allbrook FM (1957) Movements of the lumbar spinal column. *Journal of Bone and Joint Surgery (Br.)* 39: 339.

Alund M, Larsson S (1990) Three-dimensional analysis of neck motion. A clinical method. *Spine* 15: 87–91.

Barnett CH, Davies DV, MacConaill MA (1961) *Synovial Joints – Their Structure and Mechanics*. Longman, London, Ch. 4, pp. 260–268.

Ben-Haim SA, Saidel GM (1990) Mathematical model of chest wall mechanics: a phenomenological approach. *Annals of Biomedical Engineering* 18: 37.

Bogduk N (1988) Biomechanics of the cervical spine. In: Grant R (ed.) *Physical Therapy of the Cervical and Thoracic Spine*, 2nd edn. Churchill Livingstone, Edinburgh, p. 28.

Bogduk N, Engel R (1984) The menisci of the lumbar zygapophyseal joints: a review of their anatomy and clinical significance. *Spine* 9: 454.

Bogduk N, Twomey LT (1987) *Clinical Anatomy of the Lumbar Spine*. Churchill Livingstone, Edinburgh.

Campbell DG, Parsons CM (1944) Referred head pain and its concomitants. *Journal of Nervous and Mental Disease* 99: 544.

Cossete JW, Farfan HF, Robertson GH, Wells RV (1971) The instantaneous centre of rotation of the third lumbar intervertebral joint. *Journal of Biomechanics* 4: 149–153.

Dalseth I (1974) Anatomic studies of the osseous craniovertebral joint. *Manual Medicine* 12: 130.

Davis PR (1955) The thoraco-lumbar mortice joint. *Journal of Anatomy* 89: 370–377.

Di Marco AF, Kelsen SG (1981) Effects on breathing of selective restriction of movement of the rib cage and abdomen. *Journal of Applied Physiology* 50: 412–420.

Dirheimer Y (1977) *The Craniovertebral Region in Chronic Inflammatory Rheumatic Diseases*. Springer-Verlag, Berlin.

Donelson R, Grant W, Kamps C, Medcalf R (1991) Pain response to sagittal end-range spinal motion: a prospective randomized multicentre trial. *Spine* 16: 5206–5212.

Dunlop RB, Adams MA, Hutton WC (1984) Disc space narrowing and the lumbar facet joints. *Journal of Bone and Joint Surgery (Br.)* 66: 706.

Dvorak J, Hayek J, Zehender R (1987) CT-functional diagnostics of the rotatory instability in the upper cervical spine. II. An evaluation on healthy adults and patients with suspected instability. *Spine* 12: 726.

Farfan HF, Cossette JW, Robertson GH, et al (1970) The effects of torsion on the lumbar intervertebral joints: the role of torsion in the production of disc degeneration. *Journal of Bone and Joint Surgery (Am.)* 52: 468.

Fielding JW (1957) Cineroentgenography of the normal cervical spine. *Journal of Bone and Joint Surgery (Am.)* 39: 1280.

Giles LGF, Singer KP (1998) Clinical Anatomy and Management of Cervical Spine Pain. Butterworth Heinemann, Oxford, Vol. 3, p. 62.

Giles LGF, Singer KP (2000). Clinical Anatomy and Management of Thoracic Spine Pain. Butterworth Heinemann, Oxford Vol. 2, p. 49.

Grahame R (1999) Joint mobility and genetic collagen disorders: are they related? *Archives of Disease in Childhood* 80: 188–191.

Grahame R, Jenkins JM (1972) Joint hypermobility – asset or liability. *Annals of the Rheumatic Diseases* 31: 109–111.

Grieve GP (1986) Movements of the thoracic spine. In: *Modern Manual Therapy of the Vertebral Column*. Churchill Livingstone, Edinburgh, Ch. 8, pp. 86–102.

Grieve GP (1988) *Common Vertebral Joint Problems*, 2nd edn. Churchill Livingstone, Edinburgh, p. 118.

Gutmann G (1960) *Die Wirbellockierung und ihr radiologischer Nachweis. Die Wirbelsäule in Forschung und Praxis.* 50. Hippocrates, Stuttgart.

Hickey DS, Hukins DWL (1980) Relation between the structure of the annulus fibrosus and the function and failure of the intervertebral disc. *Spine* 5: 100.

Hohl M, Baker HR (1964) The atlanto-axial joint: roentgenographic and anatomical study of normal and abnormal motion. *Journal of Bone and Joint Surgery (Am.)* 46: 1739.

Jirout J (1971) Pattern of changes in the cervical spine in latero-flexion. *Neuroradiology* 2: 164.

Kapandji IA (1974) *The Physiology of the Joints. 3: The Trunk and Vertebral Column*. Churchill Livingstone, Edinburgh.

Last RJ (1972) *Anatomy: Regional and Applied*, 5th edn. Churchill Livingstone, Edinburgh.

Lee D (1994) Biomechanics of the thorax. In: Grant R (ed.) *Physical Therapy of the Cervical and Thoracic Spine*, 2nd edn. Churchill Livingstone, Edinburgh, pp. 47–64.

Lee DG (1993) Biomechanics of the thorax: a clinical model of in vivo function. *Journal of Manual Manipulative Therapy* 1: 13.

Lewin T (1968) Anatomical variation in the lumbosacral synovial joints with particular reference to subluxation. *Acta Anatomica* 71: 229.

Lewit K, Krausová L, Kneidlová D (1964) Mechanismus und Bewegungsausmasz der Seitneigung in den Kopfgelenken. *Fortschr Röntgenstr.* 101: 194–201.

Loebl WY (1967) Measurement of spine and range of spinal movement. *Annals of Physical Medicine* 9: 103.

Lysell E (1969) Motion in the cervical spine. *Acta Orthopaedica Scandinavica Supplementum* 123, 1.

McNally DS, Adams MA (1992) Internal intervertebral disc mechanics as revealed by stress profilometry. *Spine* 17: 66–73.

Milne N (1991) The role of the zygapophyseal joint orientation and uncinate processes in controlling motion in the cervical spine. *Journal of Anatomy* 178: 189–201.

Moll JMH, Wright V (1971) Normal range of spinal mobility. *Annals of the Rheumatic Diseases* 30: 381.

Nowitzke A, Westaway M, Bogduk N (1994) Cervical zygapophyseal joints. Geometrical parameters and relationship to cervical kinematics. *Clinical Biomechanics* 9: 342–348.

Panjabi MM, Brand RA, White AA (1976) Mechanical properties of the human thoracic spine. *Journal of Bone and Joint Surgery (Am.)* 58: 642.

Panjabi MM, Hausfeld JN, White AA (1981) A biomechanical study of the ligamentous stability of the thoracic spine in man. *Acta Orthopaedica Scandinavica* 52: 315.

Panjabi MM, Summers DJ, Pelker RR, et al (1986) Three dimensional load displacement curves of the cervical spine. *Journal of Orthopaedic Research* 4: 152.

Panjabi M, Dvorak J, Duranceau J, et al (1988) Three-dimensional movements of the upper cervical spine. *Spine* 13: 726.

Panjabi MM, Takata K, Goel V (1991) Thoracic human vertebra. Quantitative three-dimensional anatomy. *Spine* 16: 888–901.

Pearcy MJ, Portek I, Shepherd J (1984) Three-dimensional X-ray analysis of normal movement in the lumbar spine. *Spine* 9: 294–297.

Penning L (1968a) *Functional Pathology of the Cervical Spine*. Williams and Wilkins, Baltimore.

Penning L (1968b). *Functional Pathology of the Cervical Spine*. Excerpta Medica, Amsterdam, p. 167.

Penning L (1978) Normal movements of the cervical spine. *American Journal of Roentgenology* 130: 317–326.

Penning L (1988) Differences in anatomy, motion, development and ageing of the upper and lower cervical discs and apophyseal joints. *Clinical Biomechanics* 3: 37–47.

Penning L (1992) Acceleration injury of the cervical spine by hypertranslation of the head on cervical spine motion. Part 1. Effect of translation of the head on cervical spine motion. A radiological study. *European Spine Journal* 1: 7–12.

Penning L, Wilmink JT (1987) Rotation of the cervical spine. A CT study in normal subjects. *Spine* 12: 732–738.

Porterfield JA, De Rosa C (1995) *Mechanical Neck Pain. Perspectives in Functional Anatomy*. Saunders, Philadelphia, p. 99.

Radin EL, Paul IL, Lowry M (1970) A comparison of the dynamic force transmitting properties of subchondral bone and articular cartilage. *Journal of Bone and Joint Surgery (Am.)* 52: 444.

Rauschning W (1991) Anatomy and pathology of the cervical spine. In: Frymoyer J (ed.) *The Adult Spine*. Raven Press, New York, pp. 907–928.

Saumarez RC (1986) An analysis of possible movements of human upper rib cage. *Journal of Applied Physiology* 60: 678.

Schonstrom N, Lindahl S, Willen J, Hansson T (1989) Dynamic changes in the dimensions of the lumbar spinal canal: an experimental study in vitro. *Journal of Orthopaedic Research* 7: 115–121.

Schultz AB, Benson DR, Hirsch C (1974) Force deformation properties of the human ribs. *Journal of Biomechanics* 7: 303.

Singer KP (1989) Variations at the human thoracolumbar transitional junction with reference to the posterior elements. PhD thesis. The University of Western Australia. Cited in: Giles LGF, Singer KP (eds) Clinical Anatomy and Management of Thoracic Spine Pain. (2000) Butterworth Heinemann, Oxford, pp. 100–113.

Snyder RG, Chaffin DB, Schneider LW, Foust DR, Bowman BM, Baum JK (1975) Basic biomechanical properties of the human neck related to lateral hyperflexion injury. *Highway Safety Research Institute, University of Michigan Final Technical Report UM-HRSIBI* 75-4: 455–485.

Stockwell CW (1979) Cited in: Twomey LT, Taylor JR (1987) Lumbar posture, movement and mechanics. In: *Physical Therapy of the Low Back*. Churchill Livingstone, Edinburgh.

Stoddard A (1962) *Manual of Osteopathic Technique*, 2nd edn. Hutchinson, London.

Sturrock RD, Wojtulewski JA, Dudley Hart F (1973) Spondylometry in a normal population and in ankylosing spondylitis. Rheumatology and Rehabilitation 12: 135.

Taylor JR, Twomey LT (1981) Age-related change in the range of movement of the lumbar spine. *Journal of Anatomy* 133: 473.

Taylor JR, Twomey LT (1984) Sexual dimorphism in human vertebral shape: its relation to scoliosis. *Journal of Anatomy* 138: 218–286.

Twomey L (1985) Sustained lumbar traction. An experimental study of long spine segments. *Spine* 10: 146.

Twomey LL, Taylor JR (1986) Factors influencing ranges of movement in the lumbar spine. In: Grieve GP (ed.) *Modern Manual Therapy of the Vertebral Column*. Churchill Livingstone, Edinburgh.

Twomey LT, Taylor JR (1983) Sagittal movements of the human vertebral column: a quantitative study of the role of the posterior vertebral elements. *Archives of Physical Medicine and Rehabilitation* 64: 322.

Twomey LT, Taylor JR (1987) Lumbar posture, movement and mechanics. In: Twomey LT, Taylor JR (eds) *Physical Therapy of the Low Back*. Churchill Livingstone, Edinburgh, Ch. 2.

Valencia F (1988) Biomechanics of the thoracic spine. In: Grant R. (ed.) *Physical Therapy of the Cervical and Thoracic Spine*. Churchill Livingstone, Edinburgh.

van Mameren H, Drukker J, Sanches H, Beurgens J (1990) Cervical spine motion in the sagittal plane. I. Range of motion of actually performed movements; an x-ray cinematographic study. *European Journal of Morphology* 29: 47–68.

Van Roy P, Caboor D, Boelpaep De, Barbaix E, Clarys JP (1997) Left-right asymmetries and other common anatomical variants of the first cervical vertebra. *Manual Therapy* 2: 24–36.

Weisel SW, Rothman RH (1979) Occipital atlantal hypermobility. *Spine* 4: 187.

Werne S (1957) Studies in spontaneous atlas dislocation. *Acta Orthopaedica Scandinavica Supplementum* 23: 1.

White AA (1969) Analysis of the mechanics of the thoracic spine in man. *Acta Orthopaedica Scandinavica Supplementum* 127: 1–105.

White AA, Panjabi MM (1978a) The basic kinematics of the human spine. *Spine* 3: 12.

White AA, Panjabi MM (1978b).The clinical biomechanics of the occipito-atlantoaxial complex. *Orthopedic Clinics of North America* 9: 867.

White AA, Panjabi MM (1990) *Clinical Biomechanics of the Spine*, 2nd edn. J.B. Lippincott, Philadelphia.

Worth DR (1988) Biomechanics of the cervical spine. In: Grant R (ed.) *Physical Therapy of the Cervical and Thoracic Spine*. Churchill Livingstone, Edinburgh, Ch. 2, pp. 15–25.

Worth DR, Selvik G (1986) Movements of the craniovertebral joints. In: Grant R. (ed.) *Physical Therapy of the Cervical and Thoracic Spine*. Churchill Livingstone, Edinburgh, Ch. 5, pp. 53–63.

Yang KH, King AI (1984) Mechanism of facet load transmission as a hypothesis for low-back pain. *Spine* 9: 557.

Chapter **6**

Sacroiliac joints

The sacroiliac joints are intimately associated with spinal biomechanics and pathology, and interest in the role of the sacroiliac joints in low back pain dates back to the era of Hippocrates (460–377 BC). At the beginning of the twentieth century the sacroiliac joints were considered to be a primary source of low back pain and sciatica (Goldthwait and Osgood, 1905; Albee, 1909). It was proposed that sciatica was caused by disease or subluxation of the sacroiliac joints that compromised the lumbosacral plexus as it passed over the anterior aspect of the sacrum. When the importance of the intervertebral disc in spinal pathology was identified (Mixter and Barr, 1934), interest in the sacroiliac joint as a source of low back pain started to wane. Advances in radiographic techniques have confirmed the association of disc pathology with low back pain syndromes but have also shown that not all back pain is due to the disc.

In recent years there has been renewed interest in the role of the sacro-iliac joints in low back pain.

The pelvic girdle is constructed to withstand the enormous stresses of body weight and the forces created by contraction of the pelvic musculature. It comprises two innominate bones (Fig. 6.2) – each of which consists of an ilium superiorly, an ischium posteriorly and a pubis anteriorly – and a sacrum. The pubic bones are joined anteriorly at the pubic symphysis; posteriorly, both ilia join the central sacrum at the sacroiliac joints. An osteocartilaginous ring is formed that contains and protects viscera. In adult life, the three parts of each innominate bone unite. At their junction the acetabulum articulates with the head of the femur. The extensive surfaces of the pelvis afford attachments for the muscles of the trunk and lower limbs.

Due to the interdependence of the three pelvic joints (two sacroiliac joints and the pubic symphysis), a lesion occurring in any one of them will in some way affect the other two. A large number of soft tissues (ligaments, muscles and fascia) connect or cross the spine and sacroiliac joints, and it is inevitable that abnormal pathology or biomechanics of the sacroiliac joint will result in abnormal stresses in the spine. It is not uncommon for a patient to have signs and symptoms arising from both the spine and sacroiliac joint.

SACRUM

The sacrum is triangular in shape and formed by the fusion of the five sacral vertebrae. There is considerable variation in the shape of the sacrum both between individuals and between the left and right sides. The base of the sacrum (superior surface) is formed from the first sacral vertebra with the vertebral body anteriorly and the vertebral arch posteriorly. The sacrum is angled so that its base faces downwards and forwards. The size of the angle that the superior surface makes with the horizontal plane is approximately 42–45°, increasing by approximately 8° on standing (Hellems and Keates, 1971). To compensate for this angulation and to enable the spine to be upright, the lumbar spine assumes its lordotic curve.

Figure 6.1 Left lateral aspect of sacrum.

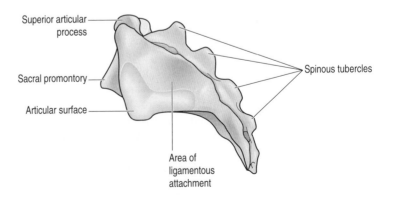

Superior articular process

Sacral promontory

Articular surface

Spinous tubercles

Area of ligamentous attachment

The spinous processes of S1–5 are fused in the midline to form the median sacral crest. The dorsal sacral foramina lie lateral to the median sacral crest and contain the dorsal sacral ramus for each sacral spinal nerve. The lateral aspect of the sacrum has an L-shaped articular surface which is contained by the costal elements of the first three sacral segments (Fig. 6.1). The short arm of the articular surface is vertical while the long arm lies in an anteroposterior direction. The shape and contours of the articular surface vary depending upon the age of the individual (Weisl, 1955; Kapandji, 1970; Vleeming et al, 1990a). There is also considerable variation in the orientation of the articular surface in both the coronal and transverse plane (Solonen, 1957; Vleeming et al, 1997).

COCCYX

The coccyx is formed by four fused coccygeal segments. In shape it is an elongated triangle with the tip facing caudally. The superior surface of the coccyx has a facet which articulates with a facet on the inferior surface of the S5 vertebral body. The first sacral segment is not always fused to the other coccygeal segments and it has two rudimentary transverse processes.

INNOMINATE (See Fig. 6.2)

The innominate is formed by the fusion of three bones, the ilium, the ischium and the pubis. The ilium is the superior portion of the innominate; it is fan shaped and the superior aspect forms the iliac crest. At either end of the iliac crest are the anterior superior iliac spine and posterior superior iliac spine. The iliac crest provides attachment for

Figure 6.2 Left innominate bone.

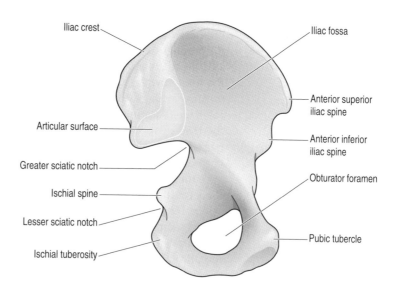

Iliac crest

Iliac fossa

Articular surface

Anterior superior iliac spine

Anterior inferior iliac spine

Greater sciatic notch

Obturator foramen

Ischial spine

Lesser sciatic notch

Ischial tuberosity

Pubic tubercle

muscles of the abdominal wall, muscles and fascia of the lower limb, and muscles and fascia of the low back. The anterior superior iliac spine and posterior superior iliac spine are often used as surface markers for palpation. Posteriorly, the ilium curves inferior to the posterior superior iliac spine and ends at the posterior inferior iliac spine.

The articular surface lies on the posterosuperior aspect of the medial surface of the ilium and is reciprocally L-shaped to articulate with the sacrum. The short arm is vertical, while the axis of the long arm is in the anteroposterior plane. The articular surface is marked by ridges, furrows and indentations that develop with age. Just above the articular surface, the surface of the ilium is roughened due to the attachment of the strong interosseous ligament.

The ischium is the lower posterior part of the innominate and comprises a body and ramus. The upper part of the body of the ischium forms the floor of the acetabulum and posteriorly approximately two fifths of the articular surface of the hip joint. The ramus runs anteromedially to join the inferior ramus of the pubis. The ischial tuberosity is a roughened area on the posteroinferior part of the ischium that provides attachment for adductor magnus, the hamstrings and the sacrotuberous ligament. An area on the medial part of the tuberosity supports the body in the sitting position.

The pubis is the anterior inferior part of the innominate and meets the opposite pubis in the midline to form a cartilaginous joint, the pubic symphysis. The pubis has a body that forms the anterior part of the acetabulum and a ramus which is directed inferiorly to join the ramus of the ischium.

SACROILIAC JOINT SURFACES

The sacroiliac joint contains synovial fluid (Bowen and Cassidy, 1981) and has matching articular surfaces: it is therefore classified as a diarthrodial joint. The sacral surface is covered with hyaline cartilage to a depth of approximately 1–3 mm (Bowen and Cassidy, 1981). The collagen fibres lie parallel to the joint surface only in the superficial zone (Mooney, 1997). The collagen fibres on the iliac surface are all orientated parallel to the joint surface; although the covering of the iliac surface is described as fibrocartilage, the collagen is Type II, which is characteristic of hyaline cartilage (Paquin et al, 1983; Bernard and Cassidy, 1991). The covering on the iliac surface is thinner and the chondrocytes are arranged in groups between bundles of collagen fibres. The hyaline cartilage on the sacral surface is thicker than the surface covering the ilium and this may be a factor in the higher incidence of sclerosis found on the iliac side of the joint than on the sacral side in osteitis condensans ilii.

An important factor to remember in spinal assessment is that the paired sacroiliac joints are normally asymmetrical to varying degrees. The paired posterior superior iliac spines are often not level, even in asymptomatic subjects. Each sacroiliac joint is unique in its structure, reflecting the forces that have been sustained by it and the individual's lifestyle.

At birth the articular surfaces are predominantly flat, but after puberty they become roughened and irregular, more so in the male. These irregularities vary to such an extent in different individuals that almost every conceivable combination of grooves, ridges, eminences and depressions may occur (Schunke, 1938; Vleeming et al, 1990a).

The grooves and depressions fit into one another to some extent, increasing stability of the joint yet allowing small degrees of movement. It is theoretically possible that the sacroiliac joints could be forced into a new position in which the ridges and grooves were no longer complementary. This would mean that the joint could be set in a 'locked' or slightly subluxed position. The amount of displacement would be so small that it could not be observed radiographically (Vleeming et al, 1990b).

The synovial membrane is surrounded by the fibrous capsule, which is attached close to the margins of both articular surfaces and is reinforced by ligaments.

LIGAMENTOUS ATTACHMENTS (Fig. 6.3)

The sacroiliac ligaments help to maintain joint integrity and offer resistance to shear forces. The toughest ligaments in the body bind the ilia to the sacrum: the interosseous sacroiliac ligament, sacrotuberous and sacrospinous ligaments. Other ligaments – the ventral and dorsal sacroiliac and the iliolumbar ligaments – also contribute to the joint's stability.

Interosseous sacroiliac ligament (Fig. 6.4)

The interosseous sacroiliac ligament is a strong, short ligament that fills the irregular space above and behind the joint. The fibres are multidirectional and can be divided into deep and superficial fibres. The deeper

Figure 6.3   Ligaments of the pelvis.

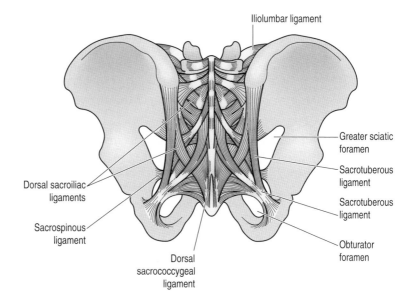

Iliolumbar ligament

Greater sciatic foramen

Sacrotuberous ligament

Dorsal sacroiliac ligaments

Sacrotuberous ligament

Sacrospinous ligament

Obturator foramen

Dorsal sacrococcygeal ligament

Figure 6.4 Horizontal section through the sacrum and sacroiliac joints.

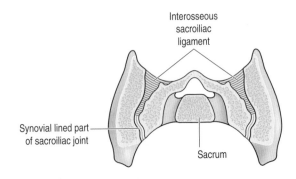

Interosseous
sacroiliac
ligament

Synovial lined part
of sacroiliac joint

Sacrum

fibres attach medially to the lateral sacral crest and laterally to the adjacent iliac tuberosity. The superficial part of the ligament is a fibrous sheet that attaches to the sacral crest laterally and to the iliac crest medially. This structure is very dense and makes intra-articular injections difficult.

Sacrotuberous ligament

The sacrotuberous ligament has a broad attachment superiorly from the posterior superior iliac spine to the upper part of the coccyx. The ligament has three large fibrous bands (Willard, 1997). The prominent lateral band extends from the posterior superior iliac spine to the ischial tuberosity and the medial band connects the coccygeal vertebrae with the ischial tuberosity. The thinner superior band connects the posterior superior iliac spines and the coccygeal vertebrae. The sacrotuberous ligament merges with the interosseous ligaments at its superior and medial borders.

The tendon of biceps femoris can extend over the ischial tuberosity to attach to the sacrotuberous ligament (Vleeming et al, 1989a,b). The tendons of the deep fibres of multifidus often attach onto the superior surface of the sacrotuberous ligament (Willard, 1997). Gluteus maximus also attaches to the sacrotuberous ligament, and contraction of the muscle increases tension in the sacrotuberous ligament (Vleeming et al, 1989a,b). The sacrotuberous ligament resists nutation (see p. 220) of the sacrum and is opposed by the long dorsal sacroiliac ligament that resists counternutation of the sacrum.

Sacrospinous ligament

The sacrospinous ligament is a triangular ligament that arises from the lateral aspect of the sacrum, coccyx and inferior aspect of the sacroiliac capsule and attaches into the ischial spine. The anterior surface of the ligament is related to the coccygeus muscle. This ligament is part of the support mechanism for the pelvic floor (Abitol, 1988).

Ventral sacroiliac ligament

The ventral sacroiliac ligament is a thickening of the anterior and inferior parts of the capsule. It is mostly thin, and is the weakest ligament of the group. When the sacroiliac joint is hypermobile, this ligament is often attenuated and a source of pain.

The long dorsal sacroiliac ligament

The long dorsal sacroiliac ligament covers the interosseous sacroiliac ligament, from which it is separated by the dorsal rami of the sacral spinal nerves and vessels. Its fasciculi pass from the intermediate and lateral crests of the sacrum to the posterior superior iliac spine and medial tip of the dorsal part of the iliac crest. The inferior fibres from the sacrum blend laterally with the sacrotuberous ligament. Medially, fibres of the dorsal sacroiliac ligament blend with the deep lamina of the posterior layer of the thoracolumbar fascia and the aponeurosis of erector spinae (Vleeming et al, 1996). Connections have also been observed at a deeper level between the long dorsal ligament and multifidus (Willard, 1997). Tension can be altered in this ligament by contraction of the muscles that attach to it or movement of the sacrum. The ligament relaxes during nutation and tightens during counternutation of the sacrum (Vleeming et al, 1996).

The skin overlying the dorsal sacroiliac ligament is a frequent area of pain in patients with lumbosacral and pelvic girdle dysfunction, but tenderness on palpation of the ligament does not necessarily incriminate this tissue given the nature of pain referral both from the lumbar spine and the sacroiliac joint (Lee, 1989).

Iliolumbar ligament

The iliolumbar ligament is a strong, complex structure that connects the transverse process of the 5th, and sometimes the 4th, lumbar vertebra to the ilium. It can have up to five parts and is described in more detail in the section on ligaments of the lumbar spine (pp. 50–51). The vertical fibres of the iliolumbar ligament pass anterior to the sacroiliac joint and contribute to its stability. Both iliolumbar ligaments sustain a great deal of tension in the upright posture when they play an important part in helping to prevent the 5th lumbar vertebra from sliding forwards on the sacrum.

FUNCTIONS OF THE SACROILIAC JOINTS

The main function of the sacroiliac joints is the transmission of forces from the head, trunk and upper limbs to the lower limbs. Body weight from the vertebral column is transmitted via the 5th lumbar vertebra to the sacrum, through the sacroiliac joints, along the alae of the sacrum and through the ischial tuberosities towards the acetabulum. The structure of this bony route reflects its weight-bearing function. Part of the reaction of the ground to the body weight is transmitted to the acetabulum by the neck and head of the femur. The rest is transmitted across the horizontal pubic ramus and is counterbalanced at the symphysis by a similar force from the other side.

The sacroiliac joints may also have an important shock-absorbing function in relation to the lumbar spine, by virtue of energy absorbed in the ligamentous tissue on translatory movements. The increased incidence of disc degeneration in the lumbar spine after deterioration of the sacroiliac joints is suggestive of this function (Wilder et al, 1980).

THE SELF–LOCKING MECHANISM OF THE PELVIS

The terms 'form closure' and 'force closure' have been used to describe the mechanisms that provide active and passive stability of the sacroiliac joints (Vleeming et al, 1990a, b). The relatively flat articular surfaces (unlike a ball and socket joint) are vulnerable to shear forces and adaptations are necessary to provide stability.

Form closure is a stable situation where joint surfaces are closely fitting and no extra forces are required to maintain the state of the system (Vleeming et al, 1990b; Snijders et al, 1993). Three factors contribute to form closure: the shape of the articular surface, the friction coefficient of the articular cartilage and the integrity of the joint ligaments. The shape of the articular cartilage with the corresponding ridges and grooves contributes to form closure. Additionally, the sacrum is wedged anteroposteriorly, helping to provide resistance to vertical and horizontal translation. However, until ossification is complete in the third decade, wedging of the sacrum is incomplete and until that time the sacroiliac joint is planar and vulnerable to shear forces. The friction coefficient of the sacroiliac joint is increased by the roughened cartilage and this contributes to the ability of the joint to resist translation. If the sacrum would fit in the pelvis with perfect form closure there would be no need for a lateral force closure.

Force closure refers to extra forces that are required to maintain the sacrum in place (Snijders et al, 1993). Forces that increase intra-articular compression will increase the friction coefficient, thereby enabling the joint to better resist translation. Force closure is affected by tension in the ligaments and muscular contraction.

A self-locking mechanism of the pelvic girdle has been described (Vleeming et al, 1990b; Snijders et al 1993). This incorporates both form and force closure. During nutation of the sacrum or posterior rotation of the innominate there is an increase in tension in the interosseous ligaments and the sacrotuberous ligaments (Vleeming et al, 1989a, b). The increase in tension of the ligaments pulls the posterior parts of the sacroiliac bones together, increasing compression of the joint. During sacral nutation there is compression of the articular structures, and the sacroiliac joints are more stable than when the sacrum is in counternutation. Hence, the sacroiliac joint can assist better with load transference if the sacrum is in nutation. Vleeming et al (1989a, b) demonstrated that nutation increased tension in the sacrotuberous ligament and they concluded that this ligament was well placed to resist nutation.

Counternutation of the sacrum or anterior rotation of the innominate has been shown to increase tension in the long dorsal sacroiliac ligament (Vleeming et al, 1996) and it is suggested that this ligament helps to control counternutation.

Muscle contraction also helps to contribute to force closure and stability of the sacroiliac joints.

MUSCLES ASSOCIATED WITH THE SACROILIAC JOINTS

An unusual feature of the sacroiliac joint is that no muscle acts as its prime mover. Movement is indirectly imposed on the joint by the actions of muscles that pass over it or those that attach the pelvis to the trunk or femora.

Various muscles are important in assisting force closure and stability of the sacroiliac joints.

Erector spinae

The lumbar paravertebral muscles are three large muscles that are each contained in their own fascial compartment. They are arranged from lateral to medial: iliocostalis, longissimus and multifidus (Bogduk, 1980). Iliocostalis and longissimus arise from the iliac crest, the posterior aspect of the posterior superior iliac spine and the thoracolumbar fascia and insert into the transverse processes and ribs in the thoracic region (see pp. 134–140). Multifidus arises from the laminae and spines of the lumbar vertebrae and has its distal attachments onto the sacral crest, interosseous sacroiliac ligaments, thoracolumbar fascia and the medial edge of the iliac crest (see pp. 132–134). The sacral section of erector spinae pulls the sacrum forward, inducing nutation of the sacrum and increasing tension in the interosseous and sacrotuberous ligaments. The section of muscle that attaches onto the iliac crests pulls the two bones towards each other, helping to maintain the sacrum in nutation. Erector spinae therefore plays an important role in force closure of the sacroiliac joints.

Gluteus maximus

Gluteus maximus is the largest muscle in the body. It is attached to the gluteal surface of the ilium, the posterior border and crest of the ilium, the posterior aspect of the sacrum, the erector spinae aponeurosis, the upper part of the sacrotuberous ligament and the thoracolumbar fascia. The majority of the muscle forms a tendinous lamina that attaches to the iliotibial tract of the fascia lata while the remaining gluteal fibres attach to the gluteal tuberosity of the femur. Gluteus maximus is coupled to the contralateral latissimus dorsi through its attachment to the thoracolumbar fascia (Vleeming et al, 1995). The fibres of gluteus maximus run parallel to the sacroiliac joint, and contraction of the contralateral latissimus dorsi and gluteus maximus acts via the thoracolumbar fascia to compress the sacroiliac joint. This compression causes the posterior aspect of the innominates to move towards each other and contributes to the force closure mechanism (Vleeming et al, 1995; Snijders et al, 1997; Vleeming et al, 1997).

The oblique system created by gluteus maximus and the contralateral latissimus dorsi provides a means of load transference during rotational activities such as running, walking and swimming (Vleeming et al, 1997).

Contraction of gluteus maximus also increases tension in the sacro-tuberous ligament.

Biceps femoris

The long head of biceps femoris arises from the ischial tuberosity and some of its fibres are continuous with the sacrotuberous ligament. Caudal traction of the long head of biceps increases tension in the sacro-tuberous ligament. The amount of tension transferred from the tendon to the sacrotuberous ligament varies in different postural positions. In cadavers, a greater percentage of force was transferred from the biceps to the sacrotuberous ligament in a flexed or stooped position than in the erect posture (Wingerden et al, 1993).

In certain positions (stooped standing, sitting with straight legs and upright sitting), the biceps femoris can act to rotate the ilium posteri-orly relative to the sacrum, thereby having a nutating effect. The nuta-tion is limited by the connections of biceps femoris to the sacrotuberous ligaments.

Transversus abdominis

The role of transversus abdominis in stabilization of the spine has been discussed in Chapter 3. Contraction of this muscle increases tension in the thoracolumbar fascia and through this mechanism it can assist in increasing tension in the posterior sacroiliac ligaments, aiding force closure.

Pelvic floor muscles

The muscles of the pelvic floor may also help to control nutation and counternutation of the sacrum. Bilateral contraction of levator ani (ilio-coccygeus and ischiococcygeus) will counternutate the sacrum while contraction of multifidus nutates the sacrum. These two muscles act as a force couple to control the position of the sacrum and form a stable base for the spine (Lee, 1999).

Rectus femoris

The biarticular muscle of the thigh can also influence the sacroiliac joints (Grieve, 1980). Through its attachment to the ilium, rectus femoris indi-rectly causes anterior rotation of the ilium in the presence of hip extension with knee flexion. This occurs at the moment of push-off in the walking cycle when the line of gravity falls anterior to the stance leg. Eccentric contraction of rectus femoris, as in descending stairs, has the same effect on the ilium.

Piriformis

Piriformis attaches to the sacrum, sacrotuberous ligament and the mar-gin of the greater sciatic foramen medially and inserts laterally to the greater trochanter of the femur. Contraction of piriformis laterally rotates the femur and helps to stabilize the femoral head in the acetabulum. It also creates a force on the sacroiliac joint capsule and posterior liga-ments, drawing the sacrum against the ilium and contributing to the self-bracing mechanism (Vleeming et al, 1989a).

NERVE SUPPLY

Anteriorly, the joints are supplied by nerves derived from L3 to S2; posteriorly, from L5 to S2. Variations may occur from one side to the other. This extensive nerve supply and the proximity of major nerves to the joints' anterior aspect have important clinical implications. The obturator and femoral nerves and lumbosacral trunk pass anterior to the joints, while the superior gluteal nerve and vessels lie lateral and distal to them, leaving the pelvis above the piriformis through the greater sciatic foramen.

Inflammation of the joints or ligamentous laxity causing malalignment of the joints' surfaces can lead to irritation of these nerves, causing referred pain and other symptoms over wide and varied areas, e.g. in the lower trunk, buttock, groin and leg.

Patients with low back disorders often complain of pain over the area of one or both sacroiliac joints but this does not necessarily identify the sacroiliac joints as the source of pain. Although the sacroiliac joint itself can be a primary source of pain, it is also the most common site of referred pain and tenderness from the lumbar spine. The examination of patients with pain in the pelvic area should always include an assessment of the lumbar spine, sacroiliac joints and hip.

MOVEMENT

Movements of the sacroiliac joints

There has been considerable interest in trying to analyse movements of the sacroiliac joints: since the middle of the 19th century a number of studies have attempted to investigate and measure movement in the joints (Sashin 1930; Weisl, 1955; Colachis et al, 1963; Wilder et al, 1980; Lavignolle et al, 1983; Sturesson et al, 1989; Vleeming et al, 1990b; Kissling and Jacob, 1997; Sturesson, 1997). These studies have shown varying degrees of movement and this is probably due to factors such as the different techniques used and whether the study used post mortem specimens or was an in vivo study. Additionally, in those studies carried out in vivo, outcome measures may have been influenced by the positions used to test movement, e.g. if the study was conducted in a weight-bearing or non-weight-bearing position. The laboratory studies have also been complemented by clinical theories and biomechanical analysis (Lee, 1989).

Most recently, roentgen stereophotogrammetric analysis (RSA) has been used to measure movement in all three planes (Sturesson et al, 1989; Sturesson, 1997). This technique involves the implantation of tantalum markers in the patient and uses a computerized system to enable precise radiographic localization of landmarks. A major drawback of this system is the exposure to radiation and it can therefore only be used on patients and not volunteers. However, RSA has been shown to measure small sacroiliac joint movements with a high degree of accuracy and specificity.

Similar results have been obtained with Kirschner wires inserted into the ilia and sacrum and stereophotogrammetry (Jacob and Kissling, 1995); although this method has the advantage of no exposure to radiation, the procedures and analysis equipment are uncomfortable for the patient (Sturesson, 1997).

Using RSA, Sturesson (1989) investigated sacroiliac joint mobility in 21 women aged 19 to 45 years and 4 men aged 18 to 45 years. The study was conducted in weight bearing, and Sturesson found only 2.5° of innominate rotation and 0.5–1.6 mm of translation. In a study of healthy individuals aged 20 to 50, Jacob and Kissling (1995) used Kirschner wires to record values of 1.8° of rotation of the innominate and 0.7 mm of translation in the men and 1.9° of rotation and 0.9 mm translation in the women. These studies show that although movements do occur at the sacroiliac joint they are very small and require sophisticated equipment for accurate analysis of the range of movement.

The pelvis can move in all three planes of the body: flexion and extension in the sagittal plane during forward and backward bending, side bending in the coronal plane during lateral flexion and axial rotation in the transverse plane during rotation of the trunk.

Movement of the sacrum

Bilateral movement of the sacrum occurs during flexion and extension of the trunk. Unilateral movement occurs at a sacroiliac joint during flexion and extension of the lower limb. When the trunk moves into flexion, the sacrum moves forwards into the pelvis about a coronal axis situated within the interosseous ligament. This movement is called *nutation* and occurs bilaterally. The articular surfaces of the sacroiliac joint are a backward-facing L shape. During nutation, the sacrum glides inferiorly down the short arm and posteriorly along the long arm of the L-shaped articular surface (Fig. 6.5). The movement is resisted by the ridges and grooves of the articular surface, the wedge shape of the articular surface, the interosseous ligament and the sacrotuberous ligament. The interosseous ligament becomes taut in nutation and the posterior superior iliac spines are drawn closer together. Only a small amount of movement (1–2 mm) occurs, but it can be palpated (Lee, 1999). The movement of nutation occurs when moving from a supine-lying position to upright standing. The sacrum is also in a position of nutation in prone-lying.

Counternutation is the backward movement of the sacrum about a coronal axis situated within the interosseous ligament. It occurs when lying supine; in some individuals it occurs at the limit of forward bending of the trunk (see p. 223). Counternutation also occurs unilaterally when the lower limb is extended. As the sacrum counternutates, it glides anteriorly along the long arm of the L-shaped articular surface and superiorly up the short arm (Fig. 6.6). The long dorsal sacroiliac ligament resists counternutation. The pelvis is relatively more unstable in a position of counternutation because the strong interosseous ligament is not taut in this position.

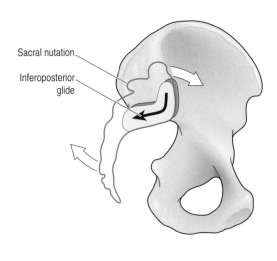

Figure 6.5 Sacral nutation. (From Lee D 1999 *The Pelvic Girdle. An Approach to the Examination and Treatment of the Lumbo-pelvic-hip Region.* 2nd Edn Churchill Livingstone, Edinburgh, Figure 5.8.)

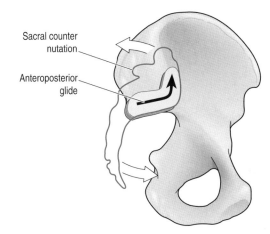

Figure 6.6 Sacral counternutation. (From Lee D 1999 *The Pelvic Girdle. An Approach to the Examination and Treatment of the Lumbo-pelvic-hip Region.* 2nd Edn Churchill Livingstone, Edinburgh, Figure 5.9.)

Rotation of the innominate

Bilateral anterior and posterior rotation of the innominates occurs during flexion and extension of the trunk. Unilateral anterior and posterior rotation of an innominate occurs during flexion or extension of the lower limb.

During forward bending of the trunk, the innominates bilaterally rotate anteriorly; there is no relative movement between the innominates because the pelvis is rotating forward as a unit on the femora. When the lower limb is extended, the innominate rotates anteriorly as the articular surface of the innominate glides inferiorly down the short arm and posteriorly along the long arm of the L-shaped articular surface (Fig. 6.7). This movement produces the same arthrokinetic motion as counternutation of the sacrum.

Posterior rotation of the innominates can occur bilaterally during extension of the trunk; there is no relative movement between the innominates as the pelvis is rotating as a unit backwards on the femora. Flexion of the lower limb rotates the innominate posteriorly as the innominate glides anteriorly along the long arm and superiorly up the short arm of

Figure 6.7 Anterior rotation of innominate. (From Lee D 1999 *The Pelvic Girdle. An Approach to the Examination and Treatment of the Lumbo-pelvic-hip Region.* 2nd Edn Churchill Livingstone, Edinburgh, Figure 5.10.)

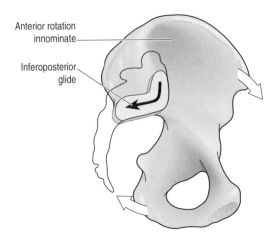

Anterior rotation innominate

Inferoposterior glide

Figure 6.8 Posterior rotation of innominate. (From Lee D 1999 *The Pelvic Girdle. An Approach to the Examination and Treatment of the Lumbo-pelvic-hip Region.* 2nd Edn Churchill Livingstone, Edinburgh, Figure 5.11.)

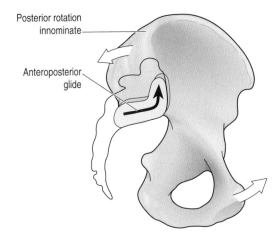

Posterior rotation innominate

Anteroposterior glide

the articular surface (Fig. 6.8). Posterior rotation produces the same arthro-kinetic motion as nutation of the sacrum (Lee, 1999).

Combined movements of the trunk and sacroiliac joints

Normal functional movements of the trunk and pelvis are not simple movements occurring only in the lumbar spine; they are a combination of complex integrated simultaneous movements at the hip, lumbar spine and sacroiliac joints. Evaluation of patients with lumbar spine and pelvic dysfunction requires an understanding of the interrelationship and inter-dependence of movement in each of these areas.

Flexion of the trunk (Fig. 6.9)

On forward bending of the trunk, the pelvis is shifted posteriorly so that the centre of gravity is moved posteriorly to maintain standing balance. The innominates rotate anteriorly on the femora and both posterior superior iliac spines should move an equal distance in a superior direction. The lumbar vertebrae rotate anteriorly and then translate anteriorly

Figure 6.9   Forward bending
relative to line of gravity.

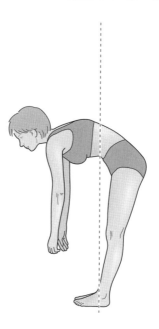

(see p. 202). The sacrum is in slight nutation in the upright standing
position, and during the initiation of trunk flexion there is a slight
increase in sacral nutation for the first 60° of forward bending (Lee,
1999). As tension increases in the sacrotuberous ligament, thoracolumbar fascia and biceps femoris the limit of sacral nutation is reached; the
innominates continue to rotate anteriorly and bilaterally on the femora
while the sacrum has relatively less flexibility. Hence, in the final stages
of forward bending of the trunk the sacrum can be in a position of relative counternutation. When the sacrum is in nutation the sacroiliac joints
are compressed, allowing better load transference of the trunk to the
legs. When the sacrum is in counternutation the sacroiliac joints are less
compressed and greater motor control is required to transfer the load of
the trunk to the legs (Lee, 1999). This effect is not seen in all individuals
and can be influenced by factors such as tight hamstrings and thoracolumbar fascia. In some individuals the sacrum remains in nutation
throughout forward bending of the trunk and this helps to maintain
good stability and transference of load (Lee, 1999).

Backward bending of the
trunk (Fig. 6.10)

During backward bending of the trunk there is an anterior shift of the
pelvic girdle and an anterior shift of the centre of gravity at the feet
to maintain standing balance. There is slight posterior sagittal rotation
of the lumbar vertebrae and a small degree of posterior translation
(see p. 202). There is no movement between the two innominates as both
rotate posteriorly together on the femora. There is a downward movement of the posterior superior iliac spine on extension that can be palpated. The sacrum remains in a position of nutation so that the sacroiliac
joints are compressed and there can be an efficient transfer of weight
from the trunk to the legs.

Figure 6.10   Backward bending.

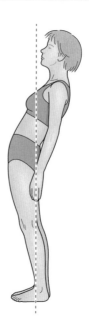

Lateral bending of the trunk (Fig. 6.11)

Lateral bending of the trunk involves lateral displacement of the upper legs and pelvis to the side opposite to the lateral bending, i.e. in lateral bending to the left, the pelvis and upper legs are displaced to the right. The line of gravity remains within the pedal base during lateral bending. In upright standing the sacrum is in nutation and the sacroiliac joints are compressed so that as the trunk bends laterally there is no movement at the sacroiliac joints.

Figure 6.11   Lateral bending.

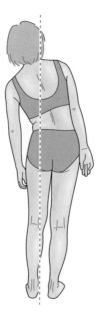

Axial rotation of the trunk   When axial rotation of the trunk occurs in the standing position, movement initially starts at the femora so that, in rotation to the right, the left femur is displaced in an anteromedial direction and the left femur is displaced in a posteromedial direction. The pelvis also moves on the femora and intrapelvic torsion is produced. The left innominate rotates anteriorly and there is a relative counternutation at the left sacroiliac joint. There is posterior rotation of the right innominate and the right sacroiliac joint nutates.

Walking   A combination of movements occurs in the pelvis and lumbar spine during walking. The entire pelvis rotates from right to left around a vertical axis and the shoulder girdle rotates in the opposite direction. Peak segmental rotation of the trunk during gait has been measured at the T6/7 level (Gregerson and Lucas, 1967). The two innominates rotate forwards and backwards synchronously in opposite directions and this creates a movement of the sacrum relative to the innominates. Movements of the lumbar spine during gait have been described and are a combination of side bending and rotation (Greenman, 1997; Lee, 1999).

When right heel strike and left toe-off occur, the right innominate is rotated posteriorly and the left innominate is rotated anteriorly. At heel strike, the posterior rotation of the right innominate increases tension in the right sacrotuberous ligament and contraction of biceps femoris will increase tension in the sacrotuberous ligament even further, preparing the sacroiliac joint to take weight. This increase in ligamentous tension contributes to force closure and augments the form closure. The pelvis as a whole rotates to the left, the sacrum is level and the lumbar spine faces forwards.

At right single-leg stance the pelvic girdle as a whole rotates to the right, translates anteriorly and adducts on the right femur. There is maximal loading of the right sacroiliac joint and hip; gluteus medius and the hip adductors on the weight-bearing leg contract to stabilize the pelvic girdle on the femur. The right innominate rotates anteriorly and the left innominate rotates posteriorly while the sacrum between the innominates is rotating to the right and side-bending to the left (Greenman, 1997). Counternutation occurs at the right sacral base and nutation at the left sacral base. There is increased activity in gluteus maximus on the weight-bearing leg together with contraction of the contralateral latissimus dorsi as the trunk counter-rotates. The contraction of gluteus maximus and latissimus dorsi facilitates the force closure mechanism at the right sacroiliac joint (Gracovetsky, 1997; Vleeming et al, 1997). At right mid stance the lumbar spine is side-bent to the right and rotated to the left.

At left heel strike the left innominate is in posterior rotation and begins to rotate anteriorly as weight is taken on the leg. The right leg is entering the swing phase and the right innominate rotates posteriorly. The sacrum has returned to being level between the two innominates, the lumbar spine is straight and the pelvis is rotated to the right.

In sacroiliac dysfunction where there is a reduction of force or form closure, changes in gait can be observed which attempt to reduce stress through the sacroiliac joint. In an uncompensated gait pattern, the pelvic girdle adducts excessively on the weight-bearing leg and the femur is laterally displaced relative to the foot so that the centre of gravity is brought closer to the sacroiliac joint, reducing the vertical shear force (Fig. 6.12). This is a non-compensated Trendelenburg gait pattern (Lee, 1997). A compensated Trendelenburg gait pattern may be observed when the patient transfers weight laterally onto the affected limb, there is abduction of the hip on the weight-bearing side and the pelvis tilts to the same side (Fig. 6.13). This action reduces the vertical shear force through the sacroiliac joints.

Figure 6.12   True Trendelenburg (uncompensated). (From Lee D 1999 *The Pelvic Girdle. An Approach to the Examination and Treatment of the Lumbo-pelvic-hip Region.* 2nd Edn Churchill Livingstone, Edinburgh, Figure 5.42.)

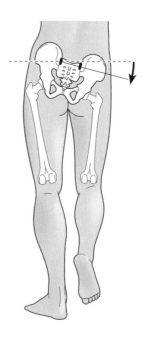

Figure 6.13   Compensated Trendelenburg. (From Lee D 1999 *The Pelvic Girdle. An Approach to the Examination and Treatment of the Lumbo-pelvic-hip Region.* 2nd Edn Churchill Livingstone, Edinburgh, Figure 5.41.)

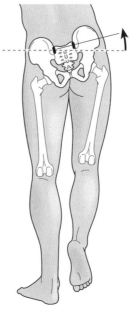

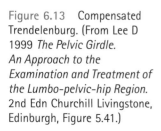

EFFECTS ON THE SACROILIAC JOINTS OF LEG LENGTH INEQUALITY

Real leg length inequality

Differences in relative leg lengths are common, the majority being minor and less than 7 mm. Greater differences are not uncommon and may be congenital or occur secondary to trauma or pathological changes in the lower limb.

Changes in the lower limb that can give a true or apparent leg length inequality

Hips
- Coxa vara
- Coxa valga
- Anteverted hips
- Retroverted hips
- Flexion contracture
- Osteoarthritis

Knees
- Hyperextended
- Flexion contracture
- Genu valgum
- Genu varum

Feet
- Equinus
- Forefoot varus
- Forefoot valgus
- Rearfoot varus

Adaptation to a short leg takes place primarily in the sacroiliac joint, where up to 7 mm can be 'absorbed', and secondarily in the lumbar spine (Stoddard, 1980).

Minor differences in leg length do not necessarily produce a lateral pelvic tilt and scoliosis. Those individuals with a more marked leg length inequality may exhibit compensatory changes. On the side of the longer leg, the ilium is often rotated posteriorly with respect to the sacrum and the sacrum is rotated towards the side of the longer leg. In minor leg length inequalities there is frequently a compensatory scoliosis affecting the lower two lumbar levels, but those with more significant leg length differences may have a compensatory scoliosis that extends into the upper lumbar and thoracic regions of the vertebral column.

The asymmetry of the pelvis and lumbar spine caused by a leg length inequality also creates asymmetrical stress at the sacroiliac joints during normal functional movements. There is a tendency for the joint on the side of the longer leg to stiffen in its posteriorly rotated position due to the stresses and strains of life (Bourdillon, 1982). Unequal leg lengths are considered to be a primary cause of sacroiliac joint dysfunction.

Apparent leg length inequality

A state of pelvic torsion can also occur through an inadequacy of force or form closure mechanisms due to a single traumatic event or repetitive minor trauma. The position of the posterior superior iliac spines relative to each other may be altered, e.g. the right posterior superior iliac spine may lie more posteriorly and caudally than the left, making the right one appear more prominent. Simultaneously, the right anterior superior iliac spine would be positioned slightly higher and more posteriorly. This pelvic asymmetry creates an apparent leg length difference and measurement taken from bony landmarks on the pelvis to estimate relative leg lengths would be inaccurate.

HYPER/HYPOMOBILITY

Hypermobility at the sacroiliac joints can be unilateral or bilateral depending on the underlying cause. Laxity of sacroiliac ligaments can occur as part of joint hypermobility syndrome and during pregnancy and post partum. Hypermobility can also result from trauma to the joint. In the hypermobile state excess movement occurs at the sacroiliac joints; if this is accompanied by weakness of the muscles that contribute to force closure the joints are liable to strain.

A state of apparent *hypomobility* can occur in hypermobile individuals, when the lax ligaments allow a joint to override and then become 'locked' in an abnormal position. The affected joint may or may not be painful, but the consequence of this type of fixation is that it puts strain on the other joints of the pelvis and also the lumbar spine.

Fibrous adhesions may form across the sacroiliac joints as a result of maturation or pathological changes. Obliteration of the synovial cavity can occur in both sexes, more so in males, and has been reported to occur in 24% of individuals (Cohen et al, 1967). In these circumstances a true state of hypomobility exists.

THE PUBIC SYMPHYSIS

The integrity of the pelvic ring depends not only upon the stability of the sacroiliac joints, but also on that of the pubic symphysis, a cartilaginous joint that holds the pelvic bones firmly together anteriorly. This acts as a compression strut, resisting the medial thrust of the femoral heads (Williams and Warwick, 1980). The adjacent surfaces of the joint are lined with hyaline cartilage and connected by an interpubic disc of fibrocartilage. It is supported by strong superior and inferior ligaments, which contribute to the stability of the joint.

Movement cannot take place at one sacroiliac joint without affecting the symphysis pubis. Movement at the symphysis is normally only minimal. During weight bearing on one leg, there is forward displacement of the pubic bone at the symphysis on the weight-bearing side. In the abnormal joint, other movements may occur such as translation (upward on one side, downward on the other) and separation.

THE EFFECT OF PREGNANCY ON THE SACROILIAC JOINTS

An increase in laxity of the pelvic ligaments is a normal and essential accompaniment of pregnancy. It renders the joints capable of more extensive movement, but it can make them susceptible to being strained. Overriding of a sacroiliac joint can occur so that the joint becomes 'locked' and apparently hypomobile. As the ligaments return to their normal post partum condition the affected sacroiliac joint may remain in an offset position and this can give rise to symptoms. Some ligamentous laxity also occurs during the menstrual cycle, although to a lesser degree.

Widening of the pubic symphyseal joint margins from the normal 4 mm to as much as 9 mm has been noted in some pregnancies (Young, 1940) and this, together with lax sacroiliac ligaments, may contribute to the instability which can develop and persist post partum.

Ligamentous laxity begins in the first half of pregnancy and increases during the last 3 months with a subsequent return to normal that starts soon after delivery and is complete within 3–5 months. These changes correlate with levels of the hormone relaxin, which increase tenfold during pregnancy, reaching a maximum at 38–42 weeks. It is possible that other hormones, including the progesterones and endogenous cortisol, may also play a part (Calguneri et al, 1982). In the second pregnancy, laxity is more marked than in the first and these mothers are at a greater risk of straining their sacroiliac joints, especially if they normally have hypermobile joints. Laxity does not continue to increase with third and subsequent pregnancies. Levels of hormones in twin pregnancies are higher than in singleton pregnancies.

A comparison of the relaxin levels in pregnant women complaining of severe pelvic pain with a control group suggested that there is an association between high relaxin levels and pelvic pain and joint laxity during late pregnancy. The highest relaxin levels during pregnancy were found in patients who were the most incapacitated clinically (MacLennan et al, 1986). However, not all patients with pelvic pain have obvious joint laxity and there are many other causes of this type of pain such as pressure from the gravid uterus, urinary tract infection, pain referred from higher levels in the spine, or nerve root irritation.

Not all pregnant women with moderately high relaxin levels have symptoms and it is thought that relaxin receptors in the connective tissues of the sacroiliac joints and pubic symphysis may be more significant than relaxin levels. It may be that some women are more susceptible to circulating or local concentrations of relaxin if a high level of receptors has been induced in these tissues. Induction of relaxin receptors is believed to be influenced by oestrogen (MacLennan et al, 1986).

In the latter stages of pregnancy a woman has to lean backwards to maintain her equilibrium in standing. This results in disequilibrium of the vertical alignment of the vertebral column with subsequent changes in the spinal curvatures. These changes in standing posture have been associated with weakness of the gluteal abductors and an unstable gait (Abitol, 1997).

References

Abitol MM (1988) Evolution of the ischial spine and of the pelvic floor in the Hominoidea. *American Journal of Physical Anthropology* 75: 53–67.

Abitol MM (1997) Quadrupedalism, bipedalism, and human pregnancy. In: Vleeming A., Mooney V, Dorman T, Snijders C, Stoeckart R (eds) *Movement, Stability and Low Back Pain*. Churchill Livingstone, Edinburgh, Ch. 31, pp. 395–404.

Albee FH (1909) A study of the anatomy and the clinical importance of the sacroiliac joint. *Journal of the American Medical Association* 53: 1273–1276.

Bernard TN, Cassidy JD (1991).The sacroiliac joint syndrome: pathophysiology, diagnosis and management. In: Frymoyer JW (ed.) *The Adult Spine, Principles and Practice*. Raven Press, New York, pp. 2107–2130.

Bogduk N (1980) A reappraisal of the anatomy of the human lumbar erector spinae. *Journal of Anatomy* 131: 525–540.

Bourdillon JF (1982) *Spinal Manipulation*, 3rd edn. William Heinemann Medical Books, London.

Bowen V, Cassidy JD (1981) Macroscopic and microscopic anatomy of the sacroiliac joint from embryologic life until eighth decade. *Spine* 6: 620–628.

Calguneri M, Bird HA, Wright V (1982) Changes in joint laxity occurring during pregnancy. *Annals of the Rheumatic Diseases* 41: 126.

Cohen AS, McNeill M, Calkins E, et al (1967) The 'normal' sacroiliac joint: analysis of 88 sacroiliac roentgenograms. *American Journal of Roentgenology* 100: 559.

Colachis SC, Worden RE, Bechtol CO, Strohm BR (1963) Movement of the sacroiliac joint in the adult male: a preliminary report. *Archives of Physical Medicine and Rehabilitation* 44: 490.

Goldthwait JE, Osgood RB (1905) A consideration of the pelvic articulations from the anatomic and pathologic and clinical standpoint. *Boston Medical and Surgical Journal* 152: 293–601.

Gracovetsky S (1997) Linking the spinal engine with the legs: a theory of human gait. In: Vleeming A., Mooney V, Dorman T, Snijders C, Stoeckart R (eds) *Movement, Stability and Low Back Pain*. Churchill Livingstone, Edinburgh, Ch. 20, pp. 243–251.

Greenman PE (1997) Clinical aspects of the SIJ in walking. In: Vleeming A., Mooney V, Dorman T, Snijders C, Stoeckart R (eds) *Movement, Stability and Low Back Pain*. Churchill Livingstone, Edinburgh, Ch. 19, pp. 235–242.

Gregersen GG, Lucas DB (1967) An in vivo study of the axial rotation of the human thoracolumbar spine. *Journal of Bone and Joint Surgery (Am.)* 49: 247–262.

Grieve E (1980) *The Biomechanical Characterization of Sacro-iliac Joint Motion*. Thesis, University of Strathclyde.

Hellems HK, Keates TE (1971) Measurements of the normal lumbosacral angle. *American Journal of Roentgenology* 113: 642.

Jacob HAC, Kissling RO (1995) The mobility of the sacroiliac joints in healthy volunteers between 20 and fifty years of age. *Clinical Biomechanics* 10: 352–361.

Kapandji IA (1970) *The Physiology of the Joints II: The Lower Limb*, 2nd edn. Churchill Livingstone, Edinburgh.

Kissling RO, Jacob HAC (1997). The mobility of the sacroiliac joints in healthy subjects. In: Vleeming A, Mooney V, Dorman T, Snijders C, Stoeckart R (eds) *Movement, Stability and Low Back Pain*. Churchill Livingstone, Edinburgh, Ch. 12, pp. 177–185.

Lavignolle B, Vital JM, Senegas J, Destandau J, Toson B, Bouyx P, Morlier P, Delorme G, Calabet A (1983) An approach to the functional anatomy of the sacroiliac joints in vivo. *Anatomica Clinica* 5: 169–176.

Lee D (1989) *The Pelvic Girdle. An Approach to the Examination and Treatment of the Lumbo-pelvic-hip Region*. Churchill Livingstone, Edinburgh, p. 25.

Lee D (1997) Instability of the sacroiliac joint and consequences for gait. In: Vleeming A, Mooney V, Dorman T, Snijders C, Stoeckart R (eds) *Movement, Stability and Low Back Pain*. Churchill Livingstone, Edinburgh, Ch. 18, pp. 231–233.

Lee D (1999) *The Pelvic Girdle. An Approach to the Examination and Treatment of the Lumbo-pelvic-hip Region*. Churchill Livingstone, Edinburgh, 2nd Edn Ch. 5, pp. 43–72.

MacLennan AH, Green R, Nicolson R, et al (1986) Serum relaxin and pelvic pain of pregnancy. *Lancet* ii: 243.

Mixter and Barr, 1934

Mooney V (1997) Sacroiliac joint dysfunction. In: Vleeming A, Mooney V, Dorman T, Snijders C, Stoeckart R (eds) *Movement, Stability and Low Back Pain*. Churchill Livingstone, Edinburgh, Ch. 2, p. 37.

Paquin JD, Van der Rest M, Mort MJ, et al (1983) Biochemical and morphological studies of cartilage from the adult human sacro-iliac joint. *Arthritis and Rheumatism* 26: 887.

Sashin D (1930) A critical analysis of the anatomy and pathological changes of the sacroiliac joints. *Journal of Bone and Joint Surgery* 12: 891.

Schunke GG (1938) The anatomy and development of the sacro-iliac joint in man. *Anatomical Record* 72: 313.

Snijders CJ, Vleeming A, Stoeckart R (1993) Transfer of lumbosacral load to the iliac bones and legs.

1: Biomechanics of self-bracing of the sacro-iliac joints and its significance for treatment and exercise. *Clinical Biomechanics* 8: 285–294.

Snijders CJ, Vleeming A, Stoeckart R, Mens JMA, Kleinrensink GJ (1997). Biomechanics of the interface between spine and pelvis in different postures. In: Vleeming A, Mooney V, Dorman T, Snijders C, Stoeckart R (eds) *Movement, Stability and Low Back Pain*. Churchill Livingstone, Edinburgh, Ch. 6, pp. 103–113.

Solonen KA (1957) The sacro-iliac joint in the light of anatomical roentgenological and clinical studies. *Acta Orthopaedica Scandinavica Supplementum* 27: 1–127.

Stoddard A (1980) *Manual of Osteopathic Technique*, 3rd edn. Hutchinson, London.

Sturesson B (1997) Movement of the sacroiliac joint: a fresh look. In: Vleeming A, Mooney V, Dorman T, Snijders C, Stoeckart R (eds) *Movement, Stability and Low Back Pain*. Churchill Livingstone, Edinburgh, Ch. 11, pp. 171–176.

Sturesson B, Selvik G, Uden A (1989) Movements of the sacroiliac joints: a roentgen stereophotogrammatic analysis. *Spine* 14: 162–165.

Vleeming A, Stoeckart R, Snijders CJ (1989a) The sacrotuberous ligament: a conceptual approach to its dynamic role in stabilizing the sacroiliac joint. *Clinical Biomechanics* 4: 204–209.

Vleeming A, Wingerden JP van, Snijders CJ, Stoeckart R, Stijnen T (1989b) Load application to the sacrotuberous ligament: influences on sacroiliac joint mechanics. *Clinical Biomechanics* 4: 204–209.

Vleeming A, Stoeckart R, Volkers ACW, Snijders C (1990a) Relation between form and function in the sacroiliac joint. 1: Clinical anatomical aspects. *Spine* 15: 130–132.

Vleeming A, Volkers ACW, Snijders CJ, Stoeckart R (1990b) Relation between form and function in the sacroiliac joint. 2: Biomechanical aspects. Spine 15: 133–136.

Vleeming A, Pool-Goudzwaard AL, Stoeckart R, van Wingerden JP, Snijders CJ (1995) The posterior layer of the thoracolumbar fascia: its function in load transfer from spine to legs. *Spine* 20: 753–758.

Vleeming A, Pool-Goudzwaard AL, Hammudoghlu D, Stoeckart R, Snijders CJ, Mens JMA (1996) The function of the long dorsal sacroiliac ligament: its implication for understanding low back pain. *Spine* 21: 556–562.

Vleeming A, Snijders CJ, Stoeckart R, Mens JMA (1997) The role of the sacroiliac joints in coupling between spine, pelvis, legs and arms. In: Vleeming A, Mooney V, Dorman T, Snijders C, Stoeckart R (eds) *Movement, Stability and Low Back Pain*. Churchill Livingstone, Edinburgh, Ch. 3, p. 53.

Weisl H (1955) The movements of the sacroiliac joint. *Acta Anatomica* 23: 80.

Wilder DG, Pope MH, Fromoyer JW (1980) The functional topography of the sacro-iliac joints. *Spine* 5: 575.

Willard FH (1997) The muscular, ligamentous and neural structure of the low back and its relation to back pain. In: Vleeming A, Mooney V, Dorman T, Snijders C, Stoeckart R (eds) *Movement, Stability and Low Back Pain*. Churchill Livingstone, Edinburgh, Ch. 1 p. 17.

Williams PL, Warwick R (1980) *Gray's Anatomy*, 36th edn. Churchill Livingstone, Edinburgh.

Wingerden JP van, Vleeming A, Snijders CJ, Stoeckart R (1993) A functional-anatomical approach to the spine-pelvis mechanism: interaction between the biceps femoris muscle and the sacrotuberous ligament. *European Spine Journal* 2: 14144.

Young J (1940) Relaxation of the pelvic joints in pregnancy. *Journal of Obstetrics and Gynaecology of the British Empire* 47: 493.

Chapter 7

Innervation of the vertebral column

CHAPTER CONTENTS

The nervous system plays an important role in normal function of the spine and consequently an understanding of neural influences on spinal function and pain mechanisms is essential. Investigations into low back pain have largely focused on mechanical causes, e.g. a prolapsed intervertebral disc compressing a nerve root or degenerate facet joints with osteophytosis. The presence of structural abnormalities in the spine poorly correlates with painful spine disorders, and there is evidence that inflammatory, vascular and immunological factors are also important causes of spinal pain (Porterfield and DeRosa, 1998). This chapter reviews the neuromechanical and neurochemical bases of spinal pain and in particular:

- Innervation of the spinal tissues
- Tissues that are a source of back pain
- Referred pain

- The influence of structural, mechanical, inflammatory, vascular and immunological factors on back pain
- The role of the autonomic nervous system
- Concomitant signs and symptoms (other than pain) which are due to malfunction of the nervous system
- Abnormalities of posture, and changes in range and quality of movement associated with neurological signs and symptoms.

SPINAL NERVES

Thirty-one pairs of spinal nerves attach to the spinal column. They are short nerves that lie within the intervertebral foramina. Each spinal nerve divides into an anterior and posterior portion and connects with the spinal cord via ventral and dorsal nerve roots (Fig. 7.1). The ventral roots attach on each side in a longitudinal series to the anterolateral aspect of the cord, while the dorsal roots pass bilaterally to the posterolateral aspect of the cord. Each ventral and dorsal root then divides into a number of small branches called rootlets (see Fig. 8.3, p. 278) that form the junction with the spinal cord. The ventral and dorsal nerve roots act as the pathway that links the central nervous system to the spinal nerves.

The dorsal roots carry only sensory fibres from the spinal nerves to the spinal cord; the ventral nerve roots transport mostly motor fibres, but may transport a small number of sensory fibres (Bogduk and Twomey, 1987). Near the junction of the dorsal and ventral roots, the dorsal root has a swelling known as the *dorsal root ganglion*. It is a collection of cell bodies of all the sensory fibres that run in the related spinal nerve. Dorsal root ganglia are usually situated in the intervertebral foramina, but the ganglia of the 1st and 2nd nerves lie on the vertebral arches of the

Figure 7.1 Formation of a spinal nerve – cervical region. (Adapted from Williams PL, Warwick R 1980 *Gray's Anatomy*, 36th edn. Churchill Livingstone, Edinburgh, p. 1088.)

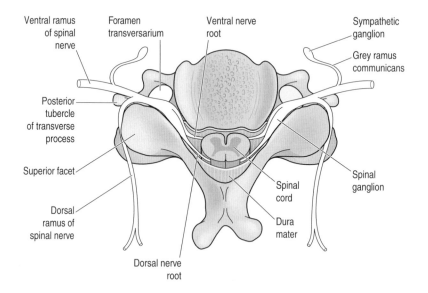

atlas and axis, the ganglia of the sacral nerves are within the vertebral canal and that of the coccygeal is within the dura.

Degenerative changes may affect the dorsal and ventral roots separately and irritation of the separate roots has been shown to produce different symptoms. Frykholm (1971) stimulated the ventral and dorsal roots in subjects with existing cervical spine disorders; stimulation of the cervical dorsal root gave pain within a dermatomal distribution, but stimulation of the ventral root produced a more diffuse pain in the neck, shoulder and upper arm.

The 31 pairs of spinal nerves are named according to the vertebra to which they are related. There are 8 cervical, 12 thoracic, 5 lumbar and 5 sacral pairs and 1 coccygeal pair of spinal nerves. The first cervical nerve (suboccipital nerve) passes out from the vertebral canal between the occipital bone and the atlas and, consequently, the cervical spinal nerves lie above the cervical vertebra with the same number. The exception to this is the 8th cervical nerve, which emerges *below* the 7th cervical vertebra. Caudal to this level the remaining spinal nerves lie below the correspondingly numbered vertebra. Through its connections with the ventral and dorsal roots and their branches, each nerve attaches to a discrete part of the spinal cord and, hence, the spinal cord is divided into a series of imaginary segments, each numbered according to the spinal nerve which attaches to it (Fig. 7.2). In the lumbosacral region the nerve roots are very long and form the cauda equina.

Each nerve is covered by pia mater and loosely invested with arachnoid mater up to the point where the nerve roots pierce the dura. The thin arachnoid adheres to the inner surface of the dura thereby creating the subarachnoid space. This space contains cerebrospinal fluid, which bathes the nerve roots and assists in nutrition of the nerve root structures. The two roots pierce the dura separately and receive a sheath from it. The ganglia receive a covering from the dura, and the dura then becomes continuous with the epineurium of the spinal cord.

DIRECTION OF THE NERVE ROOTS

The anatomical pathway of the nerve roots from the dural sac to the intervertebral foramen is termed the nerve root canal. Degenerative changes may cause a narrowing of this space: the terms *lateral canal stenosis* and *lateral recess stenosis* are used to describe narrowing of the nerve root canals. The nerve root canals may be narrowed by disc bulges or herniation, thickening of ligaments, tumours, osteophytosis and segmental instability.

Direction and length of the nerve roots varies at each segmental level. In the early development of the central nervous system, the spinal cord and bony vertebral column are the same length. At this stage, each spinal nerve runs transversely to its corresponding intervertebral foramen. However, due to the disproportionate rate of growth of the bony and neural elements, in the adult the spinal cord ends at the level of the L1/2 disc. Consequently, for the spinal nerves to remain attached to their

Figure 7.2 Diagrammatic representation of spinal nerves in relation to vertebral levels (Adapted from Grieve GP 1988 *Common Vertebral Joint Problems*, 2nd edn. Churchill Livingstone, Edinburgh.)

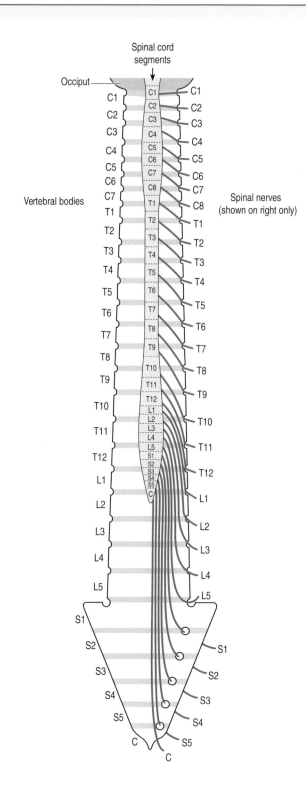

respective spinal cord segments and emerge through the corresponding intervertebral foramen, the length and obliquity of the roots increase caudally (see Fig. 7.2). The 1st and 2nd cervical nerve roots are almost horizontal as they exit from the canal. The 3rd–8th roots are directed obliquely downwards. The obliquity and length of the roots successively increases. The distance of the roots from their attachment to the spinal cord to their exit from the vertebral canal is no greater than one vertebral level in this region.

In the lower cervical and upper thoracic spine, the rootlets descend a variable distance within the dura and, on piercing it, are angled upwards in their course to the intervertebral foramen (Fig. 7.3). At the cervico-thoracic junction, the roots may descend intradurally for several milli-metres below the margin of the intervertebral foramen and then become sharply angulated to pass upwards in order to emerge through it (Nathan and Fuerstein, 1974). The spinal nerve emerges through the intervertebral foramen to pass downwards again. Some roots may undergo two marked angulations, particularly those at vertebral junction regions. The degree of angulation may be as much as 30–45°, with the roots of C6–T9 being most affected; those of T2 and T3 have the greatest degree of angulation. The roots may be further distorted by degenerative changes.

Figure 7.3 Schematic drawing of the angulated cervicothoracic nerve roots. (From Nathan H, Fuerstein M 1974 Angulated course of spinal nerve roots. *Journal of Neurosurgery* 32: 349–352, with permission.)

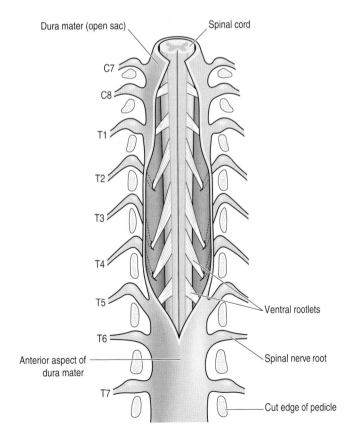

The thoracic roots are small and increase in length caudally. Upper thoracic nerve roots travel approximately one segmental level to emerge through their respective intervertebral foramina; however, in the lower thoracic spine, the roots descend in contact with the spinal cord for approximately two vertebral levels before leaving the vertebral canal.

The lumbar, sacral and coccygeal nerve roots descend with increasing obliquity. The degree of angulation of the first and second lumbar nerve roots is 70–80°; the third and fourth, 60°; the fifth, 45°; and the first sacral nerve root, 30° (Bose and Balasubramaniam, 1984). The spinal cord ends at the level of the L1/2 disc, so that the upper lumbar roots travel 9 cm and the lower lumbar roots 16 cm before emerging through the intervertebral foramina. The collection of nerve roots below the 1st lumbar vertebra is called the *cauda equina*.

In the cervical spine, the nerve root is anterior and superior to the apophyseal joint; in the thoracic spine, it is directly anterior to the joint. In the lumbar spine, the nerve root is anterior and inferior to the apophyseal joint and also in close proximity to the posterior and posterolateral aspect of the numerically corresponding intervertebral disc. The spinal nerve roots are vulnerable to trespass or irritation from degenerative changes at the apophyseal joints and, particularly in the lumbar spine, bulging or prolapse of the intervertebral discs. The spinal nerves may be compressed or irritated at any point in their course from the spinal cord to their exit through the intervertebral foramina. Rydevik (1992) found that the spinal nerves do not have the same amounts of connective tissue sheath as the more peripheral nerves, so that the spinal nerves have less protection and may be more vulnerable to mechanical deformation than the peripheral nerves.

The nerve roots have a degree of inherent elasticity that allows them to accommodate to changes in vertebral movement. Disease of the vertebral column may adversely affect the mobility of the nerve roots and this is a feature of many spinal pain syndromes.

COMPONENTS AND BRANCHES OF THE SPINAL NERVES

A typical spinal nerve contains both somatic and visceral fibres. The somatic components are both afferent and efferent fibres. The somatic efferent fibres innervate skeletal muscle, while somatic afferent fibres carry impulses to the spinal cord from receptors in the skin, subcutaneous tissue, muscle, joints, ligaments and fascia. The visceral components of the spinal nerves are afferent and efferent autonomic fibres. They include sympathetic and parasympathetic fibres at different levels (see pp. 264–269).

The paravertebral plexus (Stillwell, 1956) is a dense network of fibres in the region of the somatic nerve roots and sympathetic ganglia. Fibres interconnect between the grey rami communicantes, the sympathetic ganglia and the anterior and posterior primary rami. Mixed branches of the plexus pass externally to supply the periosteum and ligaments at the front, sides and backs of the vertebral bodies. Some fibres join the medial branch of the posterior primary rami of each spinal nerve root to supply the receptors of the apophyseal joints.

Sinuvertebral nerves

The sinuvertebral nerve is also known as the meningeal or recurrent meningeal nerve or the nerve of von Luschka. There is more than one sinuvertebral nerve at each level: an intervertebral foramen can contain between two and six sinuvertebral nerves (Groen et al, 1990). The nerves are of varying size, and an intervertebral foramen contains a number of nerves of different sizes, e.g. one large and four small nerves.

The sinuvertebral nerves originate from one or two rami communicantes close to the connection with the spinal nerve, just distal to the dorsal root ganglion and ventral to it. The sinuvertebral nerve contains small and moderately large myelinated fibres. It has mainly unencapsulated free nerve endings that are thought to have a nociceptive and proprioceptive function (Parke, 1992). The larger fibres are somato-sensory and viscero-sensory and the sinuvertebral nerve is primarily afferent, carrying sensory information back to the central nervous system. The smaller fibres are probably postganglionic sympathetic fibres and give an efferent motor supply to the smooth muscle of the vascular structures in the spinal canal.

The sinuvertebral nerve re-enters the spinal canal through the intervertebral foramen, passing anterior to the dorsal root ganglion. On entering the canal, the nerve has a variable course that may be long, short, ascending, descending, transverse or oblique and it connects with the sinuvertebral nerves of the other side and neighbouring segments. Some branches of the sinuvertebral nerve are particularly long and can extend over the two adjacent levels inferiorly and superiorly (Groen et al, 1990) with consequent implications for segmental innervation patterns. The sinuvertebral nerve supplies the dura mater and the walls of the blood vessels; it forms a dense plexus over the posterior longitudinal ligament and a more irregular plexus over the anterior longitudinal ligament (Jackson et al, 1966; Groen et al, 1990) supplying both ligaments, the outer annular fibres and the periosteum of the vertebral body. In the thoracic spine, the sinuvertebral nerve gives a branch that crosses the upper border of the neck of the nearby rib and supplies the periosteum of the neck.

In the cervical region, the branches may wander up and down the canal for two or rarely three segments before terminating in receptor endings. The ascending branches of the upper three cervical sinuvertebral nerves are relatively large and supply the cerebral dura mater of the posterior cranial fossa; if irritated, as in a whiplash injury, they may cause cervical headaches.

Cervical dorsal rami

The dorsal (posterior primary) rami of all the cervical spinal nerves, with the exception of the first, divide into medial and lateral branches. All these branches innervate muscles, but only the medial branches of C2–4 and sometimes C5 supply cutaneous areas.

The 1st cervical dorsal ramus (suboccipital nerve) arises from the C1 spinal nerve and emerges superior to the posterior arch of the atlas and inferior to the vertebral artery. It pierces the suboccipital triangle and supplies the muscles which bound this region.

The 2nd cervical dorsal ramus arises from the C2 spinal nerve dorsal to the atlanto-axial joint and deep to the inferior oblique muscle. It divides into medial, lateral, superior communicating and inferior communicating branches. The medial branch is called the *greater occipital nerve* and, with a branch of the C3 spinal nerve, it ascends into the occipital area where it divides into branches that communicate with the lesser occipital nerve to supply the skin of the scalp as far as the vertex of the skull. The lateral branch supplies the posterior neck muscles.

The 3rd cervical dorsal ramus arises from the C3 spinal nerve in the C2/3 intervertebral foramen. It passes posteriorly around the articular pillar of the 3rd cervical vertebra and divides into medial, lateral and communicating branches. There are two medial branches; the larger is called the *3rd occipital nerve* and ends in the skin of the lower part of the occipital region. The 3rd occipital nerve has been implicated in headache syndromes. Trevor-Jones (1964) found the nerve trapped by osteophytes of the C2/3 joint in three patients with severe headaches. Surgical release of the entrapment relieved the symptoms.

The dorsal rami of C4–8 arise from their respective spinal nerves just outside the intervertebral foramina. The nerves pass backwards around the articular pillar and divide into medial and lateral branches. The medial branches of C4 and C5 supply the skin, while the lateral branches of C4–8 supply the posterior neck muscles.

The atlanto-occipital and lateral atlanto-axial joints are innervated by branches of the ventral rami of C1 and C2. The C2/3 apophyseal joint receives an articular branch from the C3 *dorsal* ramus. Articular branches to the C3/4 apophyseal joint arise from the medial branch of the C3 dorsal ramus.

The medial branches of the C4–8 dorsal rami supply articular branches to the apophyseal joints above and below them. Articular branches from adjacent segmental levels may communicate with one another to form a communicating loop posterior to the apophyseal joints (Bogduk, 1982).

Thoracic dorsal rami

The thoracic dorsal (posterior primary) rami arise from their respective spinal nerves just outside the intervertebral foramina. Stolker et al (1994) reported that the dorsal ramus originated directly lateral to the dorsal root ganglion and perpendicular to the long axis of the spinal nerve. Rami communicantes connect the sympathetic trunk with the spinal nerve, thereby forming a pathway for sympathetic vasoregulatory nerves to supply the thoracic apophyseal joint capsules. A blockade of the dorsal rami will block both the sensory nerves and these sympathetic fibres (Giles and Singer, 2000).

The *medial branches* emerge between the apophyseal joint, the medial section of the costotransverse ligament and the intertransverse muscle. The medial branches of T1–6 run between semispinalis thoracis and multifidus, which they supply. They pierce rhomboids and trapezius, and the cutaneous branches descend for some distance before reaching the skin by the sides of the vertebral spines.

The medial branches of the T7–12 dorsal rami supply multifidus, longissimus thoracis and the zygapophyseal joints; they only occasionally supply the skin. The thoracic zygapophyseal joints are innervated by the medial branches of the dorsal rami of the two segments cephalad. Hence, the apophyseal joints of T4 and T5 are supplied by the T4 and T3 spinal nerves (Chua and Bogduk, 1995).

The lateral branches run between the superior costotransverse ligament and the intertransverse muscle before inclining posteriorly on the medial side of levator scapulae. They supply longissimus thoracis, iliocostalis thoracis and levatores costarum. The lateral branches of the upper thoracic dorsal rami give a variable supply to the skin in line with the angle of the ribs. The lateral cutaneous branches may descend the breadth of four ribs before becoming superficial.

The costovertebral and costotransverse joints are both innervated by the thoracic dorsal rami as well as the related intercostal nerves (Wyke, 1975).

The courses of two thoracic dorsal rami are of particular importance. The dorsal rami of the 2nd thoracic nerve descend paravertebrally until they emerge at the level of T6. The nerve then ascends over the posterior chest wall and scapula to the acromion. Irritation of this nerve can produce pain over the posterior chest wall and shoulder area. The lateral branches of the dorsal rami of the 12th thoracic nerve descend paravertebrally in the lumbar spine to the posterolateral iliac crest. They then run laterally and supply the skin over the buttock area. Vertebral disease that causes irritation or compression of this nerve can, therefore, give pain in the low lumbar and buttock area.

Lumbar dorsal rami

The L1–4 dorsal rami of the lumbar spinal nerves pass backwards and medially to divide into medial and lateral branches at every level. Intermediate branches are sometimes present. The L5 dorsal ramus is longer and passes over the ala of the sacrum (Bogduk et al, 1982).

The lateral branches supply erector spinae and the thoracolumbar fascia. The lateral branches of the L1–3 rami give off cutaneous nerves named the superior cluneal nerves. They supply the skin over the iliac crest and the gluteal region.

Intermediate branches supply the lumbar fibres of longissimus. Medial branches of the upper four dorsal rami pass along the top of their respective transverse processes, piercing the intertransverse ligament at the base of the transverse process. The nerve passes around the base of the articular process, crosses the lamina and then divides into multiple branches which supply multifidus, interspinous muscles and ligaments, and two apophyseal joints. Each medial branch supplies the apophyseal joints above and below its course (Bogduk et al, 1982). The L5 dorsal rami supply the lumbosacral apophyseal joints.

The muscular supply of the medial branches is very specific. Each medial branch supplies only those muscles attached to the laminae and spinous process of the vertebra with the same segmental number as the nerve. Therefore, the L1 medial branch supplies only those fibres arising from the 1st lumbar vertebra. This indicates that the muscles which move a particular segment are innervated by the nerve of that segment (Bogduk and Twomey, 1987).

Sacral and coccygeal dorsal rami

The sacral dorsal rami are small and, with the exception of the 5th sacral nerve, they emerge through the dorsal sacral foramina.

The medial branches of S1–3 end in multifidus. The lateral branches join together and, with branches of L4 and L5 dorsal rami, form loops on the dorsal surface of the sacrum. These loops join with a second series of loops under gluteus maximus to form the middle cluneal nerves. They give cutaneous branches to supply the skin over the gluteal and the greater trochanter areas.

The dorsal rami of S4 and S5 do not divide into medial and lateral branches, but unite and, with the dorsal ramus of the coccygeal nerve, form loops on the dorsal surface of the sacrum. Cutaneous branches from these loops supply the skin over the coccyx.

INTERVERTEBRAL FORAMINA

The intervertebral foramina are important structures forming exits from the vertebral canal. Other terms used to describe these structures include lateral canal, nerve root canal, nerve root tunnel, radicular canal and interpedicular canal. Dommisse (1975) suggests that the term 'foramina' should only be used to describe the inner and outer boundaries of the structure, while Giles and Singer (1997) state that the term 'intervertebral canal' is anatomically more appropriate.

The boundaries of the intervertebral foramina are the intervertebral disc and adjacent vertebral bodies anteriorly, the apophyseal joints posteriorly and the pedicles inferiorly (Fig. 7.4). The foramina extend from the spinal canal where the nerve root sheath comes off the dural sac and end where the spinal nerve emerges laterally through the canal. Lee et al (1988) identified three zones that are of importance clinically: the entrance zone (lateral recess area), the mid-zone (sublaminal blind zone) and the exit zone (where the nerve leaves the foramen).

The entrance zone contains the nerve root covered with dura mater and bathed in cerebrospinal fluid (CSF). The mid-zone contains the dorsal root ganglion and ventral nerve root, which are also bathed in CSF and covered with a fibrous connective tissue extension of the dura. The exit zone contains the spinal nerve, which is covered with perineurium (Lee et al, 1988).

Other structures contained within the foramina include areolar tissue, adipose tissue, spinal artery, a plexus of small veins, the sinuvertebral nerve and its branches, and lymphatic vessels.

The spinal nerve and its sheath occupy between one third and one half of the cross-sectional area of the foramen. The foraminal contents are

Figure 7.4   Boundaries of the intervertebral foramen. A, Cervical spine. B, Lumbar spine.

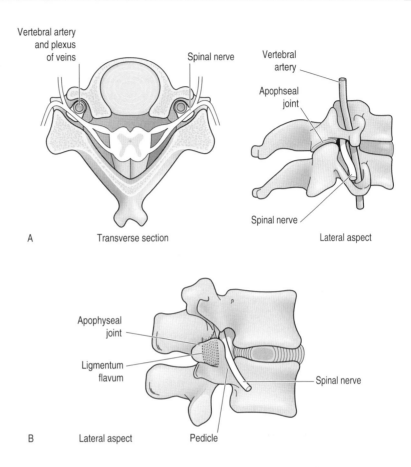

partially protected by the surrounding fat, and the CSF protects the nerve root in the entrance zone and mid-zone.

The vertical height of the foramen is greater than the anteroposterior measurement (Giles, 1993). In the cervical spine, the pedicle and posterior tubercle of the transverse process form the inferior boundary of the foramen to make a gutter for the spinal nerve. This gutter may exceed 1 cm in length. The foramina of the thoracic spine have the smallest anteroposterior dimension. In the lumbar spine, the vertical height of the foramina varies between 12 and 19 mm, while the anteroposterior measurement varies from 7 to 10 mm.

The cross-sectional area of the lumbar intervertebral foramina increases caudally from the L1–2 level, but the L5–S1 foramina is smaller than the rest, even though the 5th spinal nerve is larger than the other lumbar nerves (Hasue et al, 1983).

The spinal nerve root has been described as lying in the lateral recess (Williams and Warwick, 1980; Rydevik et al 1984; Van der Linden, 1984). The lateral recess is bounded by the medial portion of the superior articular facet and lamina above, the pedicle laterally and the vertebral body and adjacent intervertebral disc below. Peretti et al (1989) described the lumbar and first sacral nerve roots as lying immediately below the subjacent pedicle. According to Hasue et al (1989), the position of the L5–S1 spinal ganglia can vary; it may be intraspinal and lie partly within the spinal canal, it may be intraforaminal, or extraforaminal where the ganglion lies outside the intervertebral foramen.

The dimensions of the foramina may be reduced developmentally or by degenerative changes. Developmental factors such as short pedicles, shallow lateral recess or shorter interfacetal distance will result in a narrow spinal canal (spinal stenosis). The dimensions of the canal may be further reduced if degenerative changes are superimposed and the foraminal contents can then be compromised.

Direct pressure on the spinal nerve and ganglia can occur in the interpedicular zone (Giles and Kaveri, 1990). The cross-sectional area of the interpedicular zone may be reduced by a herniated disc, osteophytosis from the adjacent apophyseal joints or interbody joints, the transforaminal ligaments, hypertrophy of ligamentum flavum, or vertebral joint subluxation. Mechanical trespass of the neural structures can induce a sequence of events including a reduction of nerve root blood supply and oxygen deprivation (see Ch. 9).

The dimensions of the foramina alter with movement. The height of the intervertebral foramina tends to decrease in extension and increase in flexion. Side flexion tends to reduce the height of the foramina on the side to which movement occurs and increase the height of the foramina on the opposite side.

VERTEBRAL ARTICULAR RECEPTOR SYSTEMS

The zygapophyseal joints are richly innervated and are supplied by both myelinated and unmyelinated nerve fibres with three types of nerve endings: fine free fibres, complex unencapsulated endings and small encapsulated endings (Hirsch et al, 1963).

Wyke (1967) has classified four types of receptor nerve endings found in synovial joints. They each have individual characteristic behavioural properties and their distribution varies in different joints and in different regions of each joint capsule. Types I, II and III are corpuscular mechanoreceptors, and type IV are non-corpuscular nociceptive (pain) receptors.

Mechanoreceptors are biological transducers that react to a mechanical stimulus and convert it into electrical energy. The different types of mechanoreceptors send information about joint activity to the central nervous system (Porterfield and DeRosa, 1998).

Type I

Type I receptors are small globular mechanoreceptors which are located in the peripheral layers of the fibrous apophyseal joint capsule. They are particularly numerous in the cervical spine. These receptors are low threshold, slowly adapting and sensitive to mechanical stress. The pressure differences inside and outside joint capsules and the capsular stress produced by surrounding muscles and ligaments cause some type I receptors to discharge continuously at a low frequency. They contribute to awareness of joint position in active and static joints. These receptors are most numerous in areas subjected to the greatest stress. Other receptors are sensitive to direction, speed and degree of active and passive movement. They also monitor atmospheric pressure changes. Type I receptors have an inhibitory effect on the trans-synaptic centripetal flow of nociceptive afferent activity from type IV receptors and are, therefore, important in pain suppression.

Type II

Type II receptors are larger than type I and found mainly in the deeper layers of the capsule and on the surface of intra-articular fat pads, where they often lie in close association with blood vessels. These receptors are also more numerous in the cervical apophyseal joint capsules. They are low threshold, rapidly adapting and do not discharge at rest. They discharge at the beginning and end of movement and are sensitive to acceleration and deceleration. They are reflexogenic and do not respond to changes in joint position or movement.

Type II receptors discharge in response to vibratory stimulation and have transient inhibitory effects on the centripetal nociceptive afferent activity, thereby aiding pain suppression.

Type I and II receptor systems are operative in normal and abnormal circumstances. The reduction in pain achieved by some treatment techniques (e.g. passive oscillatory mobilization, traction, massage) is thought to be in part due to stimulation of type I and II mechanoreceptors which then have an inhibitory effect on afferent nociceptive activity.

Type III

Type III receptors occur only in intra- and extra-articular ligaments of peripheral joints, and are not present in the capsules or ligaments of vertebral joints.

Nociceptive system

The type IV receptor system is a three-dimensional plexus of unmyelinated nerve fibres. It is nociceptive (pain-provoking), high threshold and non-adaptive. The system is activated when its nerve endings are depolarized by high mechanical stress (e.g. abnormal posture, fractures, dislocations) or exposure to chemical irritants (e.g. histamine, bradykinins, lactic acid) which accumulate in the tissue fluid of acutely and chronically inflamed joints. The nociceptors are also activated by thermal stimuli (temperatures of approximately 44° or above). Type IV receptors are distributed throughout the tissues of the spine (Table 7.1).

Non-nervous tissues have the ability to stimulate nociceptive nerve endings by releasing chemical irritants. When an injury occurs there is an inflammatory reaction; mast cells, injured tissue cells and the blood vessels at the site of injury release substances such as histamine, bradykinins, prostaglandins, serotonin and leukotrienes. Some nociceptive nerve endings become sensitized to the chemical stimuli so that their threshold response to stimuli is lowered and a hyperalgesic state results (Weinstein, 1991). The nociceptors provide sensory information to the central nervous system regarding tissue injury.

Table 7.1   Distribution of type IV receptors

Tissue	Type IV receptors
Cancellous bone of vertebral bodies and arches	Blood vessels of cancellous bone are accompanied by perivascular nociceptive plexuses. The small diameter fibres are poorly myelinated or unmyelinated
Periosteum of vertebrae, tendons, fasciae, aponeuroses	Unmyelinated plexiform endings
Periarticular arteries, arterioles, epidural and paravertebral veins and venules	Plexuses of unmyelinated nociceptive nerve filaments
Deep and superficial capsule and fat pads	Plexiform nociceptive receptors. Fat pads have a very rich supply
Ligaments – longitudinal, flaval, ligamentum nuchae and intertransverse	Unmyelinated free nerve endings. Particularly numerous in the posterior longitudinal ligament
Dura mater – anterior and dural sleeves only	Unmyelinated plexiform endings
Cervical epidural adipose tissue	Unmyelinated plexiform endings

The nociceptors not only send information to the central nervous system but they also contribute to the inflammatory and repair processes. When activated by chemical irritants, the nociceptive nerve endings respond by releasing neuropeptides and neuromodulators. The function of the neuropeptides is to increase the excitability of adjacent nociceptors so that tissue repair is facilitated and inflammation modulated (Payan et al, 1987). Neuropeptides such as substance P and calcitonin gene-related peptide are synthesized in the dorsal horn of the nociceptive neuron and travel along the axon via axoplasmic flow to the terminal nerve endings. The release of the neuropeptides at the site of injury results in increased vascular permeability and cells such as polymorphonuclear leukocytes and monocytes are attracted to the area. Neuropeptides also stimulate the function of monocytes and leukocytes and contribute to repair processes in injured tissues.

There are no nociceptive nerve endings in the synovial membrane, articular cartilage or menisci.

DEGENERATIVE DISEASE AFFECTING ARTICULAR RECEPTOR SYSTEMS

Afferent impulses from the type I mechanoreceptors in periarticular tissue influence efferent impulses which control the tone of the skeletal muscles. Maintenance of normal posture and performance of voluntary movement depend on the normal afferent activity of type I receptors. Damage or irritation of the periarticular tissues in degenerative disease affects the impulses from the type I receptors so that postural and kinaesthetic sensations are impaired. Afferent (non-sensory) activity of the type I and type II mechanoreceptors exerts powerful tonic reflexogenic influences on facilitatory and inhibitory patterns in the motor neuron pools of the cervical, limb and jaw musculature (Wyke, 1979), and these underlie the functional groupings of muscles during postural control and voluntary activity. These reflexes may be important in maintaining articular congruity and assist in distributing the load on a joint (Dee, 1978).

Degenerative disease, which alters afferent input from type I and II mechanoreceptors, impairs these arthrokinetic reflexes, thereby making the joints more susceptible to damage through stresses and strains. The arthrokinetic reflexes are also disturbed when joints are immobilized (e.g. splints, collars and corsets) and, consequently, postural and kinaesthetic sense may be affected. The upper cervical apophyseal joints are particularly rich in mechanoreceptors. The latter become defective in degenerative disease and can give rise to symptoms of disequilibrium. When treating cervical dysfunction, the wealth of receptors in the neck suggests that emphasis should be placed on the rehabilitation of proprioception and dynamic function of the head and neck (Heikkila and Astrom, 1996).

If the cervical spine is immobilized in a collar, the afferent input from type I and II mechanoreceptors influences postural and kinaesthetic sense, so that the subject may find control of balance more difficult. Kinaesthetic sense is reduced in chronic whiplash-associated disorders (Jull, 2001). Postural sensation is not totally dependent on joint mechanoreceptors: cutaneous and myotatic (muscle spindle) mechanoreceptors also have a role in maintenance of posture (Wyke, 1981).

Degenerative disease that affects type IV mechanoreceptors will produce pain and abnormal patterns of muscle reflexes and also have reflexogenic effects on the respiratory and cardiovascular system.

During the ageing process, in the peripheral nerves there is a greater degeneration of the myelinated large diameter afferent mechanoreceptor neurons than the smaller pain fibres. Elderly people have a decreased pain tolerance, and it has been suggested that this may be due to the decrease in inhibitory effect of the large fibre mechanoreceptors on the dorsal horn gate mechanism (see pp. 253–254). Afferent impulses from touch and pressure receptors are conveyed by group II large diameter fibres. These fast conducting fibres are also affected by degenerative disease. Wyke (1976) believes that mechanoreceptor depletion occurs in paravertebral zones of increased sensitivity. This may be a mechanism through which such local areas of tenderness occur.

SOURCES OF PAIN

The International Association for the Study of Pain has defined pain as 'an unpleasant sensory and emotional experience associated with actual or potential damage, or described in terms of such damage' (International Association for the Study of Pain, 1986). It is important to acknowledge the term 'emotional experience' as there is increasing evidence that psychosocial factors (e.g. childhood experiences, job satisfaction) are a significant factor in chronic pain syndrome and responses to treatment.

Pain arising from the different structures in the spine varies in quality, distribution and behaviour. When assessing a patient, skilful questioning and careful listening are essential if the therapist is to develop sound clinical reasoning and the ability to understand and interpret the nature of the patient's pain.

Joint pain

The apophyseal joint capsule has both encapsulated nerve endings and free nerve endings. The free nerve endings are thought to be nociceptive. A number of experiments have shown that noxious stimulation of the apophyseal joints induces both local and referred pain in subjects (McCall et al, 1979; Marks et al, 1992). Pain arising from spinal joints is often unilateral and described as a deep diffuse ache.

Joint pain may result from an injury that causes inflammation, mechanical stress or the degenerative changes that occur with maturation of the bone. Irritation of the mechanical and chemical nociceptors in the synovial joint capsules and the innervated connective tissue of the interbody joints concurrently involved is probably a source of joint pain (Grieve, 1988, p. 314).

Small myelinated and unmyelinated nerve fibres in the epiphyseal and metaphyseal regions wind around the trabeculae and spread out on the undersurface of the articular cartilage. Compressive forces causing pressure on these plexuses may be a factor in the production of joint pain, as may engorgement of vessels in the subchondral bone. The articular cartilage of the apophyseal joints is subjected to considerable stress from repetitive loading, and different patterns of loading have been shown to increase the stress on the lumbar apophyseal joints. In lumbar hyperextension, the load between the facets and the laminae of the subjacent vertebra may exceed the joint loading capacity so that early degenerative changes may occur in the joint (Yang and King, 1984). Degenerative changes in the apophyseal joints with destruction of the articular cartilage and osteoarthritis have been attributed as a cause of spinal pain (Bough et al, 1990).

Ligamentous pain

Ligaments are rich in nociceptors that may be stimulated by mechanical stresses or chemical irritation. Various postures, positions and activities can cause an excessive stretching or deformation of the ligaments that creates a build-up of strain energy within the nerve endings embedded in the ligament. The nociceptive nerve endings are activated by mechanical stress.

Injury and degenerative changes in the joint tissues result in chemical substances being released from the affected cells. These chemical irritants diffuse into the ligaments and activate the nociceptive nerve endings.

Muscle pain

Skeletal muscle contains a large population of small myelinated and unmyelinated nerve fibres that are distributed in a plexiform network around all vessels except capillaries and respond to mechanical and chemical irritants (Mills et al, 1984). Pain from a muscle is often secondary to a variety of mechanical sources such as excessive strain of a muscle, rupture of a muscle, muscle spasm, contusions and overuse of a muscle. These factors cause biochemical changes within the muscle that are more likely to cause the pain rather than the physical disruption of the tissue itself. Muscle injuries heal by repair (scar tissue formation) rather than regeneration (Noonan and Garrett, 1992). A repaired tissue may produce an altered barrage of sensory impulses, thereby having an influence on maintenance of pain and sensitivity (Thacker, 1998).

The build-up of chemical irritants, in particular lactic acid, 5-hydroxytryptamine, bradykinin and histamine, may produce pain. Mechanical distortion of enlarged vessels in a muscle will also irritate the nociceptors of the vessel walls. Pain may also arise from the release of neuropeptides into the muscle and the accumulation of noxious chemicals when there is ischaemia.

In a normal individual, prolonged isometric contraction or repeated contractions of a muscle may cause pain, and it will be more readily felt if the person is untrained or elderly. Muscles subjected to prolonged postural stress are liable to fatigue so that pain is produced.

The relationship between pain, spasm and tenderness is complex. Pain may arise from local joint pathology rather than the muscle overlying the lesion. Both pain and muscle tenderness may be referred, and hypertonus of a muscle does not always cause pain. Muscle pain and tenderness can occur in lesions involving segmentally related viscera.

A trigger point is a hyperirritable spot within a taut band of skeletal muscle or fascia. Trigger points are characteristically painful on compression and some authors believe that they can give rise to referred pain and autonomic phenomena (Simons, 1987). There is growing evidence that trigger points are an epiphenomenon, and that they develop as a result of pain rather than being the originator of it (Cohen, 1996). Trigger points may therefore be secondary areas of hyperalgesia that do not have any significant physiological changes.

Vascular pain

Pain may be caused by arterial pressure or venous congestion. Pain that is rhythmical, surging, pounding or beating is associated with arterial pressure. Mechanoreceptors in the plexiform nervous network around the vessel walls are stimulated by vascular pulsation. They fire at the beginning or ending of movement, thereby giving rise to a throbbing sensation rather than continuous pain.

Inflammation of the soft tissues of the vertebral column is associated with venous congestion and pain may develop due to mechanical or chemical irritants. Mechanical stress of mechanoreceptors in the joint capsule or ligaments may cause pain, as will the formation of metabolites during tissue breakdown.

Arterial stenosis affecting the aortic, femoral and iliac vessels may cause low back pain and leg symptoms. The site of the stenosis affects the area of the back, buttock, thigh or lower leg where the symptoms may be referred (Szlavy and Taveras, 1995). Pain arises from the ischaemia that develops in the area distal to the stenotic lesion. Symptoms are further aggravated when the demands of muscular activity exceed the ability of the arterial flow to oxygenate the area (Laslett, 2000).

Nerve root (radicular) pain

The nerve root is often a source of pain in spinal pain syndromes. Maturation of the spine or diseases that cause intervertebral disc disorders, facet arthrosis with osteophytosis and segmental instability are all associated with nerve root pain. Pain can be caused by mechanical irritation (compression, traction) or chemical irritation of a spinal nerve (Rydevik and Garfin, 1989).

Compression or tension of a healthy nerve does not necessarily give rise to pain (Lindahl, 1966; Garfin et al, 1991), but mechanical stress placed on a nerve that is already injured produces pain (Smyth and Wright, 1958). Biochemical reactions of the inflammatory processes sensitize the nerve root so that root symptoms arise when the nerve is subjected to mechanical stress.

Experimental studies have shown that a homogenate of the nucleus pulposus acts as a chemical irritant to the nerve root with a resultant inflammatory reaction that can lead to fibrosis (McCarron et al, 1987). Inflammation or fibrosis of the nerve can cause a physical impediment to the passage of nutrients from the CSF through the membrane of the nerve. This sequence of events creates ischaemia of the nerve root complex and adversely affects normal nutrition of the nerve. Ischaemia of the nerve root and the lack of essential nutrients may result in minor damage of the axons. When an axon is damaged, the chemical reactions alter the electrical activity of the nerve root. The depolarization threshold of the nerve is reduced so that mechanical stresses that would not normally produce pain initiate a nociceptive response.

Fibrosis of the nerve root and its protective sheath can reduce its relative mobility in the nerve root canal so that it is vulnerable to certain normal and abnormal mechanical forces (see Ch. 8).

Compression of a nerve root alters its conduction capabilities and the pain may be accompanied by paraesthesiae. Clinical tests are routinely used to identify neurological involvement. Evidence of altered skin sensation, reduced muscle power or muscle wasting and absent or diminished reflexes all indicate the possibility of nerve compression.

Chemical irritation can increase the mechanical sensitivity of a nerve root. A number of clinical tests are used to evaluate the ability of the nerve root to withstand mechanical stress. The straight leg raise test is such an example. It assesses the mechanosensitivity of the lumbosacral nerve roots (see p. 282–284).

Acute nerve root pain is severe and is often described as sickening, lancinating or burning. It is generally worse distally and its distribution is clearly demarcated within the dermatome of the affected nerve root (see Figs 7.9, 7.10).

There may be a latent period to nerve root pain so that pain surges into the affected limb some seconds after the causative movement has been performed. These symptoms are usually highly irritable and great care must be taken when handling a patient with nerve root pain to ensure that the pain is not exacerbated. Two theories have been proposed to explain latency (Grieve, 1988, p. 318):

1. Compression of the nerve selectively affects fibres of different diameters, thereby influencing their rates of conduction recovery and nociceptor impulse reactivity.

2. Spinal or limb movements may displace tissue exudates into surrounding tissues, thereby causing more mechanical or chemical irritation.

Bone pain

Bone pain is often described as having an unpleasant deep throbbing quality. It may be caused by:

1. Neoplasm – primary or secondary
2. Intrinsic bone disease, e.g. Paget's disease
3. Fractures – particularly stress fractures of the spine secondary to osteoporosis
4. Venous engorgement of the vertebral veins
5. Osteomyelitis.

There is no evidence that osteophytosis and bone cysts can by themselves create pain (Harkness et al, 1984).

Disc pain

The outer annular fibres of the intervertebral disc contain free nerve endings (Bogduk et al, 1981) and the disc can be a primary source of pain (Weinstein et al, 1988). Chemical or mechanical irritation of the free nerve endings within the annular fibres may give rise to discogenic pain, which has a different quality to joint, nerve and ligamentous pain. Discogenic pain is often described as deep, nauseating and wearing. It may be bilateral but is usually unilateral and spreads across the low back and into the buttock area. The pain may extend into the upper lateral thigh and even into the anterior abdomen. Clinical trials have shown that mechanical stimulation of the outer posterior annular fibres produces low back pain (Kuslich et al, 1991).

Dorsal root ganglion pain

The dorsal root ganglion is supplied by the nervi nervorum. These nerves are mechanically sensitive nociceptors. Unlike the nerve roots, the dorsal root ganglion is sensitive to mechanical pressure even in the absence of chemical irritation (Porterfield and DeRosa, 1998). The dorsal root ganglion is vulnerable to mechanical trespass from herniated discs and osteophytes in the intervertebral foramen.

PAIN MECHANISMS

Pain is perceived as a result of the activation of specific neural pathways.

Three systems interact to produce and control pain:

1. The *sensory* system (discriminative) processes information regarding the strength, quality, intensity and location of the pain.
2. The *motivational* system (affective) determines the individual's conditioned response to pain so that there is an emotional response to every type of pain.
3. The *cognitive* (evaluative) system determines the individual's interpretation of appropriate responses to pain.

An individual's expression of pain is highly subjective and is influenced by a number of factors such as prior experience of pain, the nature of the stimulus and the context within which the noxious stimulus occurs, cultural background and gender. The perception of pain is also affected by an individual's emotional state. Response to pain varies from person to person.

The *pain threshold* is the lowest intensity of noxious stimulation at which a subject perceives pain. Experiments using stimuli such as radiant heat, electric shock and mechanical pressure have demonstrated that the pain perception threshold is fairly constant from individual to individual (Bowsher, 1988). The pain threshold does not vary in the same individual over a period of time. *Pain tolerance* is the greatest intensity of noxious stimulation an individual can tolerate before a response occurs. Pain tolerance varies greatly between individuals and in the same individual over a period of time. Factors such as stress, anger, fatigue, repeated exposure to pain and sleep deprivation can decrease pain tolerance in an individual.

The three areas of the nervous system that are involved in the generation and perception of pain are the afferent pathways (input mechanisms), the central nervous system (central mechanisms) and efferent pathways (output mechanisms).

AFFERENT PAIN PATHWAYS

There are three types of nerve fibres: A, B and C. The velocity of impulses conducted in nerve fibres is directly related to the fibre diameter: the thicker the fibre, the faster the conduction velocity. Group A fibres are myelinated and subdivided into four groups (alpha, beta, gamma, delta) with decreasing diameters and conduction velocities. Group B fibres are unmyelinated postganglionic autonomic fibres. Group C fibres are unmyelinated efferent autonomic fibres and somatic and visceral afferent fibres.

The fibres involved in perception of pain are A delta, C, and A beta fibres.

A delta nociceptors

A delta nociceptors are unmyelinated neurons that are distributed mainly in the skin, although small numbers have been located in joints and muscle. They are sensitive to high intensity mechanical stimuli and noxious temperatures. They carry impulses at an average of 15 m/s and produce sharp, pricking localized pain.

C polymodal nociceptors

C polymodal nociceptors are unmyelinated and are found in the deep layers of the skin and most tissues of the body. They remain silent unless activated by noxious stimuli and are sensitive to mechanical, thermal and chemical stimuli. They are not sensitive to different forms of energy, but to a factor common to damaged tissue, however the damage is caused. Impulses are conducted along the polymodal nociceptors at a rate of 1 m/s and reproduce a dull, aching, diffuse pain.

Following a noxious stimulus, e.g. pinching, two types of pain are normally experienced. The initial sharp pain is due to stimulation of the faster conducting A delta fibres, and the aching which develops a few seconds later is transmitted by the slower conducting C fibres.

The cell bodies of the A delta and C nociceptors are in the spinal root of the trigeminal nerve ganglia. The proximal ends of the A delta axons and 70% of the C polymodal axons enter the central nervous system through the dorsal roots. The remaining 30% of the C polymodal axons double back to the mixed nerve and enter the spinal cord through the ventral root. This arrangement partly explains why dorsal rhizotomy (cutting of the dorsal root) does not relieve pain completely.

A delta and C fibres are facilitatory to the input of pain transmission at the substantia gelatinosa.

A beta neurons

A beta neurons are large fibre, low threshold cutaneous mechanoreceptors. They carry impulses at 30 m/s and have a low threshold to noxious stimuli, a low threshold to electrical stimulation and a high threshold to chemicals. They are inhibitory to the input transmission at the substantia gelatinosa.

PERIPHERAL SENSITIZATION

The gate control theory of pain was proposed by Melzack and Wall in 1965 and has been the focus of wide-ranging research. It is known that pain perception occurs not only as a result of tissue damage but that psychosocial and environmental factors are also influential. Tissue damage triggers peripheral nociceptors, creating complex neural interactions in the nervous system. Impulses are modified by ascending pathways to the brain and by descending pain-suppressing systems which are activated by various environmental and psychological factors.

Many tissues have large numbers of nociceptors that remain silent under normal conditions. Nociceptors are found in skin, joints and muscle tissue, but their presence has not been demonstrated in muscle tissue (Mense, 1966). These nociceptors are activated when an injury occurs, the resultant tissue damage causes a release of chemical mediators and there is consequent tissue hypoxia (Schmidt, 1996). Nociceptors are activated by a variety of chemical mediators associated with the inflammatory state. These include potassium (from damaged cells), serotonin (from platelets), histamine (released from mast cells) and bradykinin (a peptide activated from a precursor in plasma). Activation of the nociceptors increases their sensitization so that they exhibit increased spontaneous discharge rates, reduced discharge thresholds and increased discharged rates in response to stimulation. Certain chemical mediators also increase the sensitivity of the nociceptors, making them more readily stimulated. These include prostaglandins, leukotrienes (released from damaged tissue and/or stimulated by bradykinin) and substance P (released from active nociceptive endings).

Nociceptor sensitivity is also influenced by the pH of the surrounding tissues. In inflammatory states, the high local proton concentrations cause a reduction in pH and this contributes to the sensitization of the polymodal nociceptors. Combinations of altered pH and chemical mediators are more influential in sensitizing nociceptors than chemical mediators on their own (Handwerker and Reeh, 1991).

Once the nociceptors have been activated by chemical changes associated with inflammation they become sensitized, so that activities such as gentle movements, gentle pressure and sustained postures that do not normally cause discomfort activate the system and trigger pain perception. The term *hyperalgesia* is used to describe an exaggerated or increased response to a noxious stimulus. The term *allodynia* is used to describe the phenomenon of pain produced by a stimulus that would not normally be painful (International Association for the Study of Pain, 1986).

CENTRAL SENSITIZATION

Following an injury there is activity in the peripheral nociceptors, with an increase in discharge of the unmyelinated sensory afferent neurons and a resultant increased input into the dorsal horn of the spinal cord. In the dorsal horn, a number of chemicals are released from the presynaptic terminals of the nociceptive afferents (excitatory amino acids, neuropeptides, neurokinin A) and these initiate a cascade of changes in the postsynaptic neurons (Duggan et al, 1990). The release of these chemicals causes complex molecular changes that increase the synaptic efficacy and neuronal excitability of the dorsal horn cells.

The sensitization of the dorsal horn cells has a number of effects. Dorsal horn neurons that normally only respond to input from nociceptors may start to respond to input from other fibre types. Consequently, a non-noxious stimulus such as light touch, which increases activity in A beta fibres, may stimulate the sensitized neurons in the dorsal horn that ascend to areas in the brain to produce pain sensation (Woolf and Doubell, 1994). The input from the A beta fibres can come from undamaged tissues so that even gentle movement and light touch can produce pain. This phenomenon is known as *secondary hyperalgesia* and can give false positive information when carrying out clinical pain provocation or 'differentiation' tests (Gifford, 1997).

When sensitized, the dorsal horn cells fire more impulses and continue to fire after the peripheral stimulus stops. If the peripheral stimulus is repeatedly applied, the sensitized cells fire even more each time. This effect is known as wind-up (Dubner and Ruda, 1992). The dorsal horn cells have a physical connection to thousands of neurons but many of these connections are inactive under normal conditions. Increased sensitivity of the dorsal horn cells enlarges their receptive fields, so that many of the connections that were sub-threshold become activated.

The altered neuronal activity is likely to influence activity in other neuronal pools with which the central nociceptive neurons make synaptic connections. Hence, changes in function of the motor and autonomic nervous systems often accompany musculoskeletal pain states (Wright, 1999).

PAIN MEMORY

It is proposed that an important factor in the ongoing nature of chronic pain is that repeated or continual nociceptive input into the central nervous system may leave a somatosensory memory or imprint (Katz and Melzack, 1990; Basbaum, 1996; Melzack, 1996). This does not imply that there is no organic basis for chronic pain, but rather there is a physiological mechanism for perpetuating pain within the central nervous system itself.

MOTOR DYSFUNCTION

Changes in sensorimotor function occur when the spinal cord neurons become hyperactive. Central sensitization is associated with facilitation of flexor withdrawal responses (Woolf, 1984). Pain may also influence the excitability of gamma motor neurons so that muscle tension and spasm are increased.

Johansson and Sojka (1991) propose that when pain affects the excitability of the gamma motor neurons a vicious cycle develops which generates pain and muscle spasm. Stimulation of the nociceptive afferents from muscles excites dynamic and static fusimotor neurons that increase the sensitivity of primary and secondary muscle spindle afferents. Increased activity in the muscle spindle afferents increases muscle stiffness; the increased muscle stiffness results in metabolite production with a consequent further increase in muscle stiffness. Additionally, increased activity in the secondary spindle afferents excites the gamma system, so that muscle stiffness is enhanced further.

REFERRED PAIN

Referred pain may be defined as: 'Pain felt at a site other than that of tissue damage'. The concept of referred pain is recognized and it is essential that the therapist is aware that the area of pain described by a patient is not necessarily the source of the pain. Pain may be referred from the spine to the periphery; from the periphery more peripherally or centrally; from the viscera to the spine; or from the spine to the viscera.

Two mechanisms have been described (Wells et al, 1994) to provide a basis for the understanding of referred pain:

1. Bifurcated axons have been identified in peripheral sensory nerves (Taylor et al, 1984). These axons have been shown to have sensory units in which one branch supplies the skin and another branch supplies muscle or some other sensory structure (Fig. 7.5). Bifurcated axons have a single cell body in a dorsal root ganglion and a single proximal axon travelling to the spinal cord from the ganglion cell.

2. The second mechanism is based on the convergence of separate peripheral sensory nerves on the same cell in the spinal cord. Therefore, nociceptors from viscera travelling to the spinal cord in sympathetic or splanchnic nerves end on the same dorsal horn cells as the nociceptors coming from the skin travelling in somatic nerves. The central cell may be more used to receiving input via one of the peripheral neurons and may interpret input from the normally less active neuron as coming from the normally more active neuron (Fig. 7.6).

Three types of referred pain are commonly recognized: somatic referred, visceral referred and radicular pain.

Figure 7.5 Referred pain due to branched sensory neurons. The primary afferent shown has branches supplying both heart and arm. (From Wells PE, Frampton V, Bowsher D 1987 *Pain: Management and Control in Physiotherapy.* Heinemann Medical Books, London, with permission.)

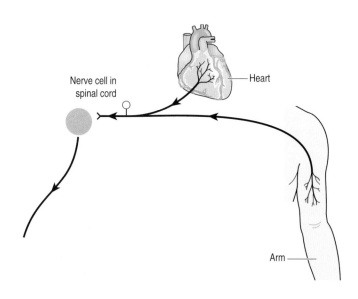

Nerve cell in spinal cord

Heart

Arm

Figure 7.6   Referred pain due to convergence. The nerve cell in the spinal cord receives input from two different peripheral neurons, one supplying the arm, the other the heart. Since the central cell is more 'used' to getting input from the arm, input from the heart may be interpreted as coming from the arm. (From Wells PE, Frampton V, Bowsher D 1987 *Pain: Management and Control in Physiotherapy.* Heinemann Medical Books, London, with permission.)

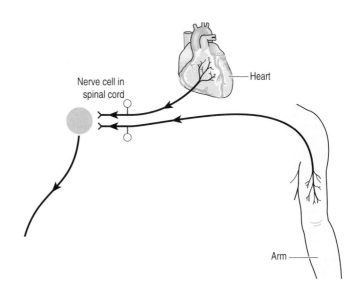

SOMATIC REFERRED PAIN

Pain can be referred from a somatic structure and felt at a location some distance from the site of origin of the pain. Noxious stimulation of non-nervous tissues in the spine may give rise to referred pain, which may be felt around the chest wall or radiating into the limbs.

Lumbar somatic referred pain

Noxious stimulation of the interspinous structures and back muscles by injecting saline into these tissues reproduces not only back pain but also referred pain and tenderness in the lower limbs (Kellgren, 1939; Feinstein et al, 1954; Hockaday and Whitty, 1967).

Attempts have been made to define specific areas of segmentally referred somatic pain, similar to the dermatomes used in the diagnosis of segmental level of nerve root compression. Segmental areas of somatic innervation have been termed sclerotomes (Inman and Saunders, 1944). Clinically, it would be useful if such information was validated, but the value of sclerotomes in determining the level of a lesion is strictly limited. In each individual there is considerable overlap in the area of referred pain from specific segments. Between different individuals there is considerable variation in the segmental pattern of referred pain (Bogduk, 1980). However, in a single subject, when the same segment is repeatedly stimulated, the area of referral of pain is consistently the same.

Somatic referred pain from the lumbar spine is most commonly experienced over the buttock area, but it may extend as far as the foot; the intensity of the stimulus is proportional to the distance of referral of pain in the leg (Mooney and Robertson, 1976). An important feature of somatic referred pain is its quality, which is often described as a deep, diffuse ache. It differs from radicular pain, which has a sharper, lancinating quality and is clearly demarcated within the dermatome of the affected nerve.

Experimental evidence has shown that the lumbar apophyseal joints may also be implicated in the production of referred pain. Noxious stimulation of the lumbar apophyseal joints has been shown to refer pain to the buttocks, groin and lower limbs (McCall et al, 1979; Fig. 7.7). Equally, in some patients, the introduction of an anaesthetizing injection into a local symptomatic apophyseal joint lesion relieves referred pain (Carrera, 1980).

The anterior dura mater is innervated and hence sensitive to pain. Traction of the dura mater can produce buttock and thigh pain (Smyth and Wright, 1958).

Thoracic somatic referred pain

The diagnosis of chest pain poses many difficulties because the pain may be of visceral or neuromusculoskeletal origin. Chest pain can be caused by pleurisy, cardiac ischaemia and disorders of the gallbladder, pancreas, oesophagus and diaphragm. Pain referred around the chest wall can also arise from a spinal or rib lesion, and this may mimic visceral disease. Potentially life-threatening diseases of the viscera must be excluded as a source of pain, but the therapist must remain aware that chest wall pain may be skeletal or somatic in origin.

Experimental noxious stimulation of thoracic interspinous structures reproduces somatic referred pain to the anterior, lateral and posterior

Figure 7.7 Areas of pain referral from lumbar apophyseal joints. A and B, Distribution of pain referral from intracapsular injections of saline solution at L1/2. C and D, Distribution of pain referral from intracapsular injections of saline solution at L4/5. (From McCall IW, Park WM, O'Brien JP 1979 Induced pain referral from posterior lumbar elements in normal subjects. *Spine* 44: 441, with permission.)

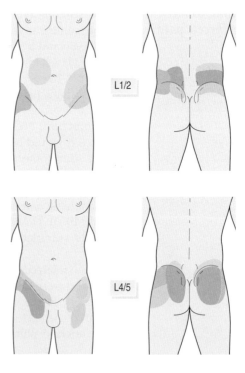

aspects of the chest wall (Kellgren, 1939; Feinstein et al, 1954; Fig. 7.8). Although there is no consistent area of referred pain from a particular segment, stimulation of the higher thoracic levels tends to refer pain to the higher parts of the chest wall. However, stimulation of a particular level may produce referred pain above or below that particular segment so that segmental level of a lesion cannot be identified from the area of referral of pain.

There has been insufficient research on pain and innervation patterns in the thoracic spine. The role of the thoracic apophyseal, costovertebral and costotransverse joints in the production of referred pain has not been verified. It is likely that the same mechanism occurs in the thoracic spine as in other areas, and future experiments on the thoracic vertebral joints may demonstrate that they are a source of referred pain.

Cervical somatic referred pain

Somatic referred pain from the cervical spine may be distributed in the head, upper chest wall (anterior, posterior or both) or upper limb. Noxious stimulation of the interspinous ligaments and muscles in

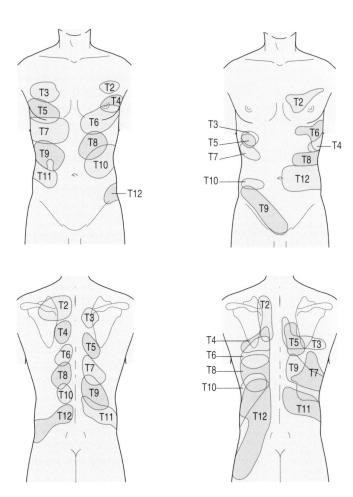

Figure 7.8 Thoracic referred pain. Shaded areas show the distribution of referred pain reported by normal volunteers after stimulation of interspinous structures at the segmental levels indicated. The figures on the left are based on the data of Kellgren (1939), those on the right are based on the data of Feinstein et al (1954). Note the differences in the distribution of pain in the two sets of figures and the extensive overlap in distribution in the figures on the right. (From Grant R, ed. 1994 *Physical Therapy of the Cervical and Thoracic Spine*, 2nd edn. Churchill Livingstone, Edinburgh, p. 85, Fig. 5.3, with permission.)

the cervical spine produces referred pain. Stimulation of the upper cervical levels (C1–3) can produce referred pain in the head and occipital area (Bogduk, 1988). Stimulation of structures innervated by C4 can cause pain in the occipital region, but stimulation of C4 and below has not been shown to cause pain in the forehead. Pain in the upper limb has been produced by stimulation of the lower cervical levels (C5–T1), while shoulder pain can be reproduced by stimulation of any level from C1 to C8 (Kellgren, 1939; Feinstein et al, 1954). Pain referred to the chest wall from the cervical spine may mimic angina.

As in other spinal regions, noxious stimulation of the interspinous spaces produces considerable overlap in the area of segmental referral of pain. There is also inconsistency in the location of pain between different subjects so that the area of referral of pain from noxious stimulation of somatic structures is not diagnostic of the affected level. Nevertheless, shoulder pain can arise from any level in the cervical spine, and the neck should be carefully examined in those patients presenting with shoulder pain.

The cervical apophyseal joints are a source of referred pain. The introduction of a local anaesthetic into the joint of patients with local apophyseal joint lesions relieved both joint and referred pain (Bogduk and Marsland, 1986; Hildebrandt and Argykaris, 1986). Experimental stimulation of cervical apophyseal joints has shown that particular segmental levels are consistently associated with characteristic patterns of referred pain (Dwyer et al, 1990) and that these patterns were found to be reliable in determining the segmental location of a symptomatic cervical apophyseal joint (Aprill et al, 1990).

Noxious stimulation of the cervical discs by electrical and mechanical means produced pain over the posterior chest wall and scapular region (Cloward, 1959). Hence, the disc can be a source of both local and referred pain (see pp. 82–84).

VISCERAL REFERRED PAIN

Visceral disease can produce pain that mimics a vertebral joint disorder. This phenomenon of referred pain is thought to be due to somatovisceral convergence, where separate nociceptors from skin and viscera converge on the same dorsal horn cells in the spinal cord. Distension, traction and, in some instances, strong contractions of a viscus may produce pain. True visceral pain from a pathological condition affecting a viscus is often difficult for the patient to localize due to the relative paucity of nerve endings. The pain may be dull, vague, cramping or stabbing, overlying the general area of the viscus.

Noxious stimulation of a viscus may produce an area of cutaneous pain that is tender to touch. This may be accompanied by cutaneous vasoconstriction and increased tone in the overlying muscles (Keele and Neil, 1971). The areas of skin on the chest wall which have the same segmental innervation as a particular viscus are termed *zones of secondary hyperalgesia*. These zones are more commonly found in acute or subacute visceral disease than in the chronic stage of visceral disease (Kunert, 1965).

Experimental stimulation of a viscus produced spasm of spinal muscles in two or three segments on the same side of the vertebral column and innervated by the same segments (Elbe, 1960). The extent of the increased tone in the vertebral segments is proportional to the intensity of the stimulus, and this irritability may spread to the contralateral side.

There is no evidence that lesions of the vertebral column can cause visceral disease, but some philosophies believe that the state of the vertebral column has a bearing on the functional status of the internal organs (Kunert, 1965; Stoddard, 1983). At present, there is no evidence to suggest that treating the spine and soft tissues can alter function of the internal organs; in clinical practice, the prime reason for treatment of the vertebral column must be treatment of a musculoskeletal disorder.

RADICULAR PAIN

Mechanical compression or chemical irritation of a nerve root is a source of referred pain. The emphasis on nerve root pain has been so great that it has been largely overlooked that somatic referred pain is an integral part of some spinal pain syndromes. Grieve (1981) states that 'all root pain is referred pain, but not all referred pain is root pain', and this is vital to our understanding of spinal pain syndromes.

Mechanical compression of a nerve root does not selectively affect the nociceptive fibres alone (Bogduk, 1987). The large diameter fibres that convey touch, vibration and proprioception are simultaneously affected and give rise to the signs and symptoms of large diameter fibre compression. Compression blocks conduction in the axons, so that true radicular pain is accompanied by particular clinical features: numbness and paraesthesiae, muscle weakness and altered reflexes. Referred pain that is not accompanied by objective neurological signs is unlikely to be due to nerve root compression.

Paraesthesiae occur as a result of ischaemia of nerves. Paraesthesiae in the presence of nerve root compression are likely to be due to compression of radicular vessels rather than compression of the nerve root itself.

Mechanical irritation of a spinal nerve cannot selectively affect those axons that innervate the vertebral column and not those supplying the limbs. Therefore, root compression is unlikely to be the pathological mechanism in patients who have local spinal pain with no area of referred pain and in the absence of neurological signs.

The 1st and 2nd cervical spinal nerve roots do not run in intervertebral foramina and do not have any structural relations that make them susceptible to trespass (Bogduk, 1988, p. 10), so compression of these roots is unlikely to be a source of upper cervical pain. At all other levels of the spine, the nerve roots lie within the intervertebral foramen and are vulnerable to compression and subsequent radicular pain with associated neurological signs. Radicular pain has a definite quality. It is described as sharp, lancinating and throbbing and follows the area innervated by the particular nerve root (Figs 7.9, 7.10). In this way, it differs from the diffuse aching of somatic referred pain.

PERIPHERAL NEUROPATHIC PAIN

The term 'peripheral neuropathic pain' is used to describe the combination of signs and symptoms in patients whose pain is due to pathological changes or dysfunction in peripheral nerves or nerve roots (Devor and Rappaport, 1989). The symptoms of peripheral neuropathic pain are categorized as negative or positive. Positive symptoms include pain,

Figure 7.9 Areas of referred pain. Dermatome charts based on areas of referred pain found in most patients who present with nerve root involvement. Variations of areas of overlap may occur when there are anomalies of the nerve supply.

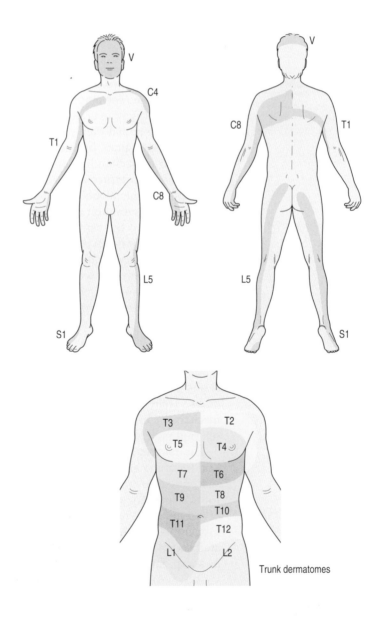

Trunk dermatomes

Figure 7.10   Areas of referred pain. Dermatome charts based on areas of referred pain found in most patients who present with nerve root involvement. Variations of areas of overlap may occur when there are anomalies of the nerve supply.

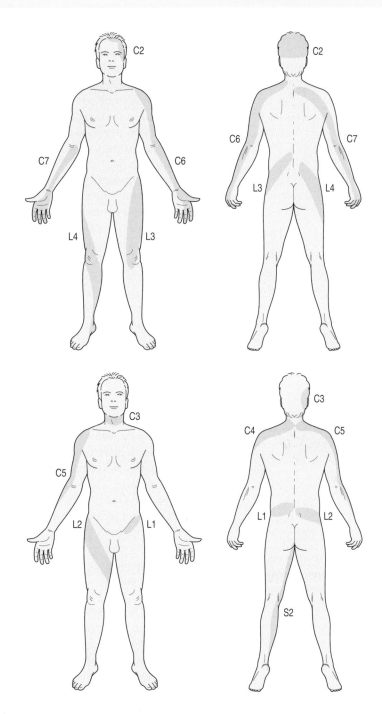

paraesthesiae and spasm; negative symptoms are anaesthesia (negative sensory) and muscle weakness (negative motor).

Two types of peripheral neuropathic pain are described: dysaesthetic pain and nerve trunk pain (Asbury and Fields, 1984). Dysaesthetic pain is felt in the peripheral sensory distribution of a sensory or mixed nerve. It is caused by impulses arising in damaged or regenerating nociceptive afferent fibres. Dysaesthetic pain has some characteristics that are not found in the deep pain of visceral or somatic pain. Features of dysaesthetic pain may include the presence of allodynia, paroxysmal shooting or stabbing, a burning or electric quality and pain in the area of the sensory deficit (Devor, 1991).

Nerve trunk pain is pain that follows the course of the nerve trunk. It is described as deep and aching or like toothache. This type of pain is aggravated by palpation, movement or stretch of the nerve trunk (Asbury and Fields, 1984). Nerve trunk pain is attributed to increased activity in mechanically or chemically sensitized nociceptors within the nerve sheaths. The nervi nervorum are afferents found within the connective tissue of the nerve trunks and they are normally capable of a mechanoreceptor function. Some of the nervi nervorum are sensitive to noxious mechanical, chemical and thermal stimuli and therefore have a nociceptive function (Bove and Light, 1995). Experimental studies have shown that the nervi nervorum are not sensitive to stretch within normal ranges of movement but they are sensitive to excessive longitudinal stretch along the entire length of the nerve and local stretch in any direction due to focal pressure (Bove and Light, 1997). Clinical studies have supported laboratory studies and shown that nerve trunks are insensitive to non-noxious mechanical deformation (Hall and Quintner, 1996).

COMBINED STATES

In many instances, particularly in the more degenerate spine, a patient's symptoms may be due to the involvement of a number of different tissues, so that both referred somatic pain and radicular pain may be present. For example, osteoarthritic changes in an apophyseal joint may be intrinsically painful and, with overriding facets or osteophytic growths, the nerve root in front of the joint may also be compressed. The patient may then present with a combination of local spinal pain, referred somatic pain, radicular pain and neurological signs.

AUTONOMIC NERVOUS SYSTEM

The peripheral nervous system consists of two systems, the autonomic and the somatic, that function as an integrated whole. The autonomic nervous system is principally concerned with the innervation of viscera, glands, the muscular walls of blood vessels and unstriated muscle, while the somatic nervous system innervates the skin, skeletal muscles and their tendons, joints and connective tissues. However, there is some overlap as autonomic fibres are present within the sinuvertebral nerve, which innervates structures within the spinal canal including the posterior longitudinal ligament and the annular fibres of the intervertebral discs (Bogduk et al, 1981; O'Brien, 1984).

The somatic and autonomic systems have nerve tracts within the spinal cord that run to and from the brain, and each spinal nerve contains both autonomic and somatic fibres. Activity of the sympathetic nervous system is a component in many severe and chronic pain states (Stanton-Hicks et al, 1995; Janig and Stanton Hicks, 1996).

The autonomic nervous system can be subdivided into the sympathetic (SNS) and parasympathetic (PNS) nervous systems. Both these systems are connected to the central nervous system by two neurons in series. Axons leave the central nervous system and synapse with a second neuron. Ganglia are collections of cell bodies of the second neurons. Axons conveying information from the central nervous system to the ganglia are called *preganglionic axons*, and axons from the ganglia travelling to the peripheral target organ are called *postganglionic axons*. In the sympathetic nervous system the ratio of preganglionic fibres to postganglionic fibres is 1:10, whereas in the parasympathetic nervous system the ratio is about 1:3. Hence, sympathetic reactions are more widespread and diffuse and a small stimulus has the potential to cause a greater response.

A major difference between the two systems is that the parasympathetic ganglia lie close to the target organ, while sympathetic ganglia lie some distance away, so that the parasympathetic postganglionic fibres are short while sympathetic postganglionic fibres are longer.

In both systems the transmission of impulses at the *synapses* between the pre- and postganglionic neurons is accomplished by the release of acetylcholine. At the *terminals* of postganglionic fibres in the sympathetic nervous system, the transmitter substance is usually norepinephrine, a catecholamine; in the parasympathetic nervous system it is acetylcholine. In the sympathetic nervous system the action of norepinephrine is terminated by reuptake of the transmitter substance by the nerve terminal. Additionally, some of the norepinephrine escapes reuptake and enters into the circulation so that sympathetic effects are spread. At the parasympathetic terminals acetylcholine is terminated by enzyme activity. These differences between the sympathetic and parasympathetic nervous systems mean that sympathetic actions are more widespread and enduring.

The adrenal medulla is innervated by preganglionic sympathetic fibres. Stimulation of the adrenal medulla by these fibres causes it to release epinephrine, which results in a general body reaction due to the circulating catecholamine. Reactions can include raised blood pressure and pulse rate, and an altered emotional state such as fear, anxiety, anger or stress.

The sympathetic nervous system is the larger subdivision of the autonomic nervous system. It can have the following effects:

- Stimulation of the sinuatrial node of the heart, thereby increasing heart rate
- Direct stimulation of cardiac muscle to increase the power of cardiac contraction

Continues

Continued

- Relaxation of smooth muscle of the alimentary tract
- Stimulation of sphincters to contract
- Relaxation of smooth muscles of the bronchi
- Acting on α-receptors, it contracts the smooth muscle of arterioles resulting in vasoconstriction
- Acting on β-receptors, sympathetic nerves cause vasodilatation
- Dilatation of the pupil
- Erection of the hairs on the skin and sweating

Broadly, the functions of the sympathetic nervous system are concerned with preparing the body for 'fight, flight, and fright' and diverting blood supply to essential areas. An increase in sympathetic activity also occurs during physiological stress (e.g. pain, fear, extreme temperature, severe muscle work). The parasympathetic nervous system has the opposite effects:

- Slowing sinuatrial node, thereby reducing heart rate
- Contraction of bronchial smooth muscle
- Contraction of smooth muscle of the alimentary canal
- Relaxation of sphincters
- Increase in secretion of salivary and lacrimal glands
- Constriction of pupil and accommodation of the lens
- Increase in mucus secretion in the respiratory system
- Acid secretion in the alimentary canal
- Vasodilatation of the internal and external carotid circulation

The parasympathetic system helps to conserve the energy resources of the body and it is the effector for visceral motor systems.

SYMPATHETIC NERVOUS SYSTEM

Two chains of nerve fibres called the sympathetic trunks (sympathetic chain) run longitudinally on either side of the vertebral column. These trunks are formed by preganglionic and postganglionic neurons of the sympathetic nervous system. At the site of synapse of the pre- and post-ganglionic neurons are swellings called sympathetic ganglia. The sympathetic trunks are situated in front of the transverse processes in the neck, anterior to the heads of the ribs, on the anterolateral aspects of the lumbar vertebral bodies, on the front of the sacrum medial to the anterior sacral foramina, and on the front of the coccyx.

Ganglia vary in number: there are approximately 2 cervical, 11 thoracic, 4 lumbar, 4 sacral and 1 coccygeal. The superior cervical ganglion lies between C1 and C3, and there is a star-shaped ganglion at the cervico-thoracic junction called the stellate ganglion. An intermediate ganglion may be present at the level of C6.

In the cervical spine, the sympathetic trunk lies within the carotid sheath on the anterolateral aspect of the neck and may be vulnerable to trauma, such as a whiplash injury. The vertebral artery has sympathetic fibres on its surface as it passes through the transverse foramen of the cervical vertebrae (Xiuqing et al, 1988).

The sympathetic preganglionic neurons originate in the thoracic and upper lumbar spinal cord and as they exit the cord they enter the adjacent sympathetic chain. The pathways of the neurons vary:

1. The neurons leave the spinal cord and synapse at the ganglion with a second neuron at the same level at which they left the spinal cord. The second neuron may then ascend or descend the sympathetic chain and leave it close to its target organ.

2. On entering the sympathetic chain, the neurons may travel up and down the trunk before synapsing with a second neuron at a ganglion. The second neuron may then leave the chain to reach its target organ.

3. On leaving the spinal cord, the neurons enter the chain and pass up or down it, to then pass through the chain and synapse with the second neuron at the target organ.

Sympathetic nerves travel to the viscera in the splanchnic nerves. Preganglionic fibres leave the spinal cord in the ventral nerve roots between the 1st and 2nd lumbar segments (Fig. 7.11). Then, in the white ramus communicans, they enter a ganglion in the sympathetic trunk. They may ascend or descend in the chain to synapse with the cells of origin of many postganglionic fibres, which travel via grey rami communicantes in the splanchnic nerves to the target organ. An exception to this are the sympathetic nerves supplying the abdominal viscera – the greater, lesser and least splanchnic nerves. These nerves are formed by preganglionic sympathetic axons which pass through the sympathetic trunk without synapsing. They synapse with ganglia surrounding the arteries that supply the abdominal viscera and then travel with the artery to the organ.

The sympathetic neurons and sympathetic chain can be compromised by osteophytes on the anterolateral intervertebral bodies, osteoarthritic changes at the costovertebral and costotransverse joints, and fibrotic thickenings of the adjacent soft tissues. Additionally, in those individuals with frank spinal deformities such as kyphoscoliosis, the pathway of the sympathetic chain may be more vulnerable to mechanical irritation.

The sympathetic nervous system is controlled by higher centres. The hypothalamus, locus ceruleus and regions of the limbic system all contribute to the functioning of the sympathetic nervous system. Many other areas of the brain are able to influence the sympathetic nervous system indirectly via the hypothalamus. The hypothalamus can act on the neurons in the thoracic and lumbar spinal cord by controlling sympathetic function through the descending tracts. It also influences the autonomic nervous system by releasing hormones that bathe the autonomic ganglia to propagate visceral responses.

Figure 7.11   Schematic representation of parasympathetic and sympathetic outflow of autonomic nervous system.

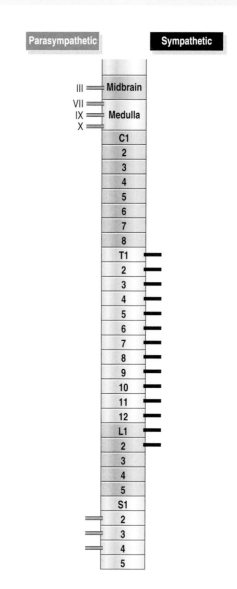

The locus ceruleus makes, stores and releases norepinephrine and may be an important area of the brain concerned with sympathetic/parasympathetic balance and modulation of emotions and psychological stress.

The sympathetic nervous system is likely to be activated or influenced by all pain states (Gifford, 1998). Pain is an emotional experience and therefore systems of the body that are involved in the regulation of emotional factors probably play an important role in pain perception. Psychological or emotional stress affects activity in systems of the body that regulate emotions (sympathetic nervous system) and thereby may influence pain perception through neurochemical changes (Porterfield and De Rosa, 1995).

PARASYMPATHETIC NERVOUS SYSTEM

The cell bodies of preganglionic parasympathetic neurons are located in the nuclei of cranial nerves III, VII, IX and X. Efferent fibres leave the central nervous system:

1. At the base of the brain with cranial nerves III (oculomotor), VII (facial), IX (glossopharyngeal) and X (vagus)
2. With somatic nerves S2, S3 and S4 to supply the rectum with visceromotor fibres, the bladder with visceromotor and its sphincter with inhibitory fibres, and the sexual organs with vasodilator fibres (see Fig. 7.11).

VISCERAL AFFERENT FIBRES

The autonomic nervous system is entirely efferent. Visceral afferent fibres share the same pathways as sympathetic and parasympathetic fibres except that they do not synapse in autonomic ganglia. The cells of origin of visceral afferent fibres lie in cranial and posterior root ganglia. Although pain evoked by visceral afferents may have a quality that distinguishes it from somatic pain, it is not strictly autonomic pain and is more correctly described as visceral pain.

Afferent impulses initiate visceral reflexes and are thought to be concerned with visceral sensations such as hunger, rectal distension and pain.

The concept of autonomic pain as a separate entity is fallacious. Investigators have shown that stimulation of autonomic elements produces pain. Gross (1974) stimulated the cervical sympathetic trunk during surgery under local anaesthetic and produced pain that did not correspond to a dermatomal distribution; also, under conditions of lumbar anaesthesia, cutting of the splanchnic nerves produced severe pain in a patient. Grieve (1988, p. 319) states that 'pure autonomic pain' is a meaningless term. Somatic roots carry autonomic efferent neurons and 'autonomic pain' produced by experiments is accompanied by somatic changes such as muscle spasm and cutaneous hyperalgesia.

Some of the more obscure symptoms that patients complain of – such as throbbing or burning pain, formication, fullness, puffiness, nausea and changes in temperature – may be due to altered autonomic nervous system activity. The terms 'sympathetically maintained pain' (SMP) and 'reflex sympathetic dystrophy' (RSD) have been used to describe signs and symptoms thought to be caused by ongoing activity in the sympathetic nervous system. However, there is no definitive way to diagnose SMP on the basis of clinical signs and symptoms. The use of techniques that block the receptors on the nociceptors that are responsive to the norepinephrine secreted by the sympathetic terminals is the only method available to diagnose SMP (Campbell, 1996). Many pain states labelled as SMP or RSD show no response to sympathetic/receptor blocking and these conditions have been termed 'sympathetically independent pain' (SIP) (Campbell et al, 1993).

References

Aprill C, Dwyer A, Bogduk N (1990) Cervical zygapophyseal joint pain patterns. II A clinical evaluation. *Spine* 15: 458.

Asbury AK, Fields HL (1984) Pain due to peripheral nerve damage: an hypothesis. *Neurology* 34: 1587–1590.

Basbaum AI (1996) Memories of pain. *Scientific American: Science and Medicine* Nov/Dec: 22–31.

Bogduk N (1980) Lumbar dorsal ramus syndrome. *Medical Journal of Australia* 2: 537.

Bogduk N (1982) The clinical anatomy of the cervical dorsal rami. *Spine* 7: 319.

Bogduk N (1987) Innervation, pain, patterns and mechanisms of pain production. In: Twomey LT, Taylor JR (eds) *Physical Therapy of the Low Back.* Churchill Livingstone, Edinburgh, p. 94.

Bogduk N (1988) Innervation and pain patterns of the cervical spine. In: Grant R (ed.) *Physical Therapy of the Cervical and Thoracic Spines.* Churchill Livingstone, Edinburgh.

Bogduk N, Marsland A (1986) On the concept of third occipital headache. *Journal of Neurology, Neurosurgery and Psychiatry* 134: 383.

Bogduk N, Twomey LT (1987) *Clinical Anatomy of the Lumbar Spine.* Churchill Livingstone, Edinburgh, pp. 92–102.

Bogduk N, Tynan W, Wilson AS (1981) The nerve supply to the human lumbar intervertebral discs. *Journal of Anatomy* 132: 39–56.

Bogduk N, Wilson AJ, Tynan W (1982) The human lumbar dorsal rami. *Journal of Anatomy* 134: 383.

Bose K, Balasubramaniam P (1984) Nerve root canals of the lumbar spine. *Spine* 9: 16.

Bough B, Thakore J, Davies M, Dowling F (1990) Degeneration of the lumbar facet joints. Arthography and pathology. *Journal of Bone and Joint Surgery (Br.)* 72: 275.

Bove G, Light A (1995) Unmyelinated nociceptors of rat paraspinal tissues. *Journal of Neurophysiology* 73: 1752–1762.

Bove G, Light A (1997) The nervi nervorum: Missing link for neuropathic pain? *Pain Forum* 6: 181–190.

Bowsher D (1988) Acute and chronic pain assessment. In: Wells PE, Frampton V, Bowsher D (eds) *Pain: Management and Control in Physiotherapy.* Heinemann Medical Books, London.

Campbell JN (1996) Complex regional pain syndrome and the sympathetic nervous system. In: Campbell JN (ed.) *Pain 1996: An updated review. Refresher course syllabus.* IASP Press, Seattle, pp. 89–96.

Campbell JN, Raja SN, Meyer RA (1993) Pain and the sympathetic nervous system: connecting the loop. In: Vecchiet L, Albe-Fessard D, Lindblom U, et al (eds) *New Trends in Referred Pain and Hyperalgesia.* Elsevier, Amsterdam, pp. 99–108.

Carrera GF (1980) Lumbar facet joint injection in low back pain and sciatica. *Radiology* 137: 665.

Chua WH, Bogduk N (1995) The surgical anatomy of thoracic facet denervation. *Acta Neurochirurgica (Wien)* 136: 140–144.

Cloward RB (1959) Cervical discography. *Annals of Surgery* 150: 1052.

Cohen ML (1996) Arthralgia and myalgia. In: Campbell JN (ed.) *Pain 1996: An updated review.* IASP Press, Seattle.

Dee R (1978) The innervation of the joints. In: Sokoloff L (ed.) *The Joints and Synovial Fluid I.* Academic Press, London.

Devor M (1991) Neuropathic pain and injured nerve: peripheral mechanisms. *British Medical Bulletin* 47: 619–630.

Devor M, Rappaport HZ (1989) Pain and pathophysiology of the damaged nerve. In: Fields HL (ed.) *Pain Syndromes in Neurology.* Butterworth Heinemann, Oxford, pp. 47–83.

Dommisse GF (1975) Morphological aspects of the lumbar spine and lumbo-sacral region. *Orthopedic Clinics of North America* 6: 163–175.

Dubner R, Ruda MA (1992) Activity-dependent neuronal plasticity following tissue injury and inflammation. *Trends in Neuroscience* 15: 96–103.

Duggan AW, Hope PJ, Jarrot B, Schaible HG, Fleetwood-Walker SM (1990) Release, spread, and persistence of immunoreactive neurokinin A in the dorsal horn of the cat following noxious cutaneous stimulation. Studies with antibody microbes. *Neuroscience* 35: 195–202.

Dwyer A, Aprill C, Bogduk N (1990) Cervical zygapophyseal joint pain patterns. I: A study in normal volunteers. *Spine* 15: 453.

Elbe JN (1960) Pattern of responses of the paravertebral musculature to visceral stimulation. *American Journal of Physiology* 198: 429.

Feinstein B, Langton JBK, Jameson RM, et al (1954) Experiments on referred pain from deep somatic structures with charts of segmental pain areas. *Clinical Science* 4: 35.

Frykholm R (1971) The clinical picture. In: Hirsch C, Zotterman Y (eds) *Cervical Pain.* Pergamon Press, Oxford, p. 5.

Garfin SR, Rydevik BL, Brown RA, Sartoris DJ (1991) Compression neuropathy of spinal nerve roots – A mechanical or biological problem? *Spine* 16: 162.

Gifford L (1998) Output mechanisms. In: Gifford L (ed.) *Topical Issues in Pain. Whiplash: science and management. Fear-avoidance beliefs and behaviour.* CNS Press Falmouth 5: 81–91.

Gifford LS (1997) Pain. In: Pitt-Brooke J (ed.) *Rehabilitation of Movement: Theoretical Bases of Clinical Practice.* Saunders, London, pp. 196–232.

Giles LGF (1993) A histological investigation of human lower lumbar intervertebral canal (foramen) dimensions. *Journal of Manipulative and Physiological Therapeutics* 15: 551–555.

Giles LGF, Kaveri MJP (1990) Some osseous and soft tissue causes of human intervertebral canal (foramen) stenosis. *Journal of Rheumatology* 17: 1474–1481.

Giles LGF, Singer KP (1997) *Clinical Anatomy and Management of Low Back Pain.* Butterworth-Heinemann, Oxford, pp. 97–113.

Giles LGF, Singer KP (2000) *Clinical Anatomy and Management of Thoracic Spine Pain*. Vol. 2. Butterworth-Heinemann, Oxford, p. 134.

Grieve GP (1981) *Common Vertebral Joint Problems*. Churchill Livingstone, Edinburgh, p. 195.

Grieve GP (1988) *Common Vertebral Joint Problems*, 2nd edn. Churchill Livingstone, Edinburgh.

Groen GJ, Baljet B, Drukker J (1990) Nerves and nerve plexuses of the human vertebral column. *American Journal of Anatomy* 188: 282–296.

Gross D (1974) Pain and the autonomic nervous system. In: Bonica JJ (ed.) *Advances in Neurology*. Raven Press, New York, p. 92.

Hall T, Quintner J (1996) Responses to mechanical stimulation of the upper limb in painful cervical radiculopathy. *Australian Journal of Physiotherapy* 42: 277–285.

Handwerker HO, Reeh PW (1991) Pain and inflammation. In: Bond MR, Charlton IE, Woolf CJ (eds) *Pain Research and Clinical Management: Proceedings of the VIth World Congress on Pain*. Elsevier Science, Amsterdam, pp. 59–70.

Harkness JAL, Higges ER, Dieppe PA (1984) Osteoarthritis. In: Wall PD, Melzack R (eds) *Textbook of Pain*. Churchill Livingstone, Edinburgh, p. 215.

Hasue M, Kikuchi S, Sakuyama Y, Ito T (1983) Anatomic study of the interrelation between nerve roots and their surroundings. *Spine* 8: 50–58.

Hasue M, Kunoji J, Komos, Kikuchis (1989) Classification by position of dorsal root ganglia in the lumbosacral region. Spine 14: 1261–1264.

Heikkila HV, Astrom P-G (1996) Cervicocephalic kinaesthetic sensibility in patients with whiplash injury. *Scandinavian Journal of Rehabilitation Medicine* 28: 133–138.

Hildebrandt J, Argyrakis A (1986) Percutaneous nerve block of the cervical facets – a relatively new method in the treatment of chronic headache and neck pain. *Manual Medicine* 2: 4.

Hirsch C, Ingelmark BE, Miller M (1963) The anatomical basis for low back pain. *Acta Orthopaedica Scandinavica* 33: 1–17.

Hockaday JM, Whitty CWM (1967) Patterns of referred pain in the normal subject. *Brain* 90: 481.

Inman VT, Saunders JB, De C.M. (1944) Referred pain from skeletal structures. Journal of Nervous and Mental Disease 90: 666.

International Association for the Study of Pain (1986) Classification of chronic pain. Descriptions of chronic pain syndromes and definitions of pain terms. *Pain* (suppl 3).

Jackson HC, Winkelmann RK, Bickel WH (1966) Nerve endings in the human lumbar spinal column and related structures. *Journal of Bone and Joint Surgery (Am.)* 48: 1272–1281.

Janig W, Stanton-Hicks M (1996) *Reflex Sympathetic Dystrophy: A Reappraisal*. IASP Press, Seattle.

Johansson H, Sojka P (1991) Pathophysiological mechanisms involved in genesis and spread of muscular tension in occupational muscle pain and in chronic musculoskeletal

pain syndromes: a hypothesis. *Medical Hypotheses* 35: 196–203.

Jull G (2001) The physiotherapy management of whiplash associated disorders. In: Proceedings of the 2nd International Private Practitioners Association Conference, England.

Katz J, Melzack R (1990) Pain 'memories' in phantom limbs: review and clinical observations. *Pain* 43: 319–336.

Keele AC, Neil E, eds (1971) *Samson Wright's Applied Physiology*, 12th edn. Oxford University Press, Oxford.

Kellgren JH (1939) On the distribution of pain arising from deep somatic structures with charts of segmental pain areas. *Clinical Science* 4: 35.

Kunert W (1965) Functional disorders of internal organs due to vertebral lesions. *Ciba Foundation Symposium* 13: 85.

Kuslich SD, Ulstrom CL, Michael CJ (1991) The tissue origin of low back pain and sciatica: A report of pain response to tissue stimulation during operations on the lumbar spine using local anaesthesia. *Orthopedic Clinics of North America* 22: 181.

Laslett M (2000) Bilateral buttock pain caused by aortic stenosis: a case report of claudication of the buttock. *Manual Therapy* 5: 227–233.

Lee CK, Rauschning W, Glenn W (1988) Lateral lumbar spinal canal stenosis: classification, pathologic anatomy and surgical decompression. *Spine* 13: 313–320.

Lindahl O (1966) Hyperalgesia of the lumbar nerve roots in sciatica. *Acta Orthopaedica Scandinavica* 37: 367.

Marks RC, Houston T, Thulbourne T (1992) Facet joint injection and facet nerve block: A randomized comparison in 86 patients with chronic low back pain. *Pain* 49: 325.

McCall IW, Park WM, O'Brien JP (1979) Induced pain referral from posterior lumbar elements in normal subjects. Spine 44: 441.

McCarron RF, Wimpee MW, Hudkins PG, Laros GS (1987) The inflammatory effect of the nucleus pulposus: A possible element in the pathogenesis of low back pain. *Spine* 12: 760.

Melzack R (1996) Gate control theory. On evolution of pain concepts. *Pain Forum* 5: 128–138.

Melzack R, Wall PD (1965) Pain mechanisms: a new theory. Science 150: 971.

Mense S (1996) Group III and IV nociceptors in skeletal muscle: are they specific or polymodal? In: Kumazawa T, Kruger L, Mizumura K (eds) *Progress in Research*, Vol. 113. Elsevier Science, Amsterdam, pp. 83–100.

Mills KR, Newham DJ, Edwards RHT (1984) Muscle pain. In: Wall PD, Melzack R (eds) *Textbook of Pain*. Churchill Livingstone, Edinburgh, p. 319.

Mooney V, Robertson J (1976) The facet syndrome. *Clinical Orthopaedics and Related Research* 115: 149.

Nathan H, Fuerstein M (1974) Angulated course of spinal nerve roots. *Journal of Neurosurgery* 32: 349.

Noonan TJ, Garrett WE (1992) Injuries at the myotendinous junction. *Clinics in Sports Medicine* 11: 783–806.

O'Brien JP (1984) Mechanisms of spinal pain. In: Wall PD, Melzack R (eds) *Textbook of Pain*. Churchill Livingstone, Edinburgh, p. 240.

Parke WW (1992) Applied anatomy of the spine. In: Rothman RH, Simone FA (eds) *The Spine*. WB Saunders, Philadelphia, p. 35.

Payan PDG, McGillis JP, Renold FK, et al (1987) Neuropeptide modulation of leukocyte function. *Annals of the New York Academy of Sciences* 496: 182.

Peretti de F, Micalef JP, Bourgeon A, et al (1989) Biomechanics of the lumbar spinal nerve roots and the first sacral root within the intervertebral foramina. *Surgical and Radiologic Anatomy* II: 221–225.

Porterfield JA, DeRosa C (1995) *Mechanical Neck Pain. Perspectives in Functional Anatomy*. Saunders, Philadelphia, p. 41.

Porterfield JA, DeRosa C (1998) *Mechanical Low Back Pain. Perspectives in Functional Anatomy*. Saunders, Philadelphia, pp. 25–52.

Rydevik B, Garfin S (1989) Spinal nerve root compression. In: Szabo RM, Thorofare NJ, Slack CB (eds) *Nerve Compression Syndromes – Diagnosis and Treatment*. McGraw-Hill, New Jersey.

Rydevik B, Brown MD, Lundborg G (1984) Pathoanatomy and pathophysiology of nerve root compression. *Spine* 9: 7–15.

Rydevik BL (1992) The effects of compression on the physiology of the nerve roots. *Journal of Manipulative and Physiological Therapeutics* 1: 62–66.

Schmidt RF (1996). The articular polymodal nociceptor in health and disease. In: Kumazawa T, Kruger L, Mizumura K (eds) *The Polymodal Receptor: A Gateway to Pathological Pain. Progress in Brain Research*, Vol. 113. Elsevier Science, Amsterdam, pp. 53–81.

Simons DG (1987) Myofascial pain syndrome due to trigger points. *International Rehabilitation Medicine Association Monograph Series* 1: 1–39.

Smyth J, Wright V (1958). Sciatica and the intervertebral disc, an experimental study. *Journal of Bone and Joint Surgery (Am.)* 40A: 1401.

Stanton-Hicks M, Janig W, Hassenbusch S, et al (1995) Reflex sympathetic dystrophy: changing concepts and taxonomy. *Pain* 63: 27–133.

Stillwell DL (1956) Nerve supply of the vertebral column and its associated structures in monkeys. Anatomical Record 125: 129.

Stoddard A (1983) *Manual of Osteopathic Practice*, 2nd edn. Hutchison, London, Appendix 3, p. 242.

Stolker RJ, Vervest ACM, Groen GJ, et al (1994) On the innervation of the dorsal compartment of the thoracic spine. In: *Pain Management by Radiofrequency Procedures in the Cervical and Thoracic Spine: A Clinical and Anatomical Study*. Thesis, Utrecht, pp. 133–144.

Szlavy L, Taveras JM (1995) *Noncoronary Angioplasty and Interventional Radiologic Treatment of Vascular*

Malformations. Lea and Febiger, Philadelphia, ch 8, pp. 186–187.

Taylor DCM, Pierau Fr-K, Mizutani M (1984) Possible bases for referred pain. In: Holden AV, Winslow W (eds) *The Neurobiology of Pain*. Manchester University Press, Manchester, pp. 143–156.

Thacker MA (1998) Whiplash – Is there a lesion? In: Gifford L (ed.) *Topical Issues in Pain. Whiplash: science and management. Fear-avoidance beliefs and behaviour*. CNS Press, Falmouth pp. 27–43.

Trevor Jones R (1964) Osteoarthritis of the paravertebral joints of the second and third cervical vertebra as a cause of occipital headaches. *South African Medical Journal* 38: 392.

Van der Linden RG (1984) Subarticular entrapment of the dorsal root ganglion as a cause of sciatic pain. *Spine* 9: 19–22.

Weinstein J (1991) Anatomy and neurophysiologic mechanisms of spinal pain. In: Frymoyer J (ed.) *The Adult Spine*. Raven Press, New York, p. 602.

Weinstein J, Claverie W, Gibson S (1988) The pain of discography. *Spine* 13: 1344.

Wells PE, Frampton V, Bowsher D (1994) *Pain Management by Physiotherapy*, 2nd edn. Butterworth Heinemann, Oxford.

Williams PL, Warwick T (1980) *Gray's Anatomy*, 36th edn. Churchill Livingstone, Edinburgh.

Woolf CJ (1984) Long term alteration in the excitability of the flexion reflex produced by peripheral tissue injury in the chronic decerebrate rat. *Pain* 18: 325–343.

Woolf CJ, Doubell TP (1994). The pathophysiology of chronic pain – increased sensitivity to low threshold Ab-fibre inputs. *Current Opinion in Neurobiology* 4: 525–534.

Wright A (1999) Recent concepts in the neurophysiology of pain. *Manual Therapy* 4: 196–202.

Wyke BD (1967) The neurology of joints. *Annals of the Royal College of Surgeons of England* 41: 25.

Wyke BD (1975) Morphological and functional features of the innervation of costovertebral joints. *Folia Morphologica* 23: 296.

Wyke BD (1976) Neurological aspects of low back pain. In: Jayson M (ed.) *The Lumbar Spine and Back Pain*. Sector, London, p. 189.

Wyke BD (1979) Neurology of the cervical spinal joints. *Physiotherapy* 65: 72.

Wyke BD (1981) The neurology of the joints: a review of general principles. *Clinics in Rheumatic Diseases* 7: 23.

Xiuqing C, Bo Sun, Shizhen Z (1988) Nerves accompanying the vertebral artery and their clinical relevance. *Spine* 13: 1360–1364.

Yang KH, King AI (1984) Mechanism of facet load transmission as a hypothesis for low back pain. *Spine* 9: 557.

Chapter **8**

Biomechanics of the spinal cord and meninges

During normal movement, the spinal cord and nerve roots are able to adapt to changes that occur within the vertebral canal. The central nervous system (CNS) has both elastic and plastic properties that allow it to respond dynamically to forces while maintaining the ability to transmit impulses. The mechanical, electrical and physiological components of the CNS are interdependent (Shacklock et al, 1994) and altered mechanics may therefore affect both the CNS and the target tissues that the CNS innervates.

The CNS consists of the brain and spinal cord and is contained within the cranium and spinal canal. The CNS is continuous with the peripheral nervous system both mechanically and physiologically so that changes within either the CNS or peripheral nervous system can have repercussions for the nervous system as a whole.

The term *neuraxis* is used synonymously with the CNS. It is a biome-chanical term that highlights the fact that the brain and spinal cord have a longitudinal axis, like a bone or joint (Bowsher, 1988).

THE BRAIN

The brain is protected by the skull and the meninges: the pia, arachnoid and dura mater. The pia mater closely envelops the brain; the pia and arachnoid mater are separated by the subarachnoid space, which is filled with cerebrospinal fluid (CSF). The ventricles of the brain are spaces which connect with the subarachnoid space. The CSF is able to flow between the ventricles and subarachnoid spaces that communicate and thus provides some shock absorption for the brain.

The three main parts of the brain are the forebrain, midbrain and hind-brain. These structures are continuous and provide a mechanism for brain tissue to respond to stresses exerted from the cord (Shacklock et al, 1994).

THE SPINAL CORD

The spinal cord lies within the bony vertebral canal. It is almost cylin-drical in shape, although slightly flattened anteroposteriorly. As a con-tinuation of the medulla oblongata, the spinal cord extends from the foramen magnum to the level of the L1/2 disc. Below this level, the lum-bar and sacral nerve roots occupy the spinal canal, and they form the col-lection of nerve roots known as the cauda equina. Caudally, the spinal cord is cone-shaped and is attached to the coccyx by the filum terminale. This is a fibrous, non-nervous structure, which is an extension of the pia mater and is covered by dura mater.

The neurons in the spinal cord are arranged in three vertical columns: dorsal, ventral and lateral. The axis of movement at the spinal motion segment is further away from the dorsal column than the ventral and lat-eral columns and this causes differential loading of the columns during spinal movements (Breig, 1978).

SPINAL MENINGES (Fig. 8.1)

Three membranes surround the spinal cord: the dura mater, the arach-noid and pia mater.

DURA MATER

The dura mater is the outermost layer of the spinal meninges. The outer endosteal layer of the cranial dura mater is continued as the periosteum of the vertebral canal, whereas the inner meningeal layer of the cerebral dura mater becomes continuous with the dura mater of the spinal cord.

The spinal dura mater extends from the foramen magnum to the 2nd sacral segment and then continues caudally, covering the filum

Figure 8.1   Schematic diagram
of the spinal meninges.

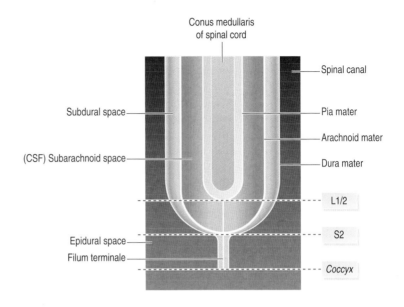

terminale, eventually blending with the periosteum on the dorsal surface of the coccyx. It is attached superiorly to the foramen magnum
and the posterior surface of the 2nd and 3rd cervical vertebral bodies.
As the dura is connected to the bony skeleton, movement of the vertebral canal results in forces being transmitted to the meninges (Troup,
1986). Small fibrous strips attach the dura to the posterior longitudinal
ligament, particularly in the lumbar spine. In the cervical spine the dura
is attached to the spinal canal wall and the intervertebral foramen by
epidural and periradicular connective tissue (Sunderland, 1974; Tencer
et al, 1985).

Laterally, the dura envelops the nerve roots as they pass through the
intervertebral foramen. In the upper spine, the dural sheaths are short,
but they increase in length caudally because of the obliquity of the nerve
roots. At the dorsal root ganglion or slightly distal to the intervertebral
foramen, the dura is continued as the perineurium of the spinal nerve.
Hence, traction forces on the spinal nerve are transmitted directly to the
spinal dura and arachnoid mater and then via the dentate ligaments
to the spinal cord (see p. 278). The epidural tissue of the spinal cord
and nerve roots is continued as the epineurium of the spinal nerve
(Sunderland, 1974).

In the cervical spine, the paired root sleeves of dura and arachnoid are
attached loosely to the cervical foramina. Nerve roots of C4–6 are stabilized in the gutter of the transverse process by myofascial slips and
fusion with the adventitia of the vertebral artery (Sunderland, 1974).
These attachments become firmer with increasing age and degenerative
change.

Throughout the rest of the spine, with the possible exception of S1,
the nerve roots are not attached to the intervertebral foramina, thereby
allowing the nerve roots to move in and out of the foramina. Attachment

of the 1st sacral nerve to the wall of the foramen was described by Hollinshead (1969).

The dura consists mainly of white fibrous tissue with a fine network of elastic fibres. Collagenous fibres lie in longitudinal bundles which are straight when stretched and wavy when relaxed. Experiments on dogs have shown that the dura is under longitudinal strain due to the attachment of the dural sheaths (Tunturi, 1977). It was observed that the elastic network was stretched almost to the limit and that it was the collagenous fibres that contributed to the elasticity of the spinal dura. The dura has great axial strength but is weaker in the transverse direction. There are also regional differences in the dura. The dorsal cervical dura is thicker and stronger than in other areas but the ventral dura is stronger in the thoracic spine (Haupt and Stopft, 1978). These differences may be due to the mechanical demands of specific spinal regions.

Anteriorly, the dura is innervated by free nerve endings from the sinuvertebral nerve (Edgar and Nundy, 1966).

Epidural (or extradural) space

The epidural space lies between the vertebral canal and dura and is bounded by the posterior longitudinal ligament anteriorly, the ligamenta flava and the periosteum of the laminae posteriorly, and the pedicles and intervertebral foramina laterally. Superiorly the space is closed at the foramen magnum where the spinal dura mater attaches with the endosteal dura of the cranium. Caudally, the epidural space ends at the sacral hiatus where it is closed by the sacrococcygeal ligament. The space communicates freely with the paravertebral space through the intervertebral foramina. It contains semi-liquid fat, areolar tissue, lymphatic vessels, the internal vertebral venous plexus, the spinal arteries and the spinal nerve roots as they exit the dural sac and pass through the intervertebral foramina.

Veins forming the venous plexus are large and valveless (see pp. 168–169). They are easily compressed and their volume changes with spinal movement (Dommisse, 1975).

Subdural space

The subdural space is a potential space between the dura mater and the arachnoid, containing serous fluid. Local anaesthetics can distribute through this space via a misplaced spinal needle or epidural catheter. When bleeding occurs in the cranium, blood may collect in the subdural space and push down on the lower layers of the meninges.

ARACHNOID

The arachnoid is a thin, delicate membrane lying between the dura and pia mater. It is continuous above with the intracranial arachnoid membrane and ends caudally at the base of the subdural cavity at the 2nd sacral segment. In some areas the arachnoid projects into sinuses formed by the dura mater: these areas are known as arachnoid granulations or villi. Their function is to aid transfer of CSF back into the bloodstream.

Laterally, the arachnoid lines the dural sleeves but, unlike the dura mater, it does not become continuous with the peripheral nerve covering. Between the ventral and dorsal nerve roots, the arachnoid links the adjacent dural layers, thereby contributing to the interradicular septum (Fig. 8.2).

Structurally, it is a loose, irregular connective tissue network made up of collagen, elastin and reticulum fibres. The fibres are arranged in a lattice pattern which permits lengthening and shortening (Breig, 1978). The arachnoid is relatively avascular but provides support for blood vessels passing from pia to dura. Tight cells within its structure form a mechanical barrier to diffusion into the CNS from the subarachnoid and subdural spaces. A network of delicate trabeculae crosses the subarachnoid space, connecting the arachnoid and pia mater and providing support for small vessels.

Subarachnoid space

The subarachnoid space lies between the arachnoid and pia mater and contains the CSF. This fluid supports the meninges and helps to disperse forces acting through it. It also brings nutrients to the brain and spinal cord and removes waste products from the system. The CSF has a definite pattern of movement. It is made in the ventricles of the brain and moves from the lateral ventricle to the third ventricle and then to the fourth ventricle. The CSF then passes into the subarachnoid space where it circulates around the outside of the brain and spinal cord and eventually works its way to the superior sagittal sinus via the arachnoid granulations or villi. In the superior sagittal sinus the CSF is reabsorbed into the bloodstream. The CSF of the neuraxis is regenerated several times every 24 hours.

PIA MATER

The pia mater is the innermost layer of the meninges and adheres closely to the spinal cord. It has an outer layer, the epipia, which supports large blood vessels, and an inner layer, the pia intima, which is continuous

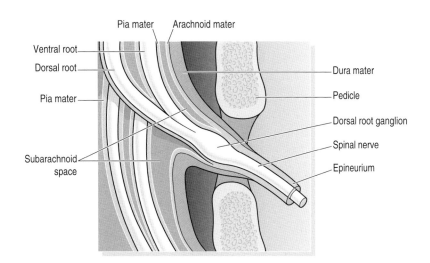

Figure 8.2   The disposition of the meningeal sheaths of spinal nerve roots. (From Palastanga N, Field D, Soames R 1989 *Anatomy and Human Movement: Structure and Function.* Heinemann Medical, Oxford, with permission.)

Pia mater   Arachnoid mater

Ventral root

Dorsal root

Pia mater

Subarachnoid space

Dura mater

Pedicle

Dorsal root ganglion

Spinal nerve

Epineurium

with nervous tissue of the spinal cord. It forms a sheath for the ventral and dorsal nerve roots as far as the interradicular septum. The pia mater ends with the termination of the spinal cord (the conus medullaris) at the level of the L1/2 disc, and is continued as the filum terminale to attach to the first coccygeal segment.

DENTATE LIGAMENTS

The dentate ligaments form a narrow fibrous sheet on each side of the spinal cord (Fig. 8.3). There are 21 pairs bilaterally between the C1 spinal nerve root and the level of exit of the L1 nerve root. These triangular, tooth-like processes lie between the ventral and dorsal nerve roots with their medial border continuous with the pia. Laterally, their points attach to the inner aspect of the dura. Upper ligaments are almost perpendicular. The tips of the ligaments act as universal joints, permitting swivelling of the dentate ligaments (Epstein, 1976). In their normal state the dentate ligaments are under a degree of tension and, if cut at their dural attachments, they contract down to the cord (Epstein, 1966). It is thought that tension on the spinal nerves is conveyed from the dura via the dentate ligaments to the spinal cord. Equally, movement of the cord is quickly transmitted to the dura so that the spinal cord and its meninges are biomechanically interdependent.

The dentate ligaments prevent excessive elongation of the cord during flexion (Tani et al, 1987).

NERVE ROOT COMPLEX

The nerve root complex comprises the two nerve roots, the dorsal root ganglion, spinal nerve and connective tissue coverings. The nerve roots

Figure 8.3 The dentate ligaments. A, Horizontal section through spinal cord and meninges. B, Anterior aspect of spinal cord.

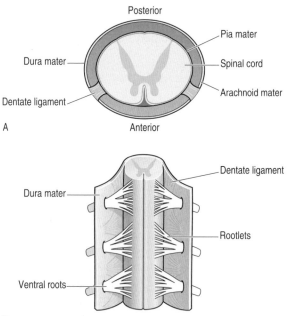

leave the dural theca through openings in the root pouch, and the dura and arachnoid form a tubular sleeve that surrounds each root. In the lumbar region the lumbosacral nerves are free to move intrathecally, but extrathecally they are attached by strips of connective tissue to the dura and arachnoid (Spencer et al, 1983). The nerve root complex is the region where forces are transmitted between the neuraxis and the spinal nerve. Movements of the limbs or spine induce forces that are transmitted along the peripheral and spinal nerves via the nerve root complex to the dura. The dura distributes the tension along its surface and to the dentate ligaments (Luttges et al, 1986). This mechanism helps to prevent a concentration of force within the nerve rootlets, peripheral nervous system and the neuraxis.

BIOMECHANICS OF THE VERTEBRAL CANAL AND THE PAIN-SENSITIVE STRUCTURES

In the normal spine, the spinal cord, meninges and nerve roots adapt freely to changes of vertebral movement, postures and pressure differences (Breig, 1960). As the dura has bony attachments both cephalad and caudad, any change in the bony vertebral canal is accommodated for by changes in the shape or position of the neuraxis. Gravity will also affect the neuraxis.

The neuraxis is highly plastic, and during normal movement it may change in length, diameter, shape and direction. Breig (1978) proposed that osteomeningeal relations are maintained due to the inherent plasticity of the tract. The collagen network of the pia mater has a rhomboid nature that allows a concertina action in the pial fibres by changes in angle between fibres at their intersection. When the fibres are placed under tension they have a more parallel arrangement and are better able to resist longitudinal forces. During compression, the pial fibres buckle so that the dura and meninges wrinkle.

The filum terminale is extensible and elongates in a linear fashion when pulled caudally (Tani et al, 1987). It helps to protect the neuraxis from longitudinal stress by taking up the slack in positions of low tension and by elongating when the neuraxis is in positions of high tension (Tunturi, 1977).

NEUTRAL POSITION

The neutral position is midway between full flexion and extension and takes into account the spinal curves. In this position the neuraxis is relaxed in the spinal canal and the blood vessels and perivascular spaces are patent, allowing blood, lymphatic and CSF flow.

FLEXION

On forward flexion of the spine, there is an increase in the length of the vertebral canal and the elongation of the posterior border of the canal is greater than that of the anterior border. Extensive experiments in cadavers have shown that the cervical and lumbar spines can lengthen by

28 mm each, but the thoracic spine only increases in length by 3 mm (Louis, 1981). An important function of the spinal cord and meninges is the ability to adapt to the increase in length of the vertebral canal as it moves from neutral to flexion while maintaining normal nerve conduction. The neuraxis and meninges adapt to spinal flexion in a number of ways: ventral displacement, lengthening/strain, axial sliding and angulation of nerve roots.

During flexion the cord and meninges 'bowstring' forwards because of their inherent elasticity. There is an increase in tension in the cord and dura, and they become drawn out and smooth, so that there is a small decrease in the cross-sectional area of the cord. Gravity will also tend to displace the cord anteriorly when flexion occurs in a sitting or standing position. As the cord moves anteriorly, it may become stretched over any osteocartilaginous bar or disc protrusion that is present.

Longitudinally, axial tension is increased in the neuraxis as the spine is lengthened during flexion of the canal. This tension in the neuraxis is created by dural fixation at the foramen magnum pulling the pons and medulla rostrally and the filum terminale pulling caudally due to its attachment to the sacrum. The tension is transmitted as far as the midbrain rostrally and the sciatic nerve caudally (Breig, 1978; Louis, 1981).

The strain on the neuraxis and meninges alters segmentally and is highest where there is greatest joint mobility in the sagittal plane. In the cervical spine, the greatest dural strain is at C5–6; in the lumbar spine the dural strain at L5–S1 reaches 30% whereas at L1–2 it is only 15% (Louis, 1981).

Louis observed in flexion and extension studies that most movement of the cord and dura occurred in the cervical and lumbar regions, and that very little movement occurred in the thoracic spine. He also noted that during flexion at C6 there is some caudal sliding of the dura at C5 and rostral movement at C6–7. At the L4 spinal level, during flexion the dura moves caudally by up to 3 mm, whereas at L5 there is rostral displacement of 3 mm. There is also rostral movement above T5 and caudal movement below, causing a relative divergence or 'tension point' in the mid thoracic region.

The term 'relative displacement' is used to describe the paradoxical lengthening and convergence of neural tissues. The neural tissues are able to lengthen but movement takes place relative to the neural structures and the interface (spinal canal). When the neuraxis moves, for example rostrally, it does so relative to the bony canal; if the canal moves around a stationary neuraxis, opposite relative displacement occurs as the canal moves rostrally relative to the neuraxis. A component of the interface (e.g. vertebra) can also move with the neural tissues so that there is no relative displacement although both have moved. These phenomena can occur simultaneously at different levels within the spine, so that at some levels different movements can occur and at other segments no relative movement takes place.

Analysis of changes in the dural sac during movements shows that changes in dural length are smaller than length changes in the bony canal (Penning and Wilmink, 1981). This may be due firstly to the anchorage of the root sheaths and secondly to the limited elasticity of the dura.

Flexion of the spine places tension on the nerve roots and their sleeves. Thoracic roots above T6 tend to follow a more vertical course, while those between T6 and T12 become more horizontal. In the lumbar region, the nerve roots above L3 become lax during flexion and follow a wavy course. Their direction becomes more horizontal and they move away from the pedicle. The L3 nerve roots remain the same length during flexion, while those below L3 are stretched by up to 16% and become more vertical in direction, so that they move into contact with the medial border of the superior pedicle (Louis, 1981).

Flexion of the cervical spine alone causes elongation of the cord and dura. Tension is transmitted throughout the spine, so that there is very slight upward movement of the thoracic cord and cauda equina, and a decrease in the cross-sectional area of the sacral cone. Cervical flexion affects the lumbar nerve roots, causing them to become more vertical so that they move into contact with the pedicles.

EXTENSION

In general, the opposite effects occur when the vertebral column is extended. In extension, the vertical height of the column is shortened by as much as 38 mm and there is a decrease in the anteroposterior dimensions of the canal (Breig, 1960). In the lumbar spine there is inward bulging of the intervertebral discs, and the ligamenta flava may bulge anteriorly into the canal, further reducing the available space (Penning and Wilmink, 1981). Tension in the neuraxis is reduced so that folds form on its posterior aspect and there is an increase in the transverse diameter of the cord. There is posterior movement of the dural sac and the lower part of the dura moves caudally by up to 2 mm. The nerve roots follow a wavier course, moving away from the pedicles.

Extension of the cervical spine alone creates slight slackening of the thoracic and lumbar dura. The lumbar and sacral nerve roots also slacken and move out of contact with the pedicles. The microcirculation of the neuraxis is more patent in extension than flexion.

LATERAL FLEXION

Lateral flexion of the vertebral column in standing causes lengthening of the canal on the convex side and shortening of the canal on the concave side. Likewise, in this position, the dura on the convex side is elongated, while the dura on the concave side forms transverse folds (Breig, 1978). For example, in right lateral flexion, the dura on the left side of the cord is lengthened, becoming smooth, but the dura of the right side of the cord forms transverse folds. Lumbosacral nerves on the concave side follow a wavier course; those on the convex side become stretched and have a more vertical pathway.

In the side-lying position, the changes in the dura vary according to which side the trunk is laterally flexed, rather than being directly influenced by the side on which the subject lies. For example, in right side-lying, if the trunk is laterally flexed to the *left*, the dura on the underside (right) is elongated and that on the left slackens. The caudal sac is held close to the centre of the canal by the dentate ligaments, but the nerve roots of the cauda equina sag towards the dura on the right. Nerve roots of the cauda equina on the left are relaxed. Alternatively, if the trunk is laterally flexed to the *right*, in the right side-lying position, the dura, dentate ligaments and nerve roots on the left become stretched, and the lumbosacral cord moves towards the centre of the canal. The left lumbosacral nerves are stretched in this position (Massey, 1986).

ROTATION

There is no significant alteration in length of the vertebral column during rotation. In the cervical spine, dorsal roots on the side to which rotation occurs are stretched and anterior roots are relaxed; opposite effects occur on the opposite side (Grieve, 1988).

LIMB MOVEMENTS

The nervous tissues of the body are continuous from the skull to the distal areas of the limbs. Movement of the limbs will, therefore, increase tension within the nerve roots and this is transmitted to the dura and cord.

BIOMECHANICS OF NEURAL TISSUE PROVOCATION TESTS

Passive neck flexion

Passive neck flexion is used to test the thoracic and lumbosacral nerve roots. When the neck is passively flexed in the supine position, minor shifts occur in the lumbar dura and tension increases in the lumbosacral nerve roots so that they become slightly elongated. This is the least sensitive test of the lumbar nerve roots. If the test reproduces the patient's low back or leg pain, it is often indicative of significant spinal pathology such as a large, central lumbar disc prolapse.

Straight-leg raising test (SLR, Laségue's sign)

The straight-leg raising test has been used in the assessment of patients with a suspected lumbar disc protrusion and also as a neural provocation test. Although biomechanical tests have shown that straight-leg raising causes movement of the lumbosacral nerve roots, it also provokes other structures in addition to the neural tissue (Kleynhans and Terrett, 1986) and therefore the findings of the SLR test must be interpreted within the context of other clinical findings.

The SLR causes a posterior pelvic rotation within a few degrees of lifting the leg from the horizontal (Fahlgren Grampo et al, 1991) and also affects the hamstring muscles, the lumbar facet joints, lumbar intervertebral ligaments, the intervertebral discs and muscles of the low lumbar spine.

Nervous tissue and the meninges have different mechanical properties. The nervous tissue of the sciatic nerve has some elasticity and it can therefore sustain a slow stretch. However, sudden stretching of the nerve or a stretch which goes beyond the elastic limit of the nervous tissue can be injurious. The circumferential arrangement of the fibres of the meninges limits stretching along the long axis of the tract and the meninges become taut within 5% of their normal length.

During the SLR test, the leg is passively raised in supine lying, so that the hip flexes and the knee remains extended. The effects of the SLR test on the lumbosacral nerve roots have been investigated (Goddard and Reid, 1965). The greatest amount of movement induced is more distally in the sciatic nerve at the greater sciatic notch and it commences when the heel is elevated 5–15 cm from the horizontal. As elevation continues, this movement is transmitted proximally and almost immediately affects the lumbosacral cord as it passes over the ala of the sacrum. At 20–30°, movement occurs in the intervertebral foramina and the lumbosacral nerve roots and dura are pulled downwards; after 70° there is little additional movement, but an increase in tension (Fig. 8.4).

The course of the individual nerve roots varies, thereby influencing the movement that occurs within them. L4 and L5 run a tortuous course through the intervertebral foramina, so that there is slack to be taken up. S2 and S3 curve in a marked manner and also have slack to be taken up. S1 runs in a direct and vertical course and moves the greatest distance (4–5 mm) on straight-leg raising. No downward movement of L3 has been noted during this test.

The low lumbar and sacral nerve roots move caudally within their intervertebral foramina and the force is transmitted via these nerves to the neuraxis. The tension is transmitted as far as the midbrain (Smith, 1956).

A positive finding of the SLR test in a patient is a reproduction of familiar leg pain during leg elevation (Shiging et al, 1987).

Sensitizing additions are additional movements that increase the tension within the neural structures being evaluated. Additions which increase the sensitivity of the SLR test are:

1. Ankle dorsiflexion: pulls distally on the tibial nerve, which increases neural tension during straight-leg raising (Smith, 1956; Breig and Troup, 1979)
2. Ankle plantarflexion with inversion: pulls distally on the common peroneal nerve (Kopell and Thompson, 1976)
3. Medial rotation of the hip: pulls caudolaterally on the lumbosacral nerve roots (Breig and Troup, 1979)
4. Hip adduction (Sutton, 1979)
5. Passive neck flexion (Breig, 1960)

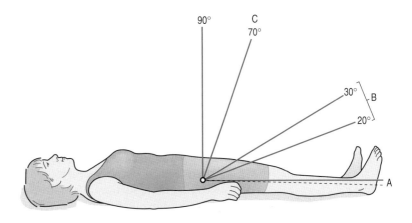

Figure 8.4   Effects of straight-leg raising: (a) movement of sciatic nerve begins at greater sciatic notch; (b) movement of roots begins at intervertebral foramen; (c) minimal movement only, but increase in tension.

6. Slump test, which combines total spinal flexion with straight-leg raising (Maitland, 1986; Butler and Gifford, 1989).

Distal movements of the sciatic nerve during straight-leg raising have been studied in monkeys (Smith, 1956). Proximal to the knee, the tibial nerve moves caudad in relation to its mechanical interface; distal to the knee, the tibial nerve moves cranially in relation to its surrounding tissues. Hence, there is a point behind the knee where the nerve and its surrounding tissues remain constant during straight-leg raising, so that this is a 'tension point'. The attachment of the common peroneal nerve to the head of the fibula is also a tension point (Butler and Gifford, 1989).

Components of the sciatic nerve are subject to pressure at various points, in particular against the greater sciatic notch and also over the convexity of the ala of the sacrum and, to a lesser extent, in the intervertebral foramina of L4 and L5. There are a large number of soft tissue connections between the sciatic nerve, and its roots, to the adjacent fascia and bone. Development of soft tissue adhesions at any point along the length of the sciatic nerve or its roots will adversely affect neural mobility.

Many people have a normal discrepancy of 5–10° between limits of right and left straight-leg raising: a normal healthy range may vary between 50° and 120° (Troup, 1986).

Well–leg raising test (cross–over Laségue)

Straight-leg raising causes the nerve roots on the opposite side to move towards the side of the straight-leg raise (Louis, 1981). Likewise, the spinal cord shifts towards the side of the limb being raised (Woodhall and Hayes, 1950). Hence, testing straight-leg raising on the symptom-free side may produce the patient's symptoms on the side affected by pathology and has been shown to be an indicator of disc pathology (Khuffash and Porter, 1989).

Slump test

The slump test combines straight-leg raising with head, neck and trunk flexion. This is a sensitive test which increases tension in the dura, nerve roots and the sciatic nerve to its distal termination in the foot (Maitland, 1978). The test consists of thoracic and lumbar flexion in the sitting position, followed by cervical flexion, extension of the knee/s, ankle dorsiflexion and hip flexion.

Maitland (1978) observed the response to this test in normal subjects aged 19 to 24. He concluded that it was unusual to find full pain-free range of movement during the test and he recorded the following responses:

1. Pain/discomfort in the mid thoracic spine to T9 on trunk and cervical flexion
2. Pain/discomfort behind the knee on trunk and cervical flexion with knee extension, increased by ankle dorsiflexion
3. Bilateral reduction in range of ankle dorsiflexion in cervical and trunk flexion with knee extension

4. Reduction of pain/discomfort with release of the neck flexion component
5. Increase in range of knee extension or ankle dorsiflexion with release of neck flexion.

A further study of 25 normal subjects showed that on a slump test 7 subjects lacked full knee extension and 16 had limitation of full dorsiflexion (Maitland, 1985). Medial rotation of the hip, dorsiflexion of the foot and cervical flexion have been shown to significantly reduce knee extension during the slump test in normal subjects (Johnson and Chiarello, 1997).

The slump test has been used to differentiate between low back pain due to involvement of neural structures from low back pain due to other causes. It has also been used to differentiate between posterior thigh pain caused by neural involvement and pain due to hamstring injury. In asymptomatic subjects, Lew and Briggs (1997) found that, during the slump test, cervical movement did not change hamstring tension and the change in experimentally induced pain during cervical flexion was not due to changes in tension in the hamstring muscle. Their study supports the view that posterior thigh pain caused by the slump test and relieved by cervical extension arises from neural structures rather than the hamstring.

The slump test has been shown to be more effective in reproducing symptoms than passive neck flexion, straight-leg raising or dorsiflexion added to the SLR test in patients with low back pain, with or without referred pain (Massey, 1982).

Prone knee bend (femoral nerve test)

The test is performed with the patient in prone-lying. The hip and thigh are stabilized and the knee is passively flexed. Flexion of the knee moves, and increases tension in, nerves and roots related to the L3 and L4 spinal segments (O'Connell, 1951). Sensitizing additions of this test are:

1. Cervical flexion
2. Spinal flexion in a side-lying position (slump in side-lying); this consists of neck and trunk flexion with the hip in extension (Davidson, 1987)
3. Alterations in hip abduction, adduction and rotation (Butler and Gifford, 1989).

Upper limb neural tissue provocation tests

Certain upper limb movements produce movement and tension in both the peripheral nerves and the neuraxis. Movement of the upper limbs causes movement of the peripheral nerves, and the effects are translated to the neuraxis due to mechanical continuity of the nervous system (McLellan and Swash, 1976; Elvey, 1980).

Depression of the shoulder girdle causes the neurovascular bundle to become taut at this point (Frykholm, 1955). As this happens, movement occurs in the C4–8 and T1 nerve roots in their intervertebral foramina. The 4th cervical nerve is involved due to its relationship with the shoulder girdle as it leaves the C3/4 foramen and travels to the shoulder as the supraclavicular nerve. Roots from C5 to T1 are affected because of their relationship with the brachial plexus. An increase in tension occurs throughout the length of the neural tissues between the shoulder and the cervical spine. The subclavian artery and vein also move and sustain tension during shoulder girdle depression (Elvey, 1988).

When the shoulder is fixed and the cervical spine is laterally flexed to the opposite side, tension increases in the C4–8 nerve roots and the T1 root. Greater movement occurs at C4–7 and there is minimal movement at C8 and T1. No alteration in movement of the subclavian artery or vein occurs, because there is no direct attachment of these vessels to the cervical spine.

Abduction of the arm at the glenohumeral joint with the shoulder girdle fixed causes most movement of the C5–7 nerve roots, less movement of the C8 and T1 roots and no movement of the subclavian artery or vein (Elvey, 1988).

Neural tissue provocation tests are passive tests that are applied in a selective manner for the examination of the compliance of different neural tissues to functional positions (Elvey and Hall, 1997). The test with a median nerve bias comprises slight shoulder girdle depression, 90° glenohumeral abduction, elbow extension, supination and wrist and finger extension. A normal response may include a stretching sensation across the anterior aspect of the shoulder, extending into the forearm and hand, and a tingling sensation in the hand (Kenneally, 1985; Bell, 1987). Normal responses are symmetrical between sides and independent of age and gender (van der Heide et al, 2001).

The normal responses to the upper limb tension test in 100 normal subjects were (Keneally, 1983):

1. Extension, abduction and lateral rotation of the glenohumeral joint – mild stretch across the anterior aspect of the shoulder joint
2. Addition of supination and elbow extension – deep painful stretch extending down the forearm and stretch across the anterior shoulder
3. Test position of extension, abduction, lateral rotation of shoulder, forearm supination, wrist and finger extension – deep stretch or ache in the cubital fossa extending down the anterior and radial aspects of forearm and occasionally on to the dorsum of the hand
4. Tingling of the thumb and first three fingers.

Studies have reported varying amounts of normal range of elbow movement during an upper limb neural tissue provocation test with a median nerve bias. Some have found full range of elbow extension (Kenneally et al, 1988) whereas others report a deficit of elbow extension of between 16° and 53° (Pullos, 1986). The differences recorded may be the result of the same movements being performed in a different sequence.

Abnormal responses to a neural tissue provocation test are:

1. Reduced range of movement of the upper limb (Kenneally et al, 1988)

2. Increased resistance to passive movement (Butler, 1991)
3. Reproduction of the patient's symptoms (Butler, 1991).

In the upper limb, sensitizing additions are:

1. Cervical movements – flexion, lateral flexion to the opposite side, rotation to the opposite side (Elvey, 1988; Selvaratnam, 1987)
2. Upper limb movements of the opposite arm (Rubenach, 1985)
3. Straight-leg raising (Bell, 1987).

Provocation tests can only be carried out within available ranges of passive movement and are affected by the severity of the pain associated with the condition. The major nerve trunks in the upper limb are likely to be affected by the following movements (Kenneally et al, 1988);

1. The *median nerve* (C5–T1) runs slightly medial to lateral in the upper arm, anteriorly across the elbow, and down the forearm to the wrist and hand. A neural tissue provocation test to assess the median nerve includes abduction and lateral rotation of the glenohumeral joint and extension of the elbow, wrist and hand.

2. The *musculocutaneous nerve* (C5–7) runs medial to lateral in the upper arm and across the anterior aspect of the elbow to become the lateral cutaneous nerve of the forearm. The physiological movements of abduction, lateral rotation of the glenohumeral joint and elbow extension cause movement of the musculocutaneous nerve.

3. The *ulnar nerve* (C7–T1) runs posterior to the medial epicondyle of the elbow and passes into the anterior forearm through the two heads of flexor carpi ulnaris. In its upper part, the nerve is affected by abduction and lateral rotation of the glenohumeral joint, while in the forearm the physiological movements of elbow flexion, forearm pronation, wrist and finger extension create movement of the ulnar nerve.

4. The *radial nerve* (C5–T1) has a posterior course in the arm and can be assessed using the movements of glenohumeral abduction and medial rotation, forearm pronation, elbow extension and wrist and finger flexion (Elvey and Hall, 1997).

FACTORS AFFECTING MOBILITY OF THE SPINAL CORD AND NERVES

Any pathological change affecting the spinal cord, meninges, nerve roots or tissues in close relationship to them is likely to alter the mobility and tension in these structures. The pain-sensitive structures may be subjected to compressive, tensile or bending stresses. They may be subjected to mechanical or chemical irritation or become adherent at any point along their length.

The inherent plasticity of the meningeal tissues decreases with ageing and these tissues are less able to sustain tension stresses. As maturation and degenerative changes occur within the vertebral column, the intervertebral discs lose height and the vertebral bodies approximate so that the neural canal becomes shorter. Folds develop within the dura to accommodate the decrease in vertical height. Degenerative changes may also lead to a decrease in the size of the bony canal. Spondylotic ridges and osteophytes may intrude into the canal, reducing the space available for the cord and meninges.

There are many sites within the body where the neural structures are particularly susceptible to compromise because of the anatomy of the interfacing tissues, such as in the fibro-osseous (e.g. carpal tunnel) or osseous (e.g. intervertebral foramen) tunnels. Additional factors such as anatomical anomalies and pathological changes can combine to result in there being insufficient room for the nerve to move freely through the non-neural adjacent tissues. Other common sites of compromise include:

- The lower portions of the brachial plexus (C7–T1) at the thoracic outlet (Edgelow, 1997)
- The median, ulnar and radial nerves at the elbow and wrist
- The T5–7 spinal canal, which is particularly narrow and has little room for adaptive displacement of the neural tissues
- L4/5, where the neural structures are firmly tethered by dural ligaments (Blikra, 1969)
- The common peroneal nerve at the head of the fibula and the posterior tibial and superficial peroneal nerves at the ankle (Mackinnon and Dellon, 1988)
- The sciatic nerve between the two heads of piriformis (Shacklock et al, 1994).

Sunderland (1976) describes a pressure gradient which must exist in the intervertebral foramen for normal neural function:

- Pressure in the epineurium of the nutrient artery→
- Pressure in endoneurial capillaries→
- Pressure in veins in epineurium→
- Intrafunicular pressure→
- Intraforaminal pressure.

Increase in the intraforaminal pressure could lead to venous congestion and stasis. Sunderland (1976) identifies three stages that may occur with persistent pressure in the carpal tunnel – hypoxia, oedema and fibrosis – and considers that similar events could occur in other tunnel sites. In the hypoxic state, decreased intrafunicular circulation impairs nerve fibre nutrition and may lead to local pain. Continuation of this situation will lead to damage of the capillary endothelium so that leakage of protein-rich fluid occurs, causing oedema. The oedema is unable to disperse because the perineurium is not crossed by lymphatics (Lundborg, 1975) and there is a subsequent increase in intrafunicular pressure.

The protein-rich oedema enhances fibroblast formation so that intraneural fibrosis develops. Such increases in connective tissue raise the intraneural pressure so that a self-perpetuating cycle is established. At this stage, axonal transport properties are affected and the situation no longer become reversible. The affected area becomes a 'fibrous cord', and 'friction fibrosis' may occur at other vulnerable sites along the tract (Sunderland, 1976). The fibrosis that occurs is also known as 'adhesions' or 'tethering'.

Adhesions or tethering can occur within a neural structure or between the neural structure and the adjacent tissues through which it passes. If adhesions occur inside a nerve root or axon, the scarred neural tissue is unable to elongate normally so that mechanical stresses will pass further along the nerve than normal (Tani et al, 1987). A nerve that has been tightened surgically can adapt within weeks to regain almost its original length (Bora et al, 1980) but scarred neural tissue is not able to adapt as effectively to changes in tension (Millesi, 1986). During physiological active and passive movements the nerve roots and nerve slide in relation to the structures through which they pass. When tethering occurs between the neural elements and adjacent bony, neural and soft tissue elements, the available range of physiological movement is reduced (Elvey and Hall, 1997).

Altered tension at one point along a nerve trunk will have mechanical repercussions elsewhere. A study of 115 patients with carpal tunnel syndrome or lesions of the ulnar nerve found that 70% had electrophysiological and clinical evidence of neural lesions in the cervical spine (Upton and McComas, 1973). These dual pathologies were termed 'double crush phenomenon'. Abnormal concentrations of stress on the neural structures slow the axoplasmic flow and may be the cause of double or multiple crush injuries.

References

Bell A (1987) The upper limb tension test – bilateral straight leg raising – a validating manoeuvre for the upper limb tension test. In: *Proceedings of the Fifth Biennial Conference of the Manipulative Therapists Association of Australia*, Melbourne, pp. 106–114.

Blikra G (1969) Intradural herniated lumbar disc. *Journal of Neurosurgery* 31: 676–679.

Bora F, Richardson S, Black J (1980) The biomechanical responses to tension in peripheral nerve. *Journal of Hand Surgery* 5: 474–476.

Bowsher D (1988) *Introduction to the Anatomy and Physiology of the Nervous System*. Blackwell, Oxford.

Breig A (1960) *Biomechanics of the Central Nervous System: Some Basic Normal and Pathological Phenomena*. Almquist and Wiksell, Stockholm, pp. 31–34, 60–61, 94.

Breig A (1978) *Adverse Mechanical Tension in the Central Nervous System*. Almqvist and Wiksell, Stockholm.

Breig A, Troup JDG (1979) Biomechanical considerations in the straight-leg-raising test, cadaveric and clinical studies of the effects of medial hip rotation. *Spine* 4: 242.

Butler DD (1991) *Mobilisation of the Nervous System*. Churchill Livingstone, Melbourne, p. 162.

Butler DS, Gifford L (1989) The concept of adverse mechanical tension in the nervous system. Part 1. Testing for dural tension. *Physiotherapy* 75: 622.

Davidson S (1987) Prone knee bend – a normative study and investigation into the effect of cervical flexion and extension. In: *Proceedings of the Manipulative Therapists Association of Australia*. 5th Biennial Conference, Melbourne.

Dommisse G (1975) Morphological aspects of the lumbar spine and lumbosacral region. *Clinical Orthopaedics and Related Research* 115: 22.

Edgar MA, Nundy S (1966) Innervation of the spinal dura mater. *Journal of Neurology, Neurosurgery and Psychiatry* 23: 251.

Edgelow PI (1997) Neurovascular consequences of cumulative trauma disorders affecting the thoracic outlet; a patient centred treatment approach. In: Donatelli R (ed.) *Physical Therapy of the Shoulder*, 3rd edn. Churchill Livingstone, New York, pp. 153–178.

Elvey R (1980) Brachial plexus tension tests and the pathoanatomical origin of arm pain. In: Idczak R (ed.) *Aspects of Manipulative Therapy*. Lincoln Institute of Health Sciences, Melbourne.

Elvey R, Hall T (1997) Neural tissue evaluation and treatment. In: Donatelli R (ed.) *Physical Therapy of the Shoulder*, 3rd edn. Churchill Livingstone, New York, pp. 131–152.

Elvey RL (1988) The clinical relevance of signs of adverse brachial plexus tension. In: *Proceedings of the International*

Federation of Orthopaedic Manipulative Therapists Congress, Cambridge.

Epstein BS (1966) An anatomic, myelographic and cinemyelographic study of the dentate ligaments. *American Journal of Roentgenology* 98: 704.

Epstein BS (1976) *The Spine – a Radiological Text and Atlas,* 4th edn. Lea & Febiger, Philadelphia, pp. 44–47.

Fahlgren Grampo J, Reynolds HM, Vorro J, Beal M (1991) 3-D motion of the pelvis during passive leg lifting. In: Anderson PA, Hobart DJ, Dnaoff JV (ed.) *Electromyographical Kinesiology.* Elsevier Science, Amsterdam, pp. 119–122.

Frykholm R (1955) Cervical nerve root compression resulting from disc degeneration and root sleeve fibrosis. A clinical investigation. *Acta Chirurgica Scandinavicum Supplementum* 160.

Goddard MD, Reid DJ (1965) Movements induced by straight-leg-raising in the lumbosacral nerve roots, nerves and plexus, and in the intrapelvic portion of the sciatic nerve. *Journal of Neurology, Neurosurgery and Psychiatry* 28: 12.

Grieve GP (1988) *Common Vertebral Joint Problems,* 2nd edn. Churchill Livingstone, Edinburgh, pp. 314, 324.

Haupt W, Stopft E (1978) Über die Dehnbarkeit und Reibfestigkeit der Dura Mater Spinalis des Menschen. *Verhandlungen Anatomische Gesallschaft* 72S: 139–144.

Hollinshead WH (1969) *Anatomy for Surgeons,* 2nd edn, Vol. 3. Harper and Row, New York, p. 176.

Johnson EK, Chiarello CM (1997) The slump test: the effect of head and lower limb extremity position on knee extension. *Journal of Orthopaedic Sports Physiotherapy* 26: 310–317.

Keneally M (1983) The upper limb tension test. An investigation of responses amongst normal, asymptomatic subjects. Unpublished thesis. Cited in: Grant R (ed.) *Physical Therapy of the Cervical and Thoracic Spines,* 1988. Churchill Livingstone, Edinburgh, p. 188.

Kenneally M (1985) The upper limb tension test. In: *Proceedings of the Fourth Biennial Conference of the Manipulative Therapists Association of Australia,* Brisbane, pp. 259–273.

Kenneally M, Robenach H, Elvey R (1988) The upper limb tension test; the SLR test of the arm. In: Grant R (ed.) *Physical Therapy of the Cervical and Thoracic Spines.* Churchill Livingstone, Edinburgh, p. 10.

Khuffash B, Porter RW (1989) Cross leg pain and trunk list. *Spine* 14: 602–603.

Kleynhans AM, Terrett AGJ (1986) The prevention of complications from spinal manipulative therapy. In Glasgow EF, Twomey LT (eds) *Aspects of Manipulative Therapy.* Churchill Livingstone, Melbourne, pp. 171–174.

Kopell H, Thompson W (1976) *Peripheral Entrapment Neuropathies.* Robert Kreiger, Malabar, Florida.

Lew PC, Briggs CA (1997) Relationship between the cervical component of the slump test and change in hamstring muscle tension. *Manual Therapy* 2: 98–105.

Louis R (1981) Vertebroradicular and vertebromedullar dynamics. *Anatomica Clinica* 3: 1.

Lundborg G (1975) Structure and function of the intraneural microvessels as related to trauma, oedema formation and nerve function. *Journal of Bone and Joint Surgery (Am.)* 57: 938.

Luttges M, Stodieck L, Beel J (1986) Postinjury changes in the biomechanics of nerves and nerve roots in mice. *Journal of Manipulative and Physiological Therapeutics* 9: 89–98.

Mackinnon S, Dellon A (1988) *Surgery of the Peripheral Nerve.* Thieme, New York.

Maitland GD (1978) Movement of pain-sensitive structures in the vertebral canal in a group of physiotherapy students. *Proceedings, Inaugural Congress of Manipulative Therapists Association of Australia,* Sydney.

Maitland GD (1985) The Slump test. *Australian Journal of Physiotherapy* 31: 215–219.

Maitland GD (1986) *Vertebral Manipulation,* 5th edn. Butterworth Heinemann, London, p. 68.

Massey AE (1982). The slump test: an investigation of the movement of pain sensitive structures in the vertebral canal in subjects with low back pain. Dissertation presented in partial fulfilment of the Graduate Diploma in Advanced Manipulative Therapy, South Australian Institute of Technology.

Massey AE (1986) Movement of pain-sensitive structures in the neural canal. In: Grieve GP (ed.) *Modern Manual Therapy of the Vertebral Column.* Churchill Livingstone, Edinburgh, pp. 182–193.

McLellan D, Swash M (1976) Longitudinal sliding of the median nerve during movements of the upper limb. *Journal of Neurology, Neurosurgery and Psychiatry* 39: 566–570.

Millesi H (1986) The nerve gap. *Hand Clinics* 2: 651–663.

O'Connell JEA (1951) Protrusions of the lumbar intervertebral discs. *Journal of Bone and Joint Surgery (Br.)* 33: 8.

Penning L, Wilmink JT (1981) Biomechanics of the lumbosacral dural sac: a study of flexion/extension myelography. *Spine* 6: 398.

Pullos J (1986) The upper limb tension test. *Australian Journal of Physiotherapy* 32: 258–259.

Rubenach H (1985) The upper limb tension test. The effect of the position and movement of the contralateral arm. *Proceedings of the Manipulative Therapists Association of Australia 5th Biennial Conference,* Brisbane.

Selvaratnam P (1987) The discriminative validity and reliability of the brachial plexus tension test. *Proceedings of the Manipulative Therapists Association of Australia 5th Biennial Conference,* Melbourne, pp. 325–350.

Shacklock MO, Butler DS, Slater H (1994) The dynamic central nervous system: structure and clinical neurobiomechanics. In: Boyling JD, Palastanga N (eds) *Grieve's Modern Manual Therapy Vertebral Column.* 2nd edn. pp. 21–38.

Shiging X, Qanzhi Z, Dehao F (1987) Significance of the straight leg raising test in the diagnosis and clinical evaluation of lower lumbar intervertebral disc protrusion. *Journal of Bone and Joint Surgery (Am.)* 69: 518.

Smith C (1956) Changes in length and position of the segments of the spinal cord with changes in posture of the monkey. *Radiology* 66: 259–265.

Spencer D, Irwin G, Miller J (1983) Anatomy and significance of fixation of the lumbosacral nerve roots in sciatica. *Spine* 8: 672–679.

Sunderland S (1974) Meningeal-neural relations in the intervertebral foramen. *Journal of Neurosurgery* 49: 756–776.

Sunderland S (1976) The nerve lesion in carpal tunnel syndrome. *Journal of Neurology, Neurosurgery and Psychiatry* 39: 615.

Sutton JL (1979) The 'straight-leg-raising test'. Unpublished thesis. South Australian Institute of Technology, Adelaide.

Tani S, Yamada S, Knighton RS (1987) Extensibility of the lumbar and sacral cord: pathophysiology of the tethered spinal cord in cats. *Journal of Neurosurgery* 66: 116–747.

Tencer A, Allen B, Ferguson R (1985) A biomechanical study of thoracolumbar spine fractures with bone in the canal. *Spine* 10: 741–747.

Troup JDG (1986) Biomechanics of the lumbar spinal canal. *Clinical Biomechanics* 1: 31.

Tunturi A (1977) Elasticity of the spinal cord dura in the dog. *Journal of Neurosurgery* 47: 391–396.

Upton ARM, McComas AJ (1973) The double crush in nerve entrapment syndromes. *Lancet* ii: 359.

van der Heide B, Allison GT, Zusman M (2001) Pain and muscular responses to a neural tissue provocation test in the upper limb. *Manual Therapy* 6: 154–162.

Woodhall B, Hayes GH (1950) The well-leg raising test of Fajersztajin in the diagnosis of ruptured lumbar intervertebral disc. *Journal of Bone and Joint Surgery (Am.)* 32: 786.

Chapter **9**

Embryology, development, ageing and degeneration

EMBRYOLOGY AND DEVELOPMENT

Prenatal life is divided into embryonic and fetal periods: the embryonic period comprising the first eight postovulatory weeks and the fetal period extending to birth.

By the third week of development, the embryo has taken the form of a flat disc consisting of two layers of cells: the ectoderm and the endoderm. Cells from the ectoderm give rise to a third layer, the mesoderm. At the end of the fourth week, a solid rod of cells called the notochord grows in the midline and forms a framework around which the primitive vertebral column will develop. Cells of the notochord induce the ectoderm posterior to it to initiate formation of the neural plate, from which develops the brain, spinal cord and most of the remainder of the nervous system.

SEGMENTATION OF THE MESODERM

The mesoderm forms three columns on both sides of the axis formed by the notochord and neural plate: a medial, thickened paraxial mesoderm, an intermediate mesoderm and a lateral plate.

The paraxial mesoderm becomes segmented into a longitudinal series of blocks or somites, commencing in the region of what will be the head and proceeding distally. By 30 days of development, 42–44 pairs of somites can be identified in the embryo, 11–12 pairs of which regress or participate in the formation of the occipital region of the skull. Variations in the number of somites may occur such as an additional or a missing one, which is often compensated for by a variation in an adjacent region.

The cells in each somite gradually change into loosely arranged tissue called mesenchyme. Cells in the anteromedial part of the somite constitute the sclerotome; those in the posterolateral part constitute the dermatome.

DEVELOPMENT OF THE VERTEBRAL COLUMN

The development of the vertebral column occurs in three stages: the mesenchymal stage, the cartilaginous stage and the ossification stage. These stages are not entirely distinct; they merge into one another.

1. Mesenchymal stage

During the mesenchymal stage, changes occur in the mesenchyme that result in the formation of a primitive model of the vertebral column. The mesodermal column re-segments into alternate light and dark bands. The dark bands are relatively slow growing fibroblastic structures that will develop into the intervertebral discs. The light bands develop into cartilage models of the vertebrae. The aorta, lying anterior to the notochord, sends intersegmental branches around the middle of each light band. The light bands grow in height more rapidly than the dark bands (Verbout, 1985).

In the sclerotome, the developing spinal nerve grows laterally into the dermomyotome and, in time, is surrounded by perineural tissue formed from the cranial half of the somite.

The remainder of the somite participates in the formation of the vertebral column. Two processes develop in the caudal half of each somite: a dorsal process, which grows to form the neural arch, and a ventrolateral process, which forms the costal element. Less dense condensations of mesenchyme join the neural arches of adjacent segments and eventually give rise to ligaments.

Meanwhile, multiplying and surrounding the notochord is a continuous column of cells called the axial mesenchyme. This forms the centrum, which is the greater part of the vertebral body, the remainder of it being formed by the third process from the sclerotome. A zone of increased density in the lower end of the cranial part of the axial mesenchyme forms the predecessor to the future intervertebral disc (Verbout, 1985).

The dermomyotome divides into the myotome, which is the forerunner of striated muscle, and the dermatome, which gives rise to the skin and subcutaneous tissues.

At about the 40th day of development, the spinal nerve divides into a ventral and a dorsal ramus. The myotome splits into two portions, the posterior of which is innervated by the posterior ramus, and the anterior by the anterior ramus.

2. Cartilaginous stage

The cartilaginous stage is a short one, commencing at about the sixth week of development in the cranial end of the column. Each light band differentiates into a cartilaginous model of a vertebra at about two months' gestation. Two centres of chondrification appear in each vertebral centrum and one in each half of the neural arch. The latter expand posteriorly to complete the neural arch and a cartilaginous spinous process develops at their union. Expansion also occurs laterally into the transverse process and anteriorly to blend with the chondrifying centrum.

The cylindrical notochord swells within each dark band or primordial intervertebral disc and gradually disappears from each cartilaginous vertebra. The notochord segment will form a nucleus pulposus at the centre of each disc, and at the periphery of each primordial intervertebral disc, fibroblasts lay down collagen fibres in outwardly convex lamellae.

3. Ossification stage

Primary ossification centres begin to appear by the ninth fetal week at the sites where blood vessels grow into the cartilaginous vertebrae. An ossification centre first appears in each half of the neural arch, the earliest centres being in the cervicothoracic region. In the vertebral body, the most common pattern is a single ossification centre (Bagnall et al, 1984). Ossification starts at different times in the vertebral arches and bodies in different areas of the spine, but by the seventh month, centres have established in all areas.

As the primary ossification centre in the vertebral body expands, it does not extend to the superior and inferior surfaces, which remain cartilaginous to ensure continuing growth. The laminae and the bulk of the spinous process become fully ossified during the first year of life.

Certain areas remain cartilaginous until secondary ossification centres appear during puberty in the cartilaginous tips of the spinous process, the tips of the transverse processes and the cartilaginous mamillary processes (Carpenter, 1961; Williams and Warwick, 1980). These areas are separated from the rest of the vertebra by a narrow interval of cartilage, and remain so during the final periods of spinal growth. This cartilage is gradually replaced with bone by the age of 25.

FORMATION OF THE INTERVERTEBRAL DISC

In the mesenchymal intervertebral disc, central cells are loosely arranged around the notochord and peripheral cells are arranged in a radial pattern. The cells closer to the notochord gradually transform into embryonic cartilage (Peacock, 1951). Towards the end of the second month of embryonic life, the notochord enlarges between the developing vertebrae. The collagen fibres formed from the peripheral cells become laminated at a very early stage and insert into the cartilage plates covering the superior and inferior parts of the vertebral bodies. The cartilage cells closer to the annulus undergo transition to fibrocartilage. At this stage, the disc has three zonal compartments: the notochord centrally, the collagenous annulus peripherally and fibrocartilage in between. The notochordal cells of the nucleus multiply rapidly and produce a proteoglycan-rich mucoid matrix that enlarges the nucleus pulposus. The growing nucleus pulposus is entirely enveloped by the annular fibres and the cartilage end plates. At birth, some of the notochord cells may persist in the disc, but these eventually atrophy and disappear during infancy.

The fetal and infant disc has plentiful blood vessels in the annulus and cartilage end plates, but they do not usually penetrate into the nucleus pulposus. Most of the blood vessels have disappeared by 4 years of age, although there remain a few small vascular buds that project from the vertebral marrow into the vertebral aspect of the end plate and some capillaries that supply the outer annular layers (Taylor et al, 1992). The notochordal cells are unable to survive an avascular environment and they are replaced during childhood by chondrocytes and fibroblasts that are better able to survive in these conditions (Giles and Singer, 1997).

GROWTH OF THE VERTEBRAL BODY

The vertebral body grows horizontally by periosteal ossification, and longitudinally by proliferation of the cartilages on the whole of its superior and inferior surfaces. The cells nearest to the vertebral body become ossified and are replaced by cells from the cartilage end plate.

The shape of the vertebral bodies changes through an increase in their anteroposterior growth rate with the assumption of the erect posture in infants and corresponding increase in lordosis. There are related changes in the shapes of the intervertebral discs and vertebral end plates, and the position of the nucleus pulposus. The end plates are convex in fetal and infant vertebrae, and become concave in children, adolescents and adults. During adolescence, the dimensions of the vertebral bodies in females are somewhat smaller than in males, but by adulthood they more closely approach dimensions in males (Bogduk and Twomey, 1987).

Ossification ceases by the age of 25 and the growth plates become thinner. They are separated from the vertebral body by a calcified layer of cartilage and a subchondral bone plate. The other part of each cartilage plate, which becomes the end plate of the intervertebral disc, does not ossify during life except for an outer bony rim or apophysis which is apparent by the age of 12 years. This fuses with the vertebral body when longitudinal growth ceases, although it does not itself contribute to growth. The ring apophysis provides a bony attachment for the peripheral annular fibres.

GROWTH IN LENGTH OF THE VERTEBRAL COLUMN

The vertebral column grows most rapidly before birth. The rate of growth decreases during infancy and childhood until there is a final growth spurt during adolescence. Vertebral column length is assessed by taking sitting height measurements. Sitting height increases by 5 cm in the second year of life and then the growth rate decreases to 2.5 cm per annum between the ages of 4 and 7 years (Taylor and Twomey, 1986). It decreases further between the ages of 9 and 10 to 1.5 cm per annum. In the preadolescent years, the rate of growth is disproportionate throughout the body: there is greater increase in length of the limbs relative to the trunk, and the centre of gravity moves more caudally (Porter, 1989).

During adolescence the peak velocity of growth height occurs approximately two years after the onset of puberty. The rate of growth peaks at 12 years in girls and 14 years in boys. During this period both girls and boys have a height growth velocity of 4 cm per annum (Taylor and Twomey, 1986). The average girl will add from 6 to 11 cm to her height, while the average boy will add from 7 to 12 cm to his height. Sitting height reaches 99% of its maximum at the age of 15 years in girls and 17 years in boys.

DEVELOPMENT OF THE APOPHYSEAL JOINTS

The dorsal processes of the mesenchymal neural arches in adjacent somites blend with one another at the sites of the future apophyseal joints. As chondrification of the articular processes proceeds, the mesenchyme recedes to form the articular capsule, any intra-articular structures and a joint space (Bogduk and Twomey, 1987). The articular processes are not completely ossified at birth.

There is a change in the orientation of the lumbar apophyseal joints, which is of particular importance. At birth all the lumbar apophyseal joints are orientated in the coronal plane, but by the age of 11 years this has changed to the adult orientation (Odgers, 1933). The reasons for this change in orientation are not known, but it has been suggested that there may be a genetic determination, or that as multifidus pulls on the mamillary process, it swings the lateral part of the superior articular process dorsally, thereby rotating the plane of the joint or imparting a curvature to it (Bogduk and Twomey, 1987).

DEVELOPMENTAL ANOMALIES

Most congenital anomalies appear during the embryonic period (Bradford and Hensinger, 1985). The principal cause of many of these anomalies has been attributed to genetic transmission (Jeffreys, 1980), other factors being metabolic, the use of drugs, irradiation, infections and maternal alcoholism (Tredwell et al, 1982).

Bony and soft tissue anomalies in the vertebral column are common; indeed, it is more rare to find true structural symmetry. It is essential to remember this when assessing an individual, particularly when observing physiological movements. Bony anomalies are likely to influence direction and range of movement at the affected motion segment and hence it may not necessarily be 'normal' for an individual to have pure symmetrical movement. Bony anomalies may also affect palpation findings in terms of both bony landmarks and accessory movements available.

While some anomalies are purely of academic interest, others may have a marked influence on biomechanics of the spine and hence its symptomatology due to the abnormal stresses they impose on joints and ligaments. Otherwise quiescent anomalies can have serious repercussions in traumatic incidents.

Structural anomalies can occur anywhere in the spine, but it is the transitional regions that are most susceptible (Schmorl and Junghanns, 1971). There is a high incidence of anomalies in the craniovertebral region and this is of particular importance to those who manipulate the upper cervical spine. Common anomalies at the craniovertebral region include posterior spina bifida of the atlas (Spillane et al, 1957), asymmetry of the superior articular facets of the atlas (Singh, 1965; Van Roy et al, 1997) and hemivertebra (Taylor and Twomey, 1994a). The relationship between developmental anomalies of the craniovertebral region and headaches has been noted (McRae, 1953). Congenital absence of the odontoid peg (os odontoideum) is a rare finding; loss of the odontoid is usually caused by trauma.

The lumbosacral region is also prone to anomalies. Of particular relevance to therapists is articular tropism, or asymmetrical orientation of the apophyseal joints, so that at one vertebral level the plane of one apophyseal joint is more inclined in the frontal or sagittal plane than that of the contralateral apophyseal joint. It is most common at the lowest two lumbar levels (Cyron and Hutton, 1980) and occurs to a varying degree in 21–37% of the population (Farfan, 1973; Grieve, 1989).

Tropism has been cited as a cause of low back pain (Cyron and Hutton, 1980; Hagg and Wallner, 1990; Cassidy et al, 1992; Vanharanta et al, 1993). Articular tropism is considered to be a factor in rotational instability when the ligaments of the apophyseal joint come under strain (Cyron and Hutton, 1980). This may also lead to a rotation strain of the disc as more stress is placed on the intervertebral disc on the side of the more obliquely orientated apophyseal joint.

When flexion occurs in the presence of tropism, it usually does so about some oblique axis X–X' (see Fig. 1.26, p. 55), so that capsular ligaments are equidistant from the axis of rotation. Flexion about X–X' causes maximal stretching of the posterolateral annulus; hence posterolateral tears usually occur at the side of the more oblique facet.

Farfan and Sullivan (1967) found a high correlation between the side of the more oblique facet and the side of sciatica but other authors have failed to corroborate this relationship (Hagg and Wallner, 1990; Cassidy et al, 1992; Vanharanta et al, 1993).

It is not within the scope of this book to describe every anomaly that can occur. The most common causes of most anomalies are failure of development of a vertebra, non-union of parts of a vertebra and failure of segmentation. Anomalies in the intersegmental branches of the dorsal aorta may result in anomalies of segmentation. In the mesenchymal stage, these vessels normally run around the centres of the loose bands and provide nutrition for the primitive vertebrae. It is conceivable that absence of such a vessel could mar the development of part of a vertebra.

Block vertebrae

Defective development of loose bands in the mesenchymal stage may give rise to block vertebrae (so-called 'fused vertebrae'). Compensatory movement and stress usually occur above and below the fused segment or segments, predisposing these levels to spondylotic changes in later life (Brain and Wilkinson, 1967).

Wedge and hemivertebrae

Interference with vertebral development can be caused by failure of condensation in the early mesenchymal stage. If partial, this can give rise to vertebral wedging; the extent of failure of formation varies and consequently so does the degree of vertebral wedging. If there is complete failure of development on one side, a hemivertebra may develop (James, 1976). These abnormal vertebrae lead to an increasing scoliosis during growth and predispose to early degenerative change (McMaster and David, 1986).

Asymmetric growth of the right and left halves of the vertebral arches commonly occurs and results in the pedicles being unequal in length. This has the effect of rotating the vertebral body towards the side of the shorter pedicle.

Schmorl's nodes
(Fig. 9.1)

During segmentation of the mesoderm, weak areas or indentations may be left in the centre of the nuclear aspect of each end plate, which remain until adolescence. These are the points at which failure occurs first on experimental compression (Brown et al, 1957).

Additionally, during fetal life, the annulus and end plates receive a blood supply from the peripheral intersegmental vessels that grow radially towards the nucleus. These vessels involute during childhood and are replaced by connective tissue, constituting channels which are weaker than the surrounding cartilage. Compressed disc material may rupture along the channels in adolescents or young adults (Taylor and Twomey, 1984).

Figure 9.1   Two types of intravertebral disc prolapse (Schmorl's nodes).

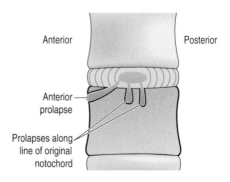

Anterior

Posterior

Anterior prolapse

Prolapses along line of original notochord

Schmorl's nodes, or intravertebral disc prolapses, can occur as a result of these weaknesses. Usually less than 2% of the disc volume is involved. These prolapses are more commonly seen along the line of the original notochord, but sometimes more peripheral prolapses occur along the radially directed channels as described above, to the anterior aspect of the vertebra (see Fig. 9.1). Anterior prolapses are usually larger and can be a source of pain through irritation of nociceptive endings in the periosteum or longitudinal ligament. Scheuermann's kyphosis occurs when the nodes are more extensive, leading to a reduction in the height of the anterior vertebral bodies so that they become wedge-shaped (Fig. 9.2). The cumulative consequence of wedging occurring at adjacent thoracic vertebra is an increase in thoracic kyphosis which is characteristic of Scheuermann's disease.

The incidence of Schmorl's nodes varies between 38% and 79%; the variation may reflect differences in study sample size, age, gender, racial characteristics and geographical distribution between the studies (Giles and Singer, 2000). The greatest incidence of Schmorl's nodes is at the thoraco-lumbar junction (Hilton et al, 1976).

Schmorl's nodes are usually a developmental event and occur during childhood or adolescence. The most common age of onset is before puberty, at a time when the spine has not finished growing. Pain may be experienced at the time the condition is developing and can be associated with 'growing pains' in adolescents. However, in many instances the condition is silent and the individual remains symptom free during his or her teenage years. Ultimately, the affected segments have increased stiffness, partially due to the effects of lack of disc height. Clinically, sites of adjacent hypermobility often develop to compensate for the hypomobile areas. The increase in thoracic kyphosis is accompanied by compensatory increases in the thoracic and lumbar lordoses. The back extensors

Figure 9.2 Wedge-shaped vertebrae in Scheuermann's kyphosis.

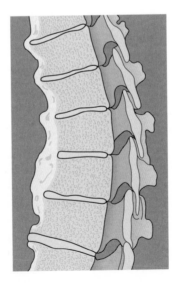

have reduced functional strength in patients with Scheuermann's disease in comparison with controls (Murray et al, 1993).

Spinal stenosis

Spinal stenosis is a narrowing of the spinal canal. Stenosis can be either developmental or degenerative and may compromise the neural structures within the central vertebral canal or nerve root canal. The shape of the vertebral canal is determined by the depth and angulation of the pedicles and laminae. Individuals with trefoil-shaped canals have a greater susceptibility to spinal stenotic syndromes.

The neural contents of the vertebral canal are at greater risk in those who have a congenitally smaller canal that is then subjected to degenerative changes. Degenerative changes that further reduce the size of the vertebral canal include disc herniation, osteophytosis, buckling of ligamentum flavum and apophyseal joint hypertrophy.

Spina bifida

Spina bifida is the most common form of non-union. It ranges from failure of the laminae to unite dorsally behind the cauda equina (spina bifida occulta), which is minor and common, to complete splitting of the skin, vertebral arch and underlying neural tube with associated neurological deficits. Some forms of spina bifida appear during the embryonic period, while others, such as spina bifida occulta, develop during the fetal period.

Sacralization and lumbarization

The lowest lumbar vertebra may become incorporated into the sacrum (sacralization) so that, in effect, there are only four mobile lumbar vertebrae. Conversely, the first sacral vertebra may be mobile (lumbarization). The incidence of transitional lumbosacral vertebrae is 4–8% of the general population (Elster, 1989). Disc herniation is nearly nine times more common at the interspace immediately above the transitional vertebra than at any other level (Elster, 1989). Spinal stenosis and nerve root canal stenosis are also more likely to occur at the interspace above the transitional vertebra.

Congenital scoliosis

Scoliosis is a lateral curvature of the spine. The congenital type develops in the fetus, either through the failure of the vertebrae to form symmetrically or through failure of the vertebrae to separate completely from each other. In some instances both these deformities are found together.

Congenital scoliosis is structural so that, in addition to a lateral curvature, there is vertebral rotation. In the individual vertebra, the bony elements on the concave side have not grown as much as on the convexity. The body is wedged on the concave side, the pedicle is shorter and narrower, and the lamina smaller than on the convex side. The spinous process is directed away from the midline towards the concavity of the curve. Ligamentous structures between the vertebrae are adapted in length. Often posterior joints are abnormal, being compressed on the concave side, where osteophytosis develops earlier than normal.

An irregular pattern of structural curves may be seen in congenital scoliosis. Usually there is a single curve, but two or even three structural curves may be visible. Thoracic curves are the most common. The ribs on the convexity are carried backwards with the vertebral body rotation and are, therefore, more prominent, whereas the ribs on the concavity are crowded together and carried forward, so that there may be an anterior protrusion of the chest wall on this side. Usually there are missing, deformed or fused ribs or a combination of all three, usually – but not always – on the concave side.

The curve is nearly always progressive because the irregular ossific centres and growth plates increase the asymmetry as growth proceeds. The scoliosis can be combined with lordosis or kyphosis depending on the site of the defect. Congenital thoracolumbar and lumbar curves tend to increase considerably; in part this is related to the difficulty of developing compensation below and the association of congenital pelvic obliquity (James, 1976).

Idiopathic scoliosis can occur in infants and young children but it is a condition that affects mainly adolescent girls. The spine is normal at birth, and the curvature usually develops during the adolescent growth spurt. The most common presentation is with a thoracic or thoracolumbar curve convex to the right and a lumbar curve convex to the left. The condition is more frequently seen in girls, the incidence ratio of girls to boys being 8:1. Although it is acknowledged that there is a genetic influence the cause of the disease remains largely unknown. Theories of causation include genetic tendencies, neuromuscular imbalances, leg length difference, hormonal imbalances and physical and emotional stresses (Goldberg et al, 1997).

Commonly associated with spinal curvature is a dropping of one shoulder, a prominent scapula, forward protrusion of the anterior chest wall on one side and prominence of one iliac crest.

A neuromuscular scoliosis develops when there is paralysis of the muscles that support and stabilize the spine. The paralysis may be caused by conditions such as poliomyelitis, cerebral palsy, muscular dystrophy and spinal injury.

Congenital kyphosis

Congenital kyphosis is a spinal deformity occurring exclusively or primarily in the sagittal plane, developing from one or more vertebral body malformations. The defect most commonly presents at the lumbar and thoracolumbar levels, although it can occur anywhere in the spine. It is always progressive. The cause can be either a failure of formation of the vertebral bodies or a failure of segmentation. If the segmentation failure is purely anterior then a kyphosis results: if it is anterolaterally located, then a kyphoscoliosis results.

Thoracic kyphosis can also result from Scheuermann's disease and osteoporosis. Patients with congenital scoliosis and kyphosis have a higher incidence (25%) of segmentation defects in the cervical spine (Winter et al, 1984).

AGEING AND DEGENERATION

As individuals age, their spines undergo fairly characteristic changes. The difficulty arises when attempting to distinguish between those changes that are part of the 'normal' ageing or maturation process and those that are due to degeneration. The same changes may occur both in ageing and in degenerative disease of, for example, the intervertebral disc; when degeneration is present these changes occur earlier than would be expected from normal ageing. 'Normal' age changes are considered to be those that conform to the standard in individuals of a particular age and ethnic group, so the changes considered 'normal' in a 20-year-old spine differ from what is 'normal' in a 70-year-old spine.

Degeneration is characterized by slow, destructive changes which are not balanced by the regeneration that occurs in younger tissues (Grieve, 1981). The normal ageing process can be accelerated by increased exposure to mechanical stresses, which then give rise to degenerative changes. Which part of a motion segment is initially affected depends on the particular mechanical stresses or postures to which the spine is subjected and the integrity of the tissues themselves. The interdependence of the joints comprising the motion segment dictates that failure of one element, either through degeneration or trauma, tends to lead sooner or later to degenerative changes in the other elements (Andersson, 1983).

Ageing and degeneration are not necessarily synonymous: a few elderly discs may behave like younger discs when subjected to compression and torsional loads. Nevertheless, the incidence of degeneration does increase with age. No correlation has been found between radiological evidence of degenerative changes in the spine and the experience of pain. Just as severe changes can be present on a radiograph in the absence of pain, an individual may have intense pain of musculoskeletal origin but a normal radiograph.

The term 'arthrosis' is used to denote degenerative changes in synovial joints, and 'spondylosis' to denote changes in the interbody joints (Fig. 9.3).

Figure 9.3   Degenerative changes in the cervical spine. A, Arthrosis of apophyseal joint. B, Spondylosis.

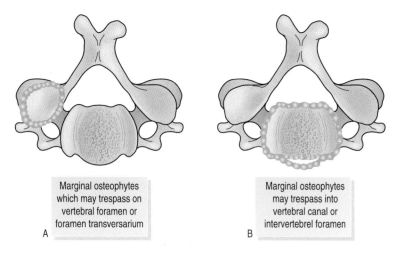

Marginal osteophytes which may trespass on vertebral foramen or foramen transversarium

Marginal osteophytes may trespass into vertebral canal or intervertebrel foramen

A

B

CHANGES IN THE VERTEBRAL BODIES

Ageing is accompanied by loss of both trabecular and cortical bone throughout the skeleton in both sexes. The most severe degree of loss is in trabecular bone, such as that found in the vertebrae (Exton-Smith, 1983). This results in a decrease in bone strength, which is more marked in women than in men. While the structural integrity of trabecular bone is preserved with age in men but not in women, the width of the trabeculae themselves is reduced with age in men (Aaron et al, 1987).

The rate at which bone loss occurs is influenced by such factors as the menopause, reduced plasma calcitonin levels, decreased adrenal androgen production, smoking, declining calcium absorption and reduced physical exercise (Francis and Peacock, 1987). Bone mass and muscle mass are closely interrelated, and exercises play an important role in preventing bone mineral loss in postmenopausal women (Twomey and Taylor, 1985b).

The height of the vertebral bodies declines in old age, principally due to the reduction of transverse trabeculae which act as 'cross-braces' to the vertical trabeculae. On compressive loading, the vertical trabeculae are then less able to withstand the stresses and some of them microfracture. This is most marked below the area of nuclear pulp. Osteoporosis is the major cause of loss of vertebral column height (Dent and Watson, 1966).

As the trabecular system weakens, a greater portion of the compressive load is borne by cortical bone. Consequently, the vertebral body becomes less resistant to deformation and injury. Lacking support from the underlying bone, the vertebral end plates also deform by microfracture and gradually bow into the vertebral body. This increased vertebral concavity leads to a disc convexity in old age.

Fractures may occur in the end plates at areas of reduced resistance, and they may be large enough to allow nuclear material to extrude into the vertebral body to form Schmorl's nodes or intravertebral disc prolapses (see pp. 299–301). Their incidence is greatest in adolescence but it does not increase thereafter (Hilton et al, 1976).

OSTEOPHYTES

Osteophytes are outgrowths of healthy bone from the vertebrae. Their development is an important defence mechanism against compressive forces which exceed the capacity of the bone to resist them. They are composed of more compact, stronger bone than the rest of the vertebral body and bear a marked similarity to the capitals and bases used in architecture which increase the resistance of pillars to compression. The vertebrae, by the formation of osteophytes, are converted into low pillars with capitals and bases.

Nathan (1962) described four successive stages in the development of osteophytes (Fig. 9.4).

1st degree: Isolated points of initial hyperostosis which may pass unnoticed on x-ray

2nd degree: Bony protrusions projecting more or less horizontally from the vertebral body

Continues

Continued

By increasing the superior and inferior surfaces of the vertebral bodies, the 1st and 2nd degree osteophytes effectively reduce the force per unit area.

3rd degree: Characteristic bird's beak shape, curving in the direction of the intervertebral disc

4th degree: Fusion of two adjacent vertebrae

A young person with normal vertebrae may develop osteophytes when the pressure on the vertebral bodies is excessive, as in heavy manual work or strenuous sports. Disc degeneration and the subsequently impaired shock-absorbing capacity of the vertebral column can also lead to their formation, as can pathological processes that weaken the vertebrae, such as osteoporosis.

In the fourth decade, most spines have osteophytes, and by the eighth decade nearly all spines are affected by 3rd or 4th degree osteophytes. They arise where the pressure is greatest, that is in the concavities of either the normal vertebral column or one where there is a deformity such as scoliosis. In relation to the curvatures in the sagittal plane, Nathan (1962) found that the highest incidence coincided with the peaks of the spinal curves (C5, T8, L3/4), whereas the lowest incidence was where the line of gravity crossed the spine (T1, T12 and L5/S1). The incidence of anterior osteophytes was found to be greater than that of posterior osteophytes.

In the different regions of the spine, osteophytes were found to predominate in the prevertebral muscles (longus capitis and longus cervicis) in the cervical spine, in the anterior longitudinal ligament in the thoracic spine, and at the origins of the psoas muscles and crura of the diaphragm in the lumbar spine. Their formation is not necessarily a pathological reaction but they can give rise to symptoms by pressing on neural tissues, e.g. in the vertebral canal or intervertebral foramina (Fig. 9.5), lumbar sympathetic ganglia, or viscera such as the oesophagus and trachea. Other factors in addition to pressure are involved, however, because symptoms can abate while osteophytes remain.

Figure 9.4   Osteophytes. (After Nathan, 1962.)

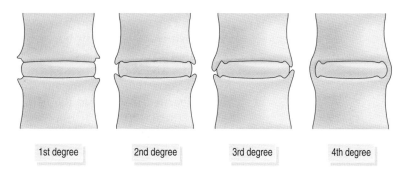

1st degree   2nd degree   3rd degree   4th degree

Figure 9.5 A, Normal vertebra. B, Arthritic vertebra. Osteophytes may impinge on neural structures as they emerge between the zygapophyseal and uncovertebral joints. (From Taylor JR, Twomey LT 1994 Functional and applied anatomy of the cervical spine. In: Grant R, ed. *Physical Therapy of the Cervical and Thoracic Spine*, 2nd edn. Churchill Livingstone, Edinburgh, Fig. 1.10, p. 20, with permission.)

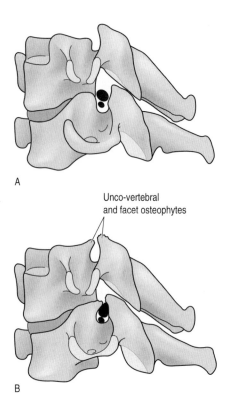

A

Unco-vertebral and facet osteophytes

B

Quite marked osteophytosis may be present without giving rise to symptoms. Depending on their size, osteophytes are associated with some degree of movement restriction. The more advanced osteophytes are often accompanied by pathological changes in the motion segment.

CHANGES IN THE END PLATES

At birth the end plate is part of the growth plate of the vertebral body. The disc side of the end plate is formed by fibrocartilage, the vertebral side being the growth zone. There is a gradual reduction in the width of the growth zone up to the age of 16–20 years, after which the end plates consist of only articular cartilage, which is directly apposed to bone (Bernick and Cailliet, 1982). Collagen fibres arise from the articular cartilage and radiate into the nucleus pulposus. These fibres are independent of the anchoring fibres of the annulus and may serve to give stability to the disc. Progressive resorption and thinning of the articular cartilage occurs, with replacement by bone, so that over the age of 60 there is often only a thin layer of calcified cartilage separating the disc from the vertebral body. The shock-absorbing capacity of the end plates is thereby reduced. A common radiographic appearance with ageing is bulging of the lumbar end plates into the vertebral bodies (Fig. 9.6), outlined by sclerosis (Roaf, 1960).

With increasing age, it is likely that there is a decrease in the diffusion of substances through the end plates. Since the cells in the disc are

Figure 9.6   Disc bulging.

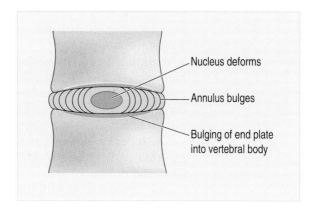

dependent on this route both for their supply of nutrients and the removal of waste products, closure of the end plate route would be expected to lead to nutritional deficiencies as well as to a build-up of metabolic products, such as lactic acid. Thus, changes in the permeability of the end plates could be one of the causes of disc degeneration (Urban and Maroudas, 1980).

CHANGES IN THE INTERVERTEBRAL DISCS

In both nucleus and annulus, the fundamental change with age is the fall in the content of proteoglycans, those that persist being smaller in size. Both of these factors are largely responsible for the progressive decrease in the water-binding capacity of the nucleus. At birth, the nucleus contains 88% water; by the age of 75 this has dropped to 65–72%, the majority of this loss occurring before early adult life (Twomey and Taylor, 1985a).

It is a commonly held belief that loss of vertebral column height with age is due to a reduction in disc height, but studies do not support this idea. Average disc height is usually maintained and may even increase in old age (Nachemson et al, 1979; Twomey and Taylor, 1985a); loss of vertebral column height is caused by loss of vertebral body height. In a normal ageing disc, the mid-sagittal disc height is greater than the small decline in anterior and posterior disc heights. These changes occur as a result of the decrease in central height of the vertebral body and an increase in the end plate concavity together with an increase in peripheral osteophytosis and marginal bony hypertrophy (Taylor and Twomey, 1994b). The intervertebral disc is able to grow and adapt to the changes in vertebral body shape.

There is a gradual increase in the relative proportion of collagen in both nucleus and annulus, possibly because of loss of other components such as proteoglycans. The nature of the collagen also changes: the diameter of the collagen fibrils in the nucleus increases (Happey, 1976) and its Type II collagen resembles the Type I collagen of the annulus. Reciprocally, there is a decrease in the average fibril diameter in the annulus, resulting in less distinction between annulus and nucleus.

The reduction in water content and relative increase in collagen in the nucleus affect its hydraulic properties, making it more rigid and less resilient.

If the disc becomes vascularized, which can occur when the end plates are damaged, disc degeneration is accelerated. The term 'brown degeneration' is sometimes used when the nucleus becomes discoloured through the breakdown of haemoglobin. Nerve fibres then accompany the blood vessels into the disc and may serve a nociceptive function (see p. 8.3).

The concentration of elastic fibres in the annulus drops, and they are replaced by large fibrous inelastic bands, causing a progressive loss of elasticity.

Disc degeneration with the subsequently impaired shock-dissipating capacity of the vertebral column leads to the formation of osteophytes along the margins of the vertebral bodies (called 'lipping'). In the cervical spine, the outgrowths may include nuclear as well as annular material and, continuous at either side with outgrowths from the uncovertebral joints, form a hard, osseocartilaginous bar which projects into the spinal canal, and in severe cases compresses the cord and its meninges into a series of horizontal corrugations.

Rolander (1966) proposed a system of classification of disc degeneration based on the morphological appearance on midline sagittal post mortem sections.

- *Grade 0:* Normal juvenile discs
- *Grade 1:* Normal adult discs, white in colour, nucleus bulges on section
- *Grade 2:* Normal changes of middle age; less distinction between annulus and nucleus, yellowish colour
- *Grade 3:* Frank disc degeneration with desiccation, thinning and fissuring

Twomey and Taylor (1982) found that 72% of all lumbar discs in a study population aged over 60 did not have the significant degenerative changes classed by Rolander as grade 3. Most of the discs were grade 2; desiccation and thinning of the disc is not universal or even the norm in an elderly spine.

ISOLATED DISC RESORPTION

Isolated disc resorption is a condition in which a single intervertebral disc is narrowed and degenerated in an otherwise normal spine. It is caused by trauma through excessive compression which fractures the cartilage end plate, exposing the antigenic proteoglycans of the nucleus to the blood supply of the vertebral body. An autoimmune reaction is thought to result, causing disc degradation. The disc space is eventually represented by a thin slit filled with fibrous tissue between the vertebral bodies. Vertebral bone on either side of the disc is sclerotic, and the disc is anchored around its circumference by peripheral osteophytes. Occasionally ankylosis occurs.

INCIDENCE OF DISC DEGENERATION

There is a strong familial predisposition to discogenic low back pain and the etiology of degenerative disc disease includes both genetic and environmental factors (Postacchini et al, 1988). The incidence of disc degeneration in the spine as a whole is highest at the lowest two lumbar levels, particularly in the lumbosacral disc. The lumbosacral disc is the largest in the spine and there are many factors which contribute to the greater degree of degeneration seen at this level. As it forms part of the first motion segment above the sacrum, a longer lever arm acts on it during movements of the trunk and arms, subjecting the disc to greater stresses. The large amount of movement at this level and the shear forces acting on the disc with the lordotic posture in the standing posture also increase the forces on the disc. The shape of the posterior aspect of the disc itself has been implicated (Hickey and Hukins, 1980). This is usually flattened or rounded rather than concave and, consequently, has fewer annular fibres to resist flexion, lateral flexion and rotation. In addition, the planes of the apophyseal joints in the lower lumbar spine, being orientated more in the frontal plane, offer less resistance to torsional stresses than those higher in the lumbar spine, whose orientation is more in the sagittal plane.

In the cervical spine, the most common sites of spondylosis are the most mobile regions, namely C5/6 and C6/7 (Bull, 1951). In the thoracic spine, the highest incidence of spondylosis is related to its kyphotic curvature: T7/8 in females and T8/9 in males.

Sustained loading on the spine due to a sedentary life style can accelerate the onset of degenerative changes. Other factors associated with early onset of degenerative changes include excessive and repetitive movements and chemical and hereditary causes. Structural factors and mechanical stresses also influence the onset and rate of degenerative changes.

STRUCTURAL FACTORS INFLUENCING THE DEGENERATIVE PROCESS IN THE LUMBAR SPINE

Degree of lumbar curvature

A study in cadavers (Farfan, 1973) showed that the site of annular damage and Schmorl's nodes varied depending on whether the spine was flat or had a marked lordotic curve. Those with a marked lordotic curve (i.e. with a lumbosacral angle of more than 35°) had the highest incidence of (a) annular damage in the L4/5 disc, and (b) Schmorl's nodes at the L3/4 level, whereas in flat spines (with lumbosacral angles of less than 20°) the distribution of both annular damage and Schmorl's nodes was more evenly distributed over the whole of the lumbar spine. The lordotic curves showed a lesser overall incidence of Schmorl's nodes, suggesting that in these spines the discs were better able to withstand compression loads.

The location of the 5th lumbar vertebra in relation to the iliac crest

The location of the 5th lumbar vertebra varies between individuals. When deeply seated in the pelvis, the lumbosacral disc was found to be less likely to prolapse (Farfan, 1973). In spines where the 5th lumbar vertebra was higher, such that the 4th lumbar vertebra was located entirely above the iliac crest, the lumbosacral disc was more vulnerable to prolapse.

Local structural anomalies

Sacralization

In the presence of complete or almost complete sacralization, the lumbosacral disc may show some degree of hypoplasia by its diminished vertical height, but it rarely shows radiographic evidence of degeneration and is usually stable with minimal or no movement. However, the stability of the 5th lumbar vertebra may induce early degeneration of the L4/5 motion segment, probably because of the reduced capacity for movement of the lumbar spine, which only has four motion segments in this instance.

Tropism (see Fig. 1.26)

One quarter of the general population has some degree of tropism of the apophyseal joints in the lumbar spine. Depending on the degree of asymmetry, there is undoubtedly an association between tropism and the pattern of degeneration in the annulus, probably related to the failure of the joints to protect the disc from torsional injury. Joints with symmetrical facets tend to develop a symmetrical pattern of degeneration: posterior midline radial fissures in discs with a rounded posterior annulus, or bilateral posterolateral radial fissures if the joint has a flattened posterior outline. The asymmetrical interbody joint develops a unilateral posterolateral degenerative pattern.

Spondylolysis and spondylolisthesis

Spondylolysis is a break or discontinuity in the pars interarticularis of a vertebra – a stress or fatigue fracture that results from repetitive hyperflexion, hyperextension and twisting (Ichikawa et al, 1982; Fredrickson et al, 1984; Hensinger, 1989). There may be an underlying genetic component in many cases (Hoshina, 1980). A separation can occur at the defect so that there is a forward shift or slip of one vertebral body on the vertebral body below, creating a *spondylolisthesis*. This condition frequently occurs during the adolescent growth spurt (Alexander, 1984) and can be exacerbated by sporting activities such as gymnastics, diving and rugby. Spondylolisthesis can also develop secondary to degeneration of the lumbar facet joints. If the facet orientation changes through degeneration and remodelling, it can become more horizontal and eventually allow movement of the vertebral bodies. In the degenerative form of spondylolisthesis there is no defect in the pars interarticularis. The presence of a spondylolysis or spondylolisthesis increases the shear forces on the intervertebral disc at the motion segment involved, accelerating degenerative changes in the disc. Segmental instability is a characteristic of spondylolysis and spondylolisthesis, and the segment will become even more unstable if there is failure of some of the annular fibres.

It should be borne in mind that spinal anomalies have been shown to be present in symptom-free individuals, indicating that the anomaly may be just one factor in the multifactorial nature of back pain.

EFFECTS OF MECHANICAL STRESSES ON THE INTERVERTEBRAL DISCS

Mechanical stresses can affect the integrity of the disc in different ways and may accelerate the normal ageing process. The changes that occur in the discs do not always follow a neat and tidy pattern, because structural as well as mechanical factors influence the degenerative process.

Injuries to ligaments either precede or accompany injuries to the discs. Hyperflexion strains in the lumbar spine have been shown to damage the supraspinous and interspinous ligaments first, then the capsular ligaments and then the disc (Adams, 1980). The supraspinous and interspinous ligaments are invariably ruptured or slack in patients with a disc prolapse (Rissanen, 1960).

The first pathological changes that occur in the disc are usually circumferential tears or separations between the laminae in the outer third of the annulus (Fig. 9.7A), the yield point being at the junction of the

Figure 9.7   Stages of disc prolapse. A, Circumferential annular tear. B, Posterolateral radial fissure. C, Annular protrusion. D, Nuclear extrusion. E, Sequestrated disc material.

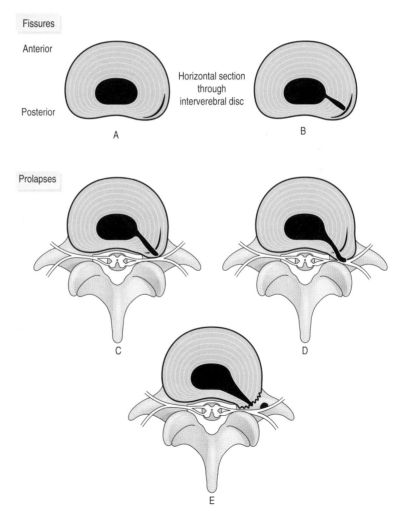

lamina with the end plate. These occur mainly in the posterolateral part of the annulus and do not initially communicate with the nucleus.

Circumferential tears are commonly thought to be caused by repetitive rotation strains. Because of the orientation of the annular fibres, during axial rotation only half of them are able to resist the movement, the outer fibres being stretched more than the inner ones. In the lumbar spine, the apophyseal joints normally protect the discs from rotation beyond a few degrees and the relevance of torsion in producing damage has therefore been questioned. In certain circumstances the apophyseal joints allow the 'safe degree' of rotation to be exceeded. If, say, the cartilage lining of the apophyseal joints is thinned by 3 mm through degeneration, it has been estimated that this would allow an extra 6° of movement (Adams and Hutton, 1981). When the apophyseal joints are more inclined towards the frontal plane, the facet orientation provides less resistance to torsion (see Fig. 1.25). Another factor which allows more rotation is flexion in the intervertebral joint in combination with rotation. The apophyseal joints are less effective in resisting the rotatory component in this combination of movements.

Circumferential tears are usually evident before radial fissures appear (Fig. 9.7B). The latter are most common in thoracic spines (Eckert and Decker, 1947). The shape of the posterior surface of the disc (see Fig. 2.5) dictates the location of the line of maximal torsional stress and hence possibly influences the site of radial fissures (Hickey and Hukins, 1980). In discs that have a concave posterior surface, such as those in the upper lumbar spine, the line of stress radiates posterolaterally. Discs at the lower two lumbar levels most commonly have flat posterior surfaces in which the line of torsional stress radiates to the medial aspect or to the middle of the pedicle, this being the most common direction of radial fissures. Discs with rounded posterior surfaces have a stress concentration in the midline posteriorly; this is often seen at the lumbosacral level.

The development of radial fissures has been attributed to circumferential tears in the annulus that become larger and coalesce to form a tear passing from the annulus into the nucleus (Kirkaldy-Willis, 1988). Farfan (1973) suggested that the radial fissures commence at the nucleus and work towards the periphery to communicate with pre-existing tears. Posterolateral and radial fissures were produced experimentally in cadaveric lumbar discs that were fatigue compression loaded while wedged in flexion and lateral flexion (Adams and Hutton, 1982). The radial fissures occurred as a result of creep deformation of the lamellae and they appeared on the side away from the component of lateral flexion. As the outer annular fibres are innervated, disruption and fissuring of the lamellae could give rise to symptoms.

Once a radial fissure has formed, it creates a pathway down which nuclear material could track in certain circumstances. Prolapse and extrusion do not inevitably follow because of this, but distortion of the lamellae in this manner has been demonstrated as the early stage of a gradual disc prolapse (Fig. 9.8; Adams and Hutton, 1985).

Once the disc has begun to fragment and be disrupted, the nucleus and its retaining annulus become less capable of transmitting axial

Figure 9.8   Distortion of annular lamellae on repeated flexion. Repeated flexion combined with lateral flexion causes the lamellae to become more distorted in the contralateral corner of the disc. (Adapted from Adams M, Hutton WC 1985 Gradual disc prolapse. *Spine* 10: 530.)

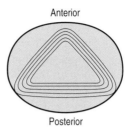

Anterior

Posterior

forces. A greater proportion of these forces are then transmitted vertically to the end plates of the subjacent vertebra.

Repetitive high-velocity movements may take ligaments and annular fibres beyond their normal elastic limits, thereby causing small tears or fissures at the attachment of the annular fibres to the vertebral rim (Osti et al, 1990; Taylor et al, 1990). The discs are particularly vulnerable to these movements if creep has occurred while the disc has been maintained in a sustained flexed or extended posture.

DISC PROLAPSE

A disc prolapse involves the displacement of nuclear material. In the lumbar spine it is most common between the ages of 30 and 50, after which the nuclei have become more fibrotic and are less likely to be expressed as a semifluid substance. Both mechanical overload and biochemical degenerative changes are involved in the mechanics of disc prolapse.

A prolapse can take one of two forms:

1. An annular protrusion (see Fig. 9.7C), when displaced nuclear material stretches the outer annulus, causing it to bulge outwards; the annulus is not completely ruptured
2. A nuclear extrusion (see Fig. 9.7D), when nuclear pulp escapes from the disc through a ruptured annulus.

The term 'disc herniation' is sometimes used when expelled nuclear material rests in a defect in the peripheral annulus and only partially protrudes into the vertebral canal.

There are several mechanisms that can cause a disc to prolapse.

Gradual prolapse

Gradual prolapse is probably the most common mechanism. The injury starts with annular lamellae being distorted to form radial fissures. Nuclear pulp then breaks through the distorted lamellae, causing the outermost lamellae and the adhering posterior longitudinal ligament to protrude. In the final stage, the pulp either extrudes from the mouth of the fissure or migrates behind the final barrier and emerges elsewhere.

Because of the insidious nature of events leading up to the prolapse, the 'final straw' which gives rise to the patient's signs and symptoms may be caused by a somewhat trivial event, such as picking up a pencil from the floor.

Gradual disc prolapses have been reproduced in cadaveric lumbar discs (Adams and Hutton, 1985). Cadaveric lumbar discs were fatigue loaded in compression and flexion, causing trauma to the disc material. The results suggested that prolapses could occur gradually over days or even months. Not all the discs prolapsed, only those that had a soft, pulpy nucleus and a posterior annulus that was thinner than the anterior annulus. Young discs at the L5/S1 level and L4/5 levels showed most internal disruption. Discs in the upper lumbar spine, where the posterior annulus tends to be thicker and stronger, rarely prolapsed. Tests on older discs with pre-existing ruptures failed to demonstrate leakage of nuclear pulp. This is probably because the nucleus in these discs consists of fibrous lumps which are too large to track down a fissure, rendering the disc more stable.

Functional activities that could lead to a gradual disc prolapse are those involving repetitive bending and lifting, not necessarily in the fully flexed position or with maximal loads. This type of prolapse may be preceded by bouts of pain in the lumbar region which the patient passes off as 'muscular'.

Sudden prolapse

Discs can also prolapse suddenly if loading of sufficient intensity is involved, especially in flexed postures. A typical example is a patient who describes having bent down to lift a heavy weight some distance away from his body, such as a battery from a car.

This type of prolapse has been produced in the laboratory on cadaveric lumbar discs (Adams and Hutton, 1982). Discs were wedged to simulate hyperflexion and lateral flexion, and compressed to a maximum that represented the likely compressive force generated by heavy lifting. Hyperflexion is flexion beyond the normal limit: approximately 1–6° of hyperflexion was required to produce the prolapses. The nucleus extruded posterocentrally or on the opposite side to the component of lateral flexion where the annulus was stretched the most. The fissure through which the nuclear pulp was extruded usually occurred at the boundary between the annulus and the cartilage end plate. When the protrusion was large and central it ruptured the posterior longitudinal ligament. Smaller extrusions either formed a bulge behind the ligament (giving the impression of a bulging annulus) or were deflected sideways and appeared on one or both posterolateral margins of the disc. Adams and Hutton described their unsuccessful attempts at pushing extruded material back into the disc as like 'trying to push toothpaste back into the tube'. The susceptibility of discs to this type of prolapse depended on age, degree of disc degeneration and spinal level. Those which were most vulnerable belonged to the 39–51 age group, had moderate degrees of disc degeneration and were from the lower two lumbar levels.

Sudden disc prolapse is quite distinct from gradual prolapse. However, sudden prolapse can occur when a disc is already in the various stages of gradual disc prolapse.

In life, the mechanism of a sudden prolapse undoubtedly varies depending on factors such as the individual's particular anatomical structure, the position of the spine when the trauma occurs and the external forces involved. Hyperflexion of the lumbar discs can occur if the posterior ligaments are first overstretched. This does not necessarily entail high angles of flexion if, for example, the intervertebral joint is stiff. Because of the viscoelastic nature of the posterior ligaments, any prolonged period in the flexed posture will produce creep in the muscles and ligaments, and increase the normal range of flexion. The supra/interspinous ligament is usually found to be ruptured or slack in patients presenting for surgery for prolapsed disc (Newman, 1952; Rissanen, 1960) suggesting that this may be a precursor of disc injury by permitting an unacceptable degree of segmental flexion. If flexion is performed quickly or it is not under adequate muscular control, a joint sprain could result (Adams and Hutton, 1982).

When an individual bends to lift a weight at some distance from the body, the following series of events can be postulated. The posterior annular fibres are stretched and thinned and become the 'weak link' of the intervertebral joint. If the lumbar spine is also laterally flexed, there is further stress on the posterolateral annular fibres on the side away from this component. If the weight is heavy, the lumbar spine flexes further before the lift is executed (see p. 338). The force required to balance and lift the weight may be considerable, and the spinal muscles contract, compressing the vertebral column and raising the hydrostatic pressure in the nucleus. When the lumbar spine is in this position of hyperflexion combined with lateral flexion, only a moderately high compressive force is necessary to produce nuclear extrusion or annular protrusion (Adams and Hutton, 1982). The addition of rotation to flexion raises the existing level of intradiscal pressure.

Cervical disc prolapse

Due to differences in structure between the cervical and lumbar discs (see pp. 81–82), nuclear herniation of the cervical discs is rare. Although early transverse fissuring occurs across the posterior aspect of the cervical disc, the nucleus accumulates collagen rapidly and there is a decrease in the central soft gel, therefore cervical disc herniations are less likely to develop. Commonly, the disc bulges or protrudes posteriorly into the spinal canal, forming a transverse osteocartilaginous bar. The presence of the uncinate processes forms a mechanical bar to posterolateral disc herniations into the intervertebral canal.

Isolated cervical disc degeneration and disc resorption occur mostly in middle-aged and elderly subjects. This is associated with marked loss of disc height, affects one or more discs, and is most frequently seen in the lower three cervical discs (Kramer, 1981; Taylor and Twomey, 1994b). The anteroposterior dimensions of the cervical spinal canal are relatively large and the cord normally only occupies approximately 60% of the available space (Penning, 1968). Hence, osteophytic bars and degenerative changes will not necessarily impinge on the spinal cord.

As the discs become thinner, the uncovertebral joints bear higher compressive loads than normal, and the cartilage lining these joints becomes more like the articular cartilage of synovial joints with osteophytic changes. Osteocartilaginous osteophytes grow out from the uncovertebral joints and can impinge on either the spinal nerve roots or the vertebral artery.

Thoracic disc prolapse

In the thoracic spine, the ratio of disc diameter to height is significantly higher than in the lumbar spine (Kulak et al, 1976) and this is said to give the thoracic discs elastic properties resembling those of solid materials (Horst and Brinckmann, 1981). The thoracic nucleus is relatively small and centrally placed and the disc is given protection from the articulation of the ribs at the costovertebral joints. This combination of factors increases the stability in the area so that thoracic disc herniations and prolapses are relatively rare (Panjabi et al, 1976). Changes in the thoracic discs resulting from road traffic accidents have been observed; Taylor and Twomey (1994b) found evidence of bleeding into thoracic discs following localized thoracic vertebral end plate fractures.

EFFECTS OF VERTICAL LOADING

When the vertebral column is stressed to failure by vertical compression tests, the site of failure depends on anatomical variations and age. In a middle-aged adult, a compression force may produce a wedge fracture of the vertebral body, depending on its mineral content. The same force applied to the spine of an adolescent or healthy young adult would produce vertical extrusions of the nucleus through the cartilage end plate into the vertebral bodies forming Schmorl's nodes or intravertebral prolapses (see pp. 299–301) (Porter, 1989).

HEALING PROCESS

In order for healing to occur following trauma or degeneration of an intervertebral disc, a good blood supply is necessary. The very outermost layers of a normal disc are penetrated by blood vessels and so, theoretically at least, circumferential tears have a chance to heal. Following trauma or as a natural process of ageing, blood vessels penetrating the end plates and annulus, and fresh granulation tissue invading the nucleus, have been seen at surgery (Haley and Perry, 1950) and provide evidence of a healing process. Initial healing by scar formation may have sufficiently different characteristics to produce a change in the mechanical behaviour of the annulus. Insufficient evidence exists of the rate of turnover of collagen in humans, but experiments in dogs suggest that any collagen repair is likely to be extremely slow. Herbert et al (1975) found that in a degenerate human disc and the disc above it there were some immature collagen cross-links, suggesting that some form of remodelling or synthesis was occurring.

SEQUESTRATION

Once a mass of nuclear material has been extruded from the disc, it may become detached or sequestrated (see Fig. 9.7E). Outside the confines of the retaining annulus, the nuclear material first swells and then later shrinks. The sequestrated fragment may migrate some distance from its origin, for example along a nerve root.

COMPRESSION OF NEURAL TISSUE

One of the most serious consequences of degenerative change is impingement or irritation of neural tissue, e.g. the spinal cord or cauda equina in the spinal canal or the nerve roots in the radicular canals or intervertebral foramina.

Pain arising from the nerve roots

Pain associated with the nerve root occurs as a result of nerve root compression or nerve root irritation. The nerves can be compressed or irritated along their course through the spinal canal, radicular canals or in the intervertebral foramina. The normal function of the nerve roots can be affected by the following:

1. Injury or mechanical irritation of the nerve root or dorsal root ganglion
2. Inflammatory conditions of the nerve root
3. Neuroischaemia of the nerve root complex
4. Adhesions and fibrotic scarring that decrease percolation of nutrients from the cerebrospinal fluid from the subarachnoid space to the nerve root
5. Reduced mobility of the spinal nerve and sheath at the nerve root canal.

The most common cause of nerve root compression in the lumbar spine is the disc, either from bulging or from an extruded mass of nuclear material. However, the nerve roots can be compressed by other structures such as osteophytes from an apophyseal joint (see Fig. 9.3A), overriding or subluxation of an apophyseal joint, a hypertrophied ligamentum flavum, an enlarged pedicle, spondylolisthesis, spinal stenosis or other pathological lesions. It is not unusual for more than one of these factors to be responsible.

Compression of a nerve root does not necessarily result in clinical signs and symptoms, as a normal nerve root is able to tolerate a certain amount of deformation, especially if the process is slow, such as the growth of an osteophyte. When a nerve root is compressed, the conduction capabilities of the axons are altered; compression of motor fibres causes weakness or sometimes paralysis of the muscles they supply, and compression of sensory fibres causes paraesthesiae and numbness in the appropriate dermatome. Simple compression of a normal nerve root does not cause pain, just as compression of the common peroneal nerve round the head of the fibula from a too tightly fitting plaster may cause weakness in the foot but does not give rise to pain.

Increased sensitivity is a direct result of an inflammatory process of the nerve root (Porterfield and DeRosa, 1998). At surgery for a recently prolapsed intervertebral disc, the nerve root is often found to be inflamed. Repeated trauma to a nerve root, rendering it fibrotic and ischaemic, may result in pain when it is stretched. Vascular oedema has also been implicated in causing additional pressure to that caused by the original lesion (Murphy, 1977). When a nerve root is compressed, the radicular veins, which are intimately related to it, are also obstructed and the resulting oedema may interfere with nerve conduction.

Chronic inflammation with reactive fibrosis caused by repeated trauma can result in ischaemia of the nerve root. Instead of appearing red and swollen, as in acute inflammation, the nerve root now appears white and tight, and with its meninges may be embedded in fibrous tissue forming adhesions which tether the root, restricting its extensibility or mobility. In this condition of nerve root fibrosis, the nerve and its meninges are unable to adapt freely to spinal and limb movements – in particular spinal flexion and lateral flexion – performed passively or actively, and there may be considerable tension resulting in pain and producing at least temporary changes in the motor, sensory and autonomic function. The proximal parts of the spinal nerves themselves may also be affected by fibrotic adhesions.

Spinal cord compression

Where the spinal canal is large, the likelihood of cord compression is very much reduced. In the cervical region, the average sagittal diameter of the spinal canal is 17 mm, and in this region the average anteroposterior diameter of the cord is 10 mm. Therefore, in the average individual, gross changes in the cervical spine need to be present before cord compression is likely. Narrowing of the canal (central stenosis) through a developmental anomaly (see p. 301) renders the individual more likely to suffer the consequences of degenerative encroachment. In patients with myelopathy due to cervical spondylosis, the average measurement of the canal was found to be 14 mm – that is, about 3 mm less than the average (Payne and Spillane, 1957). If the cervical cord is involved there will be abnormalities at or below the level involved. At the level of compression, lower motor neuron signs predominate and are often bilateral; below this level there will be upper motor neuron signs (Giles and Singer, 1998). Reflexes are brisk and abnormal reflexes may be present (Babinski's sign in the foot). In the cervical spine, cord compression is usually caused by osteocartilaginous bars formed from osteophytes and ruptured discs, calcification of ligamentum flavum, or a combination of both, rather than a simple posterior cervical disc herniation.

Narrowing of the lumbar spinal canal acquired through degenerative trespass is mainly caused by osteophytic enlargement of the two inferior facets (Kirkaldy-Willis, 1988). Other causes include a prolapsed disc, lipping of the posterior aspect of the vertebral bodies, a thickened ligamentum flavum, thickening of the neural arches, synovial cysts (Jackson et al, 1989), vertebral misalignment and trauma. Several levels may be affected. The decisive factor in the production of signs and symptoms is the available space, i.e. the relationship between the size of the canal and its contents. The cauda equina and its blood vessels are often compromised to a greater extent than individual spinal nerves.

Patients with spinal stenosis may present with a variety of signs and symptoms that can include back pain, radicular pain, neurogenic claudication and altered reflexes, power and sensation in the lower limbs. The symptoms can be unilateral but are frequently bilateral.

CHANGES IN THE SYNOVIAL JOINTS

Apophyseal joints   The apophyseal joints exhibit all the gross anatomical features of synovial joints elsewhere in the body, and may undergo degenerative changes characteristic of arthrosis (see Fig. 9.3A). Although rare under the age of 30, the incidence increases with advancing age.

The changes that occur in the hyaline cartilage of the apophyseal joints are different to those occurring in osteoarthritis. Maturation results in thinning of the articular cartilage, but there is no degradation or repair that is characteristic of osteoarthritis (Ferguson, 1975). The water content of the hyaline cartilage reduces with age, whereas in osteoarthritis water content in the hyaline cartilage remains the same or increases (Dick, 1972). Degenerative changes in the apophyseal joints may be primary and have been reported in the absence of disc degeneration or deformity (Lewin, 1964), but they are more commonly secondary to these factors (Fig. 9.9).

> ### Incidence of arthrosis
>
> In the cervical spine, the incidence is highest in the upper segments, especially in the median atlanto-axial joint (Von Torklus and Gehle, 1972). Even in the presence of marked spondylosis in the lower cervical spine, the apophyseal joints may be spared.
>
> In the thoracic spine, the two levels showing the highest incidence of apophyseal joint arthrosis are C7/T1 and T4/5 (Shore, 1935).
>
> In the lumbar spine, the incidence of arthrosis varies according to age (Lewin, 1964). Below the age of 45, early arthrosis is more common in the upper lumbar segments, while after this age the lower lumbar segments are more frequently affected.

Sustained lordotic postures such as erect standing can result in high stresses on the tips of the lumbar facets by causing them to make contact with the laminae of the subjacent vertebra. When the lumbar spine is extended by two degrees per motion segment, as in erect standing, the apophyseal joints resist most of the shear force acting on the spine (Hutton et al, 1977) as well as approximately 16% of the compressive force increasing with more extension (Adams and Hutton, 1980). Prolonged pressure depresses the nutrition of the articular cartilage, and chronic overloading may well cause arthrosis in these joints. Weak abdominal musculature predisposing to hyperextension could be a contributory factor in overloading the joints.

Acute injury or sprain of an apophyseal joint produces synovial effusion, histamine release, stretching or tearing of the capsule and ligaments, and bleeding. This limits the movements possible in the joint. Normal movement may be restored after minor injuries but some residual limitation of movement may persist following more severe injuries.

Figure 9.9 Effect of loss of height in a lumbar intervertebral disc. A, Normal disc. B, Degenerative changes in disc leading to loss of disc height and impingement of tip of facet of apophyseal joint. C, Degenerative changes in facet of lumbar apophyseal joint (shown on one side only but often bilateral).

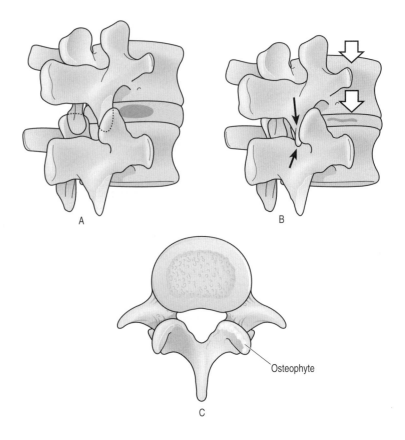

Repetitive stresses over the years can result in a chronic synovial reaction becoming established and a synovial fold may project into the joint between its articular surfaces. The surface of the articular cartilage undergoes fibrillation and becomes frayed and softened. Fragments of the cartilage may break off, forming loose bodies which can lie freely in the joint or become attached to the synovial membrane. Thinning and stiffening of the subchondral bone in middle age causes a reduction in its energy-absorbing capacity, which may hasten the changes in the articular cartilage.

The capsule later becomes lax, allowing subluxation of the joint surfaces to occur. Stresses in the capsule and periosteum result in marginal osteophytes which may encroach on the spinal canal or intervertebral foramina. Thickening or hypertrophy of the laminae may develop, which is more pronounced in the lumbar spine.

In the final stages of degeneration, there is erosion of articular cartilage from the surface with exposure of the underlying bone. Fat pads, which are mainly fibrous in the young, increase in size and become more fatty with age, acting as padding beneath the bony spurs to help attenuate forces developed at the extremes of movement. Simultaneously, changes in the capsule occur: the dorsal capsule thickens and often areas of cartilage develop within its substance. Intra-articular adhesions passing from one articular surface to the other are not uncommon and can vary from a single filmy strand to a dense mat that precludes all movement.

Uncovertebral joints

Fissuring across the posterior parts of the intervertebral disc extends between the two uncovertebral joints (see p. 82); this is accompanied by loss of disc material and a reduction in disc height so that the uncinate processes become weight-bearing.

Degenerative changes develop at the uncovertebral joints in response to the weight-bearing and shearing forces, and osteophytes grow posterolaterally into the intervertebral canals. The cervical nerve roots in the intervertebral canals are at risk from being squeezed in a pincer-type action between apophyseal and uncovertebral osteophytes (see Fig. 9.5; Taylor and Twomey, 1994a p.20). Osteophytes from the uncovertebral joints can also trespass on the vertebral artery, and indeed they are more likely to compromise the vertebral artery than osteophytes from the apophyseal joints.

Costovertebral and costotransverse joints

Studies on the costovertebral and costotransverse joints have been relatively few, but it appears that arthrosis is on the whole less commonly found in them than in other synovial joints in the spine. This may be related to the fact that slight movement occurs in them all the time during breathing. A study in cadavers showed an incidence of 48%, with peaks at T1, T6–8 and T11/12, the inferior hemifacets being more affected than the more superior hemifacets (Nathan et al, 1964).

COMBINED DEGENERATIVE CHANGES IN THE SPINE

Degenerative changes may predominantly affect the disc in some individuals, while in others they mainly affect the apophyseal joints. There is some degree of independence in these changes, at least in the initial stages. Different levels of the spine show a predisposition to either spondylosis or arthrosis. Commonly, eventually the whole motion segment is affected, and changes in the disc interact with those in the uncovertebral joints, as well as in the apophyseal joints, albeit in varying degrees.

Loss of disc height, leading to a shortening in the length of the spinal column, imposes unusual mechanical strains on the synovial joints. In some patients, the apophyseal joints may be virtually 'remade' (Farfan, 1973), new articulations forming on the articular processes where there is overlap of the true facet. These new articulations are largely osteophytic, with no true articular cartilage. In severe cases of degeneration and loss of disc height, the facets may resist up to 70% of the compressive force on the spine (Adams and Hutton, 1983). Much of this abnormally high resistance is due to extra-articular impingement of the facet tips on the adjacent lamina or pedicle (see Fig. 9.9b) (Dunlop et al, 1984).

Shortening of the spinal column also has a marked effect on the soft tissues. Bulging of the ligamenta flava into the spinal canal causing compression on the spinal cord is seen in severe cases of degeneration. Because of its attachment to the entire undersurface of the superior lamina, but only to the upper edge of the inferior lamina, the ligament can only bulge posteriorly into the spinal canal. During extension movements, the upper edge of the lower lamina forces the intervening ligamentum flavum downward in the spinal canal. Hypertrophy of ligamentum flavum may occur as a response to stiffness in adjacent motion segments. Age-related changes in ligamentum flavum result in a decrease in the elastic fibres, an increase in collagen fibres and a shift to high molecular weight proteoglycans (Kashiwagi, 1993; Okada et al, 1993). These changes favour the deposition of calcium so that ossification and hypertrophy of the ligament subsequently occur. Stenosis of the central spinal canal may occur at one or several levels.

Narrowing of an intervertebral foramen (see Fig. 9.5) and consequent compression of its nerve and other contents can be caused by many factors such as reduced disc height, a bulging or prolapsed disc, subluxation of posterior facets, a retrospondylolisthesis (backward slip) of the upper on the lower vertebra, or osteophytes projecting from the vertebral body or the apophyseal joints. Diminution of the transverse diameter of the foramen rather than its vertical height is more likely to affect the foraminal contents.

Distortion of the vertebral artery can occur through shortening of the vertebral column and it can be displaced laterally by spondylotic changes in the vertebrae. The degree of displacement depends on the size and position of the bony prominences which arise as a result of these degenerative changes: the displacement of the artery may vary from a gentle curve to a marked distortion. Obstruction of one or other vertebral arteries may occur during movements of the cervical spine, especially rotation and extension of the head (see p. 164). Atheroma commonly occurs in the vertebral artery, but the presence of these intrinsic occlusive lesions only gives rise to symptoms if the blood supply to an area is critically reduced and there is no collateral supply.

Movement becomes increasingly restricted; this can vary from loss of normal accessory movement to considerably reduced physiological movement. Stiffness at one level imposes strains on adjacent levels, as can be seen following fusion of one segment. A degenerative lesion that was previously confined to one level can spread to involve several levels (Kirkaldy-Willis, 1988).

INSTABILITY

The term 'spinal instability' is frequently used, despite the lack of a commonly agreed definition. In its simplest form, instability could be considered to be a 'loss of motion stiffness' (Pope and Panjabi, 1985). A definition of clinical relevance from the American Academy of Orthopaedic Surgeons (1985) is 'an abnormal response to loads, characterized by movements in the motion segment beyond normal constraints'.

The many causes of instability include fractures, dislocations, tumours, infections, scoliosis, spondylolisthesis and degenerative and age-related changes. Instability can result in pain and put the neural structures at risk.

Abnormal increased movement of an intervertebral joint may occur in severe disc degeneration accompanied by capsular laxity in the apophyseal joints and lack of effective muscular control. It occurs in both the cervical and lumbar spine but is less common in the thoracic spine.

In the lumbar spine, abnormal movements of the disc pull on the outermost annular fibres and cause a spur of bone – the so-called traction spur – to develop approximately 1 mm away from the discal border of the vertebral body. The traction spur differs from the claw-type osteophyte which develops at the edge of the vertebral body and curves over the outer fibres of the intervertebral disc (Macnab, 1977; Fig. 9.10). The presence of a traction spur indicates that there is or has been a lack of annular control of that particular motion segment, and the segment is or was unstable. Real instability should not be confused with hypermobility due to excessive laxity of ligaments, where the range of movement exceeds the normal but is controlled by appropriate muscle activity.

When subjected to torsion, the affected disc may have increased lateral translation (2.5–10.2 mm). Another manifestation of instability is increased forward translation of a vertebra on the one below on flexion, and increased backward translation on extension. The intervertebral joint's ability to withstand the normal strains of movement is reduced; consequently, the forces are greater on the ligamentous and joint structures. Not all degenerate joints go through this unstable phase; it is sometimes temporary, as the stiffening that eventually occurs with degeneration tends to restabilize the motion segment. Forced manipulation of joints with instability will increase the instability and is, therefore, contraindicated.

Radiological findings suggesting segmental instability include loss of disc height, traction spurs, facet arthrosis, scoliosis, spondylolysis and spondylolisthesis. At present, the correlation between radiological evidence and clinical findings of instability remains unresolved (Boden et al, 1990; Frymoyer, 1991; Rowe, 1997). It is often impossible to assess

Figure 9.10   Difference between osteophyte and traction spur. (After McNab, 1977.)

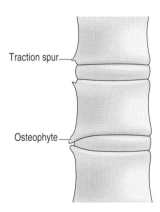

Traction spur

Osteophyte

the degree and direction of abnormal movement from radiographs due to the fact that in many individuals pure movements are not possible (Farfan, 1973); if the paravertebral muscles are in spasm when the investigations are performed, the movements possible will be limited. Flexion/extension radiographs are used to measure intersegmental motion; a combined flexion/extension translation of more than 3 mm is considered to be evidence of instability, although some believe that 4–5 mm is more appropriate (Frymoyer, 1991).

References

Aaron JE, Makins NB, Sagreiya K (1987) The histology and microanatomy of trabecular bone loss in normal ageing men and women. *Clinical Orthopaedics and Related Research* 215: 260.

Adams M, Hutton WC (1981) The relevance of torsion to the mechanical derangement of the lumbar spine. *Spine* 6: 241.

Adams M, Hutton WC (1982) Prolapsed intervertebral disc. A hyperflexion injury. *Spine* 7: 184.

Adams M, Hutton WC (1985) Gradual disc prolapse. *Spine* 10: 524.

Adams MA (1980) The mechanical properties of lumbar intervertebral joints with special reference to the causes of low back pain (PhD Thesis). Polytechnic of Central London, London.

Adams MA, Hutton WC (1980) The effect of posture on the role of the apophyseal joints in resisting intervertebral compressive force. *Journal of Bone and Joint Surgery (Br.)* 62: 358.

Adams MA, Hutton WC (1983) The biomechanics of the posterior elements of the lumbar spine. Spine 8: 326.

Alexander MJ (1984) Biomechanical aspects of lumbar spine injuries in athletics: A review. Canadian Journal of Applied Sports Science 10: 1–20.

American Academy of Orthopaedic Surgeons (1985) *A Glossary on Spinal Terminology*. American Academy of Orthopaedic Surgeons, Chicago, p. 34.

Andersson GBJ (1983) The biomechanics of the posterior elements of the lumbar spine. *Spine* 8: 326.

Bagnall KM, Harris PF, Jones PRM (1984) A radiographic study of variations of the human fetal spine. *Anatomical Record* 208: 265.

Bernick S, Cailliet R (1982) Vertebral end-plate changes with ageing of human vertebrae. *Spine* 7: 97.

Boden SD, Davis DO, Dina TS, et al (1990) Abnormal magnetic-resonance scans of the lumbar spine in asymptomatic subjects. *Journal of Bone and Joint Surgery (Am.)* 72: 403–408.

Bogduk N, Twomey LT (1987) *Clinical Anatomy of the Lumbar Spine*. Churchill Livingstone, Edinburgh.

Bradford DS, Hensinger RM, eds (1985) *The Pediatric Spine*. Thieme, New York.

Brain Lord WR, Wilkinson M (1967) *Cervical Spondylosis*. William Heinemann Medical Books, London.

Brown T, Hansen RJ, Yorra AJ (1957) Some mechanical tests on the lumbosacral spine with particular reference to the intervertebral discs. *Journal of Bone and Joint Surgery (Am.)* 39: 1135.

Bull JED (1951) In: Feiling A (ed.) *Modern Trends in Neurology*. Butterworth, London.

Carpenter EB (1961) Normal and abnormal growth of the spine. *Clinical Orthopaedics and Related Research* 21: 49.

Cassidy JD, Loback D, Yonh-Hing K, Tchang S (1992) Lumbar facet joint asymmetry. Intervertebral disc herniation. Spine 17: 570–574.

Cyron BM, Hutton WC (1980) Articular tropism and stability of the lumbar spine. *Spine* 5: 168.

Dent CE, Watson L (1966) Osteoporosis. *Postgraduate Medical Journal Suppl.* 42: 583–660.

Dick WC (1972) *An Introduction to Clinical Rheumatology*. Churchill Livingstone, London, p. 24.

Dunlop RB, Adams MA, Hutton WC (1984) Disc space narrowing and the lumbar facet joints. *Journal of Bone and Joint Surgery (Br.)* 66: 706.

Eckert G, Decker A (1947) Pathological studies of the intervertebral discs. *Journal of Bone and Joint Surgery (Am)* 29: 477.

Elster AD (1989) Bertolotti's syndrome revisited: transitional vertebrae of the lumbar spine. *Spine* 14: 1373–1377.

Exton-Smith AN (1983) Metabolic bone disease. In: Wright V (ed.) *Bone and Joint Disease in the Elderly*. Churchill Livingstone, Edinburgh, pp. 150–166.

Farfan HF (1973) *Mechanical Disorders of the Low Back*. Lea and Febiger, Philadelphia.

Farfan HF, Sullivan JD (1967) The relation of facet orientation to intervertebral disc failure. *Canadian Journal of Surgery* 10: 179.

Ferguson AB (1975) The pathology of degenerative arthritis. In: Creuss RL, Mitchell NS (eds) *Surgical Management of Degenerative Arthritis of the Lower Limbs*. Lea and Febiger, Philadelphia, pp. 3–9.

Francis RM, Peacock M (1987) The local action of oral 1,24 (OH)^2 Vitamin D3 on calcium absorption in osteoporosis. *American Journal of Clinical Nutrition* 46: 315.

Fredrickson BE, Baker D, McHolick WJ (1984) The natural history of spondylolysis and spondylolisthesis. *Journal of Bone and Joint Surgery (Am.)* 66: 699–707.

Frymoyer JW (1991) Segmental instability. Overview and classification. In: Frymoyer JW (ed.) *The Adult Spine, Principles and Practice*. Raven Press, New York, pp. 1873–1891.

Giles LGF, Singer KP (1997) *Clinical Anatomy and Management of Low Back Pain*. Butterworth Heinemann, Oxford.

Giles LGF, Singer KP (1998) *Clinical Anatomy and Management of Cervical Spine Pain*. Butterworth Heinemann, Oxford, p. 129.

Giles LGF, Singer KP (2000) *Clinical Anatomy and Management of Thoracic Spine Pain*. Vol. 2. Butterworth Heinemann, Oxford, Ch. 5, pp. 63–82.

Goldberg CJ, Fogarty EE, Moore DP, et al (1997) Scoliosis and developmental theory. Adolescent idiopathic scoliosis. *Spine* 22: 2228–2238.

Grieve GP (1981) *Common Vertebral Joint Problems*. Churchill Livingstone, Edinburgh.

Grieve GP (1989) *Common Vertebral Joint Problems*, 2nd edn. Churchill Livingstone, Edinburgh, p. 24.

Hagg O, Wallner A (1990) Facet joint asymmetry and protrusion of the intervertebral disc. *Spine* 15: 356–359.

Haley JC, Perry JH (1950) Protrusions of intervertebral discs: study of their distribution, characteristics and effects on the nervous system. *American Journal of Surgery* 80: 394.

Happey F (1976) A biophysical study of the human intervertebral disc. In: Jayson MIV (ed.) *The Lumbar Spine and Back Pain*. Grune & Stratton, New York, pp. 293–316.

Hensinger RN (1989) Spondylolysis and spondylolisthesis in children and adolescents. *Journal of Bone and Joint Surgery (Am.)* 71: 1098–1107.

Herbert CM, Lindberg KA, Jayson MIV, Bailey AJ (1975) Changes in the collagen of human intervertebral discs during ageing and degenerative disc disease. *Journal of Molecular Medicine* 1: 79–91.

Hickey DS, Hukins DWL (1980). Relation between the structure of the annulus fibrosus and the function and failure of the intervertebral disc. *Spine* 5: 106.

Hilton R, Ball J, Benn R (1976) Vertebral end-plate lesions (Schmorl's nodes) in the dorsolumbar spine. *Annals of the Rheumatic Diseases* 35: 127–132.

Horst M, Brinckmann P (1981) Measurement of the distribution of axial stress on the end-plate of the vertebral body. *Spine* 6: 217–232.

Hoshina H (1980) Spondylolysis in athletes. *Physician and Sports Medicine* 8: 75–79.

Hutton WC, Stott JRR, Cyron BM (1977) Is spondylolysis a fatigue fracture? *Spine* 2: 202.

Ichikawa N, Ohara Y, Marishita T, et al (1982) An etiological study on spondylolysis from a biomechanical aspect. *British Journal of Sports Medicine* 16: 135–141.

Jackson DE Jr, Atlas SW, Mani JR, et al (1989) Intraspinal synovial cysts: MR imaging. *Radiology* 170: 527–530.

James JIP (1976) *Scoliosis*, 2nd edn. Churchill Livingstone, Edinburgh.

Jeffreys E. (1980). Disorders of the Cervical Spine. London: Butterworth.

Kashiwagi K (1993) Histological changes of the lumbar ligamentum flavum with age. *Nippon Seikeigeka Gakkai Zasshi* 67: 221–229.

Kirkaldy-Willis WH (1988) *Managing Low Back Pain*, 2nd edn. Churchill Livingstone, Edinburgh.

Kramer J (1981) *Intervertebral Disc Lesions: Causes, Diagnosis, Treatment and Prophylaxis*. Georg Thieme Verlag, Stuttgart.

Kulak RF, Belytschko TB, Shultz AB (1976) Nonlinear behaviour of the human intervertebral disc under axial load. *Journal of Biomechanics* 9: 377–386.

Lewin T (1964) *Osteoarthrosis in Lumbar Synovial Joints*. Orstadius Boktryckeri, Aktiebolag, Gothenburg.

Macnab I (1977) *Backache*. Williams & Wilkins, Baltimore, p. 4.

McMaster MJ, David CV (1986). Hemivertebrae as a cause of scoliosis. *Journal of Bone and Joint Surgery (Br.)* 68: 588.

McRae DL (1953) Bony abnormalities in the region of the foramen magnum: correlation of the anatomic and neurologic findings. *Acta Radiologica* 40: 335.

Murphy RW (1977) Nerve roots and spinal nerves in degenerative disk disease. *Clinical Orthopaedics and Related Research* 129: 46.

Murray PM, Weinstein SL, Spratt KF (1993) The natural history and long term follow-up of Scheuermann's kyphosis. *Journal of Bone and Joint Surgery (Am.)* 75: 236–248.

Nachemson A, Schultz AB, Berkson MH (1979) Mechanical properties of the human lumbar spine motion segments. *Spine* 4: 1–8.

Nathan H (1962) Osteophytes of the vertebral column. *Journal of Bone and Joint Surgery (Am.)* 44: 243.

Nathan H, Weinberg H, Robin GC, et al (1964) The costovertebral joints: anatomico-clinical observations in arthritis. *Arthritis and Rheumatism* 7: 228.

Newman PH (1952). Sprung back. *Journal of Bone and Joint Surgery (Br.)* 34: 30.

Odgers PNB (1933) The lumbar and lumbosacral diarthrodial joints. *Journal of Anatomy* 67: 301.

Okada A, Harata S, Takeda Y, Nakamura T, Takagaki K, Endo M (1993) Age-related changes in proteoglycans of human ligamentum flavum. *Spine* 18: 2261–2266.

Osti OL, Vernon-Robertes B, Fraser RD (1990) Annulus tears and intervertebral disc degeneration: an experimental study using an animal model. *Spine* 15: 762–767.

Panjabi MM, Brand RA, White AA (1976) Three dimensional flexibility and stiffness properties of the human thoracic spine. *Journal of Biomechanics* 9: 185–192.

Payne EE, Spillane JD (1957). The cervical spine. An anatomico-pathological study of 70 specimens (using a special technique) with particular reference to the problem of spondylosis. *Brain* 80: 571.

Peacock A (1951) Observations on the prenatal development of the intervertebral disc in man. *Journal of Anatomy* 85: 260.

Penning L (1968) *Functional Pathology of the Cervical Spine*. Williams and Wilkins, Baltimore.

Pope M, Panjabi M (1985) Biomechanical definition of spinal instability. *Spine* 10: 255.

Porter RE (1989) Normal development of movement and function: Child and adolescent. In: Scully RM, Barnes MR (eds) *Physical Therapy*. JB Lippincott, Philadelphia.

Porterfield JA, DeRosa C (1998) *Mechanical Low Back Pain. Perspectives in Functional Anatomy*. 2nd edn. Saunders, Philadelphia, pp. 25–52.

Postacchini F, Lami R, Pugliese O (1988) Familial predisposition to discogenic low-back pain. An epidemiologic and immunogenetic study. *Spine* 13: 1403.

Rissanen PM (1960) The surgical anatomy and pathology of the supraspinous and interspinous ligaments of the lumbar spine with special reference to ligament ruptures. *Acta Orthopaedica Scandinavica* (Suppl.) 46.

Roaf R (1960) A study of the mechanics of spinal injuries. *Journal of Bone and Joint Surgery (Br.)* 42: 810.

Rolander SD (1966). Motion of the lumbar spine with special reference to the stability effect of posterior fusion. *Acta Orthopaedica Scandinavica* (Suppl.) 90.

Rowe L (1997) Imaging of mechanical and degenerative syndromes of the lumbar spine. In: Giles LGF, Singer KP (eds) *Clinical Anatomy and Management of Low Back Pain*, Butterworth Heinemann, Oxford Vol. 1, Ch. 18, pp. 275–313.

Schmorl G, Junghanns H (1971) *The Human Spine in Health and Disease*, 2nd edn. Grune & Stratton, New York, p. 55.

Shore LR (1935) On osteoarthritis in the dorsal intervertebral joints. *British Journal of Surgery* 22: 833.

Singh S (1965) Variations of the superior articular facets of atlas vertebrae. *Journal of Anatomy* 99: 565.

Spillane JD, Pallis C, Jones AM (1957) Developmental abnormalities in the region of the foramen magnum. *Brain* 80: 11.

Taylor JR, Twomey LT (1984). The role of the notochord and blood vessels in vertebral column development and in the aetiology of Schmorl's nodes. In: Grieve GP (ed.) *Manual Therapy, 1, The Vertebral Column*. Churchill Livingstone, Edinburgh.

Taylor JR, Twomey L (1986) Factors influencing growth of the vertebral column. In: Grieve G. (ed.) *Modern Manual Therapy*. Churchill Livingstone, Edinburgh, pp. 30–36.

Taylor JR, Twomey LT (1994a) Functional and applied anatomy of the cervical spine. In: Grant R (ed.) *Physical Therapy of the Cervical and Thoracic Spine*, 2nd edn. Churchill Livingstone, Edinburgh, Ch.1, pp. 1–25.

Taylor JR, Twomey LT (1994b). The effects of ageing on the intervertebral discs. In: Boyling J, Palastanga N (eds) *Grieve's Modern Manual Therapy. The Vertebral Column*, 2nd edn. Churchill Livingstone, Edinburgh, Ch. 14, pp. 177–188.

Taylor JR, Twomey LT, Corker M (1990) Bone and soft tissue injuries in post-mortem lumbar spines. *Paraplegis* 28: 119–129.

Taylor JR, Scott JE, Bosworth TR, Cribb AM (1992) Human intervertebral disc acid and glycosaminoglycans. *Journal of Anatomy* 180: 137–141.

Tredwell SJ, Smith DF, Macleod PJ, et al (1982) Cervical spine anomalies in fetal alcohol syndrome. *Spine* 7: 331.

Twomey LT, Taylor JR (1982) Flexion creep deformation and hysteresis in the lumbar vertebral column. *Spine* 7: 116–122.

Twomey LT, Taylor JT (1985a) Age changes in lumbar intervertebral discs. *Acta Orthopaedica Scandinavica* 56: 496.

Twomey LT, Taylor JR (1985b) Vertebral column development and its relation to adult pathology. *Australian Journal of Physiotherapy* 31: 83–88.

Urban J, Maroudas A (1980) The chemistry of the intervertebral disc in relation to its physiological function and requirements. *Clinics in Rheumatic Diseases.* 6: 1.

Van Roy P, Caboor D, Boelpaep De, Barbaix E, Clarys JP (1997) Left-right asymmetries and other common anatomical variants of the first cervical vertebra. *Manual Therapy* 2: 24–36.

Vanharanta H, Floyd T, Ohnmeiss DD, et al (1993) The relationship of facet tropism to degenerative disc disease. *Spine* 18: 1000–1005.

Verbout AJ (1985) The development of the vertebral column. Vol. 90. In: Beck F, Hild W, Ortmann R (eds) *Advances in Anatomy, Embryology, and Cell Biology*. Springer Verlag, Berlin.

Von Torklus D, Gehle W (1972) *The Upper Cervical Spine*. Butterworth, London, p. 21.

Williams PL, Warwick R, eds (1980) *Gray's Anatomy*, 36th edn. Churchill Livingstone, Edinburgh.

Winter RB, Moe JH, Lonstein JE (1984) The incidence of Klippel-Feil syndrome in patients with congenital scoliosis and kyphosis. *Spine* 9: 363.

Chapter 10

Posture

Posture is the position assumed by the body either by means of the integrated action of muscles working to counteract the force of gravity, or when supported during muscular inactivity. Many postures are assumed by an individual during the course of 24 hours, and at any given moment posture comprises the positions of all the joints of the body (Kendall et al, 1993).

Dynamically and statically, an efficient posture:

1. Is stable
2. Minimizes stress and strain on the tissues
3. Minimizes energy cost

Subtle departure from an optimal posture is common and subjects the body to routine, eccentric and increased mechanical stress (Kappler, 1982).

In a stable posture the combined centre of gravity (COG) of the various body parts must fall within a base of support (the contact area between the body and the supporting surface). Irvin (1997) states that the upright posture is dependent on the size, shape and attitude of three cardinal bases of support:

1. The supporting surface
2. The feet, as they are the lowermost support of the body
3. The base of the sacrum, as it is both the approximate centre of the body and the lowermost support of the vertebral column.

The alignment of the body parts must be maintained to ensure continual stability and it is in maintenance of posture that stress arises (Bridger, 2003, pp. 31–57). Stresses on the body may be from either intrinsic mechanisms such as muscle activity, or extrinsic factors such as the supporting surfaces. Stress can also be defined as acute or chronic: postural stress or task-induced stress. Postural stress is the term used for mechanical load on the body by virtue of its posture (Grieve and Pheasant, 1982); task-induced stress depends on the mechanical effort needed to perform the task (Bridger, 2003, pp. 31–57). Task-induced and postural stress can vary independently of each other: for example, an individual can lift a weight while maintaining a non-stressful posture.

A large number of working postures may be assumed during the day; a study of working positions in a steel factory, typical for heavy industry, yielded a classification of 72 different postures. It was observed that two workers doing the same job used different postures on a large percentage of occasions (Karhu et al, 1977).

CONTROL OF POSTURE

Postures are maintained or adapted as a result of neuromuscular coordination, the appropriate muscles being innervated by means of a complex reflex system. Afferent stimuli arise from a variety of sources all over the body, including the joints, ligaments, muscles, skin, eyes and ears, and are conveyed and coordinated in the central nervous system. The efferent response is a motor one, the antigravity muscles being the principal effector organs.

The apophyseal joints in the upper cervical region have a particularly abundant supply of these receptors, and degeneration in these joints and soft tissues can lead to alterations in the discharge of afferent impulses and disturbances in the perception of posture and balance. The head/neck relationship has an effect on the posture of the entire body (Alexander, 1932).

While it is accepted that the bony structure in individuals may vary, it is less obvious that the amount of muscle activity used when performing identical tasks may also vary, and this could account for the apparent contradictions shown in different studies of muscle activity. Although some people are able to sit comfortably and relax in many positions without a large increase in muscular activity, people who are tense show a pronounced increase in various postures and, when performing tasks, do not relax completely in more than a few positions (Lundervold, 1951). When the spinal muscles contract, they have a compressive effect on the intervertebral discs; consequently, muscular contractions in excess of normal requirements may have a detrimental effect on the nutrition of the discs, as this is dependent on imbibition of fluid, which occurs when the compression is reduced.

LYING POSITION

The lowest levels of back muscle activity and intradiscal pressure (see Fig. 2.8, p. 72) occur in the lying position. Patients with some (though not all) types of intervertebral disc pathology obtain relief from pain in this position. The position that the spine normally assumes varies according to several factors, such as the resilience of the surface, the build of the individual and the position of the limbs.

For example, a soft surface encourages the spine to flex more when supine-lying, or extend more when lying prone, than would a firmer surface. Prone-lying is a position not easily tolerated by people with stiff spines or those who have symptoms arising from degenerated apophyseal joints, usually because either the neck is in full rotation or the lumbar spine is at the end of its extension range; the apophyseal joints are under stress in both cases.

The build of an individual when lying on the side influences the degree of lateral flexion in the spine, e.g. a woman with a wide pelvis would tend to flex the lumbar spine laterally more than a man with a narrower pelvis.

The position of the limbs influences spinal posture in a manner similar to that described for the sitting position (see p. 333).

STANDING POSITION

Alignment of the body is analysed relative to the line of gravity.

In the ideal normal erect posture, in the sagittal plane, the line of gravity is located (Kendall et al, 1993):

1. Through the odontoid
2. Through the bodies of most of the cervical vertebrae
3. At a point just in front of the shoulders
4. Through the bodies of the lumbar vertebrae
5. Slightly posterior to the lateral axis of the hip joint
6. Anterior to the lateral axis of the knee joint
7. Slightly anterior to the lateral axis of the ankle

In standing, the pelvis is held in an anteriorly tilted position by the iliopsoas muscles, and the hip joint is able to extend freely during the stance phase of gait. The angle between the upper surface of the sacrum and the horizontal is approximately 50–53° (Hellems and Keates, 1971). This tilt, and compression from body weight on the lumbar spine, accentuates the lumbar lordosis. It can be further increased by pregnancy, obesity, wearing high-heeled shoes and acquired muscle imbalances.

The apophyseal joints resist most of the shear force acting on the spine in the erect posture (Hutton et al, 1977) as well as approximately 16% of the compressive force (Adams and Hutton, 1980). The resulting stress between the articular surfaces is concentrated in the lower margins of the joint (Dunlop et al, 1984).

In the upright position, the muscles and ligaments play a stabilizing role by means of the active and passive torques they exert around the joints to correct minimal displacements of movement in directions away from the joints. An efficient posture is one in which destabilizing moments are minimized and the posture is maintained by the resistance of the relatively incompressible bones (Bridger, 2003, pp. 89–120).

In quiet standing, assuming that the curvatures of the spine are in correct alignment, surprisingly little muscular activity is required to maintain this position, slight or moderate activity being present for only 5% of the time (Soames and Atha, 1981). The function of the strong antigravity muscles is not so much to maintain postures such as the upright position, but to produce the powerful movements necessary for major changes in posture.

Economical though it may be in terms of spinal muscular energy, the ideal erect posture is not usually sustained for long periods, and people often resort to standing asymmetrically, using the right and left leg alternately as the main support. They may do this in order to cope with the inadequacies of the venous and arterial circulation, or because they find a reduced lordosis, with subsequent reduction in the compressive forces on the apophyseal joints (Adams and Hutton, 1980), more comfortable, even at the expense of increasing back muscle activity. Standing with the weight supported mainly by one leg, with the other leg relaxed, increases electromyographic activity at L5 on the side of the weight-bearing leg (Dolan et al, 1988). If the curvatures are not in correct alignment due to disease, poor posture or congenital abnormalities such as idiopathic scoliosis, far greater muscular activity over the affected area is then required to maintain the upright posture.

The lumbar erector spinae are the main extensors of the trunk. In standing, approximately three times as many people exhibit slight constant or intermittent activity in erector spinae only, as those who show abdominal muscle activity (Floyd and Silver, 1951). The erector spinae are used to control flexion and come into play when the trunk is displaced even slightly forwards or when a weight is held in front of the body. There is very little abdominal muscle activity in standing and even less in sitting (Burdorf et al, 1993).

SITTING POSITION

In the sitting position, the knee and hip are flexed so that iliopsoas shortens and the hip extensors lengthen (Link et al, 1990; Bridger et al, 1992). This alters the balance of the muscles that control the pelvic tilt: in standing, the pelvis is in anterior pelvic tilt but when it moves into the sitting position it tilts posteriorly almost immediately and continues to flex in proportion to the flexion at the hip (Bridger, 2003 pp. 89–120). To allow an erect position of the head on the rest of the spine to be maintained, the lumbar spine flexes to compensate for the tilting pelvis. The mean angle of lumbar curvature of a seated individual is 34° in comparison with 47° in standing (Lord et al, 1997).

Intradiscal pressure is generally higher in the unsupported sitting position, largely due to psoas major, which is vigorously active as a stabilizer of the lumbar spine in this position and at the same time has a compressive effect on the spine (Keagy et al, 1966). Further increases or decreases in intradiscal pressure can be brought about by an alteration in either the lumbar lordosis or in the seat or backrest inclination, the lumbar support, and the chair and (if applicable) table height. Rohlmann et al (2001) found that intradiscal pressure was lower in relaxed sitting than standing, but increased in sitting if the subject extended the spine in order to sit upright. In a well-designed chair that allows the subject to recline against a backrest, the intradiscal pressure can be lower than when standing.

The ideal sitting position for most people is with the intervertebral joints somewhere in mid-range (Fig. 10.1), allowing freedom of movement with balanced anterior and posterior muscles. In this position, the stress between the articular surfaces of the apophyseal joints is lower than in the standing position, and it is concentrated in the middle and upper parts of the joint (Dunlop et al, 1984). The joints resist the shear force, but play less part in resisting the intervertebral compressive force. However, even an 'ideal' sitting posture cannot be maintained for long periods, and it is important that seat design permits changes in posture.

Deviating from the mid-range for sustained periods leads to stresses on the joint and ligamentous structures. In a normal spine, sitting in a slumped posture can lead to overstretching of the posterior intervertebral ligaments and posterior annular fibres (Fig. 10.1A), and considerably increases intradiscal pressure. Myoelectric activity in erector spinae is nil in this posture (Floyd and Silverman, 1955), which is one of the reasons people tend to find it comfortable initially. Patients with spondylolisthesis or degenerative changes in their lumbar apophyseal joints sometimes find that sitting with their spine in some degree of flexion gives them relief from pain.

In the increasingly sedentary modern lifestyle there is a tendency for people to spend long hours in the sitting position, both for work and leisure purposes. Many people suffering from backache find that this

Figure 10.1 Lumbar motion segments in different sitting positions. A, Flexion. B, Mid range. C, Extension. * Sites of stress.

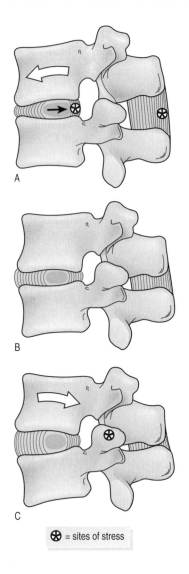

A

B

C

⊗ = sites of stress

position aggravates their problem. Evidence does not support a popular belief that sitting at work is a risk factor for low back pain (Hartvigsen et al, 2000): but prolonged sitting at work (for more than 95% of the day) is associated with back pain (Hoogendoorn et al, 2000). It is therefore probable that it is the static posture in sitting, rather than high loads on the spine, which is the important factor in low back pain aggravation. People who change their position, varying sitting with moving, have on the whole a low incidence of back pain (Magora, 1972). The reason for this may be that nutrition of the disc is dependent on movement and variation in posture. Prolonged overloading and underloading are factors in disc degeneration (Grieco, 1986). Any posture that results in sustained static muscle work induces fatigue. Therefore, when considering the optimal sitting position for a particular individual, the aim should be to reduce static muscle work to a minimum.

Postural problems can start at an early age and an increasing number of children of school age are presenting with back pain. Patterns of poor sitting posture, when started at such a young age, are difficult to improve later in life. This emphasizes the need for chairs and tables that can be adjusted to the individual's requirements, coupled with postural education in schools.

Effect of pelvic and limb positions

The position of the head, shoulders and trunk is determined by the task to be done, especially in relation to visual requirements.

For close work, such as reading or writing, the optimal distance for the work is approximately 30 cm from the eyes. As soon as the arms are moved forwards in front of the body, neck and shoulder muscle activity increases. In particular, a considerable increase in the activity levels of the upper thoracic and cervical extensors was found to be caused by arm abduction (Schuldt et al, 1986), which tends to occur when working at a table which is too high.

Activities such as typing or working at a visual display unit do not impose high loads on the neck and shoulder muscles, but they cause sustained tension. This can lead to fatigue and pain, because the capacity for sustained static muscle load is very limited (Bjorksten and Jonsson, 1977). There are considerable differences in the levels of static activity in neck and shoulder muscles in different sitting postures. The slumped posture gives higher levels of activity than does an erect posture; even lower activity levels than this have been found in subjects who sat with a slightly backward-inclined thoracolumbar spine with the cervical spine vertical, when performing light assembly work (Schuldt et al, 1986). However, this position carries with it an increased risk of extreme flexion in the lower cervical spine, and if used, instruction should be given as to how to avoid extreme positions. Schuldt et al suggested that the backward inclination should be no more than 10–15°.

The position of the lumbar spine is also affected by the angulation of the pelvis, the position of the hips and sometimes, the position of the knees.

When moving from a standing to an unsupported sitting position, as the hips move into flexion, tension in the hamstring and gluteal muscles rotates the pelvis backwards, taking with it the lumbar spine, which starts to flex. Using radiography, Schoberth (1962) found that in the 'traditional' sitting posture, i.e. with the thighs at 90° to the trunk, this was divided on average into 60° of flexion in the hips and 30° of flexion in the lumbar spine, 80–90% of which occurred at L4 and L5. There is a similarity between this position of the lumbar spine and bending forwards from the standing position (Fig. 10.2). It is not easy to maintain the 'traditional' sitting posture if the spine is unsupported, because the lumbar spine is so flexed that the tendency is for it to flex even more. Balance between the muscles anterior and posterior to the pelvis is achieved when the hip joint is in its neutral position of 45° of flexion: simultaneously the lumbar spine assumes a neutral position, which is easier to maintain.

Figure 10.2 The effects of standing, sitting and stooping on the lumbosacral curve. A, The lumbar curve is accentuated in the standing position. B, Marked flattening of the lumbosacral curve occurs when the patient is sitting in an ordinary straight chair with trunk and thighs at a right angle. C, Note how similar is the flattened lumbar curve to that of B. (From Keegan JJ 1953 Alterations of the lumbar curve related to posture and seating. *Journal of Bone and Joint Surgery (Am.)* 35: 590, with permission.)

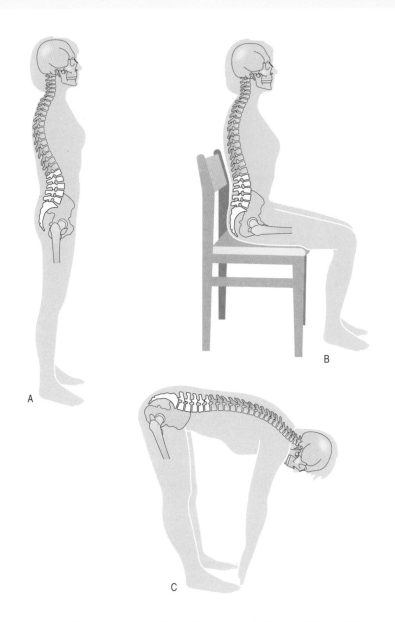

Due to the hamstring muscles acting over the hip and knee joints, the amount of knee extension may affect the position of the hips and, ultimately, the lumbar spine. When the knee is flexed to 90° or more, the lumbar mechanism is not very sensitive to small alterations in the position of the hip. However, it is extremely sensitive to any change in the hip flexion angle if the knee is flexed to 70° or less (Brunswic, 1984), an increase in knee extension of 20° corresponding roughly to a 10° increase in hip flexion. This is significant for patients when the knee position is determined by the working position, e.g. the location of pedals to operate machinery or drive a car, when knee flexion may vary between 10° and 70°, causing more flexion in the lumbar spine.

Increased intradiscal pressure has been recorded when drivers change gear (Andersson et al, 1975). This is due to an increase in knee extension and, consequently, lumbar flexion when depressing the clutch pedal, coupled with movement of the leg against gravity, and possibly also additional trunk flexion with the movement of the arm.

Seat inclination

Spinal posture in the sitting position is also influenced by degree of seat inclination (Fig. 10.3). A seat which is inclined backwards encourages the lumbar spine to flex. In order to sit upright on a 5° backward-sloping seat, the lumbar spine will be flexed to 35°. If the individual is working at a desk on this type of seat, it tilts the body away from the working surface and, to position the eyes at a suitable distance from the work, the subject compensates by flexing the spine even more. With increasing forward inclination of the seat, the lumbar spine moves into greater extension. When there is a 5° forward slope, the individual can sit upright with only 25° lumbar flexion, and this can be reduced to 15° when the seat is tilted forwards 15° (Mandal, 1984). This type of seat also tilts the body closer to the working surface and is often preferred by patients who need to avoid overflexing their spines.

Eklund and Corlett (1987) carried out laboratory studies on workers performing an assembly task when sitting on seats with two different inclinations: a 'sit-stand' seat (i.e. one with a forward inclination) and a conventional horizontal seat. The 'sit-stand' seat was found to cause substantially less loss of disc height; there was a lower biomechanical load on the spine, less discomfort from the spine, and it encouraged a slightly less flexed spinal posture.

Studies of the Balans chair, in which sitting occurs in a semi-kneeling position, show that this posture results in increased activity of both cervical and lumbar muscles when compared with the posture in a standard chair (Lander et al, 1987).

Backrest inclination and lumbar support

A backrest is usually positioned at right angles to the horizontal or sloping backwards to varying degrees. When a task is being performed at a table or bench, the body weight is usually transferred forwards and the backrest is then not used. When sitting on a horizontal seat with the backrest inclined backwards, there is a decrease in myoelectric activity in the paravertebral muscles (Andersson et al, 1979) because the need for

Figure 10.3   The backward-sloping seat increases the flexion of the lumbar region. (From *Human Factors* 1982; 24: 257–269, with permission of The Human Factors Society Inc.)

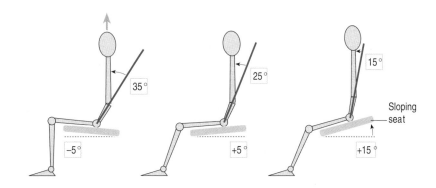

them to stabilize the spine is less as it approaches the horizontal position. Correspondingly, there is a decrease in intradiscal pressure (Fig. 10.4). This position is, of course, often sensibly chosen for relaxation.

A lumbar support was found to have a similar effect on myoelectric activity and intradiscal pressure when the body was inclined. Experimenting with lumbar supports ranging from –2 to +4 cm, the latter depth causing a lumbar lordosis which resembled that in the standing position, Andersson et al (1979) found that there was a marked effect on the degree of total lumbar extension, which changed from a mean of 9.7° to 46.8° as the lumbar support was increased.

Seat and table height

Seat and table height need to be considered as a single unit. A seat which is too low for a particular individual encourages a flexed sitting posture, especially when working at a desk. Mandal's experiments (1984) on the postures of Danish schoolchildren during a 4-hour examination highlighted this issue (Figs 10.5, 10.6); it is recommended that chair height should be at least one third of the individual's body height and the table at least half the body height.

Figure 10.4 The effect of backrest inclination and lumbar support on intradiscal pressure. (Adapted from Nachemson A 1976 The lumbar spine: an orthopaedic challenge. *Spine* 1: 59–71.)

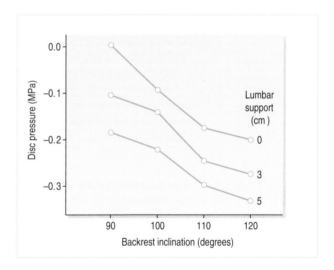

Figure 10.5 The low chair increases the flexion of the lumbar region. (From *Human Factors* 1982; 24: 257–269, with permission of The Human Factors Society Inc.)

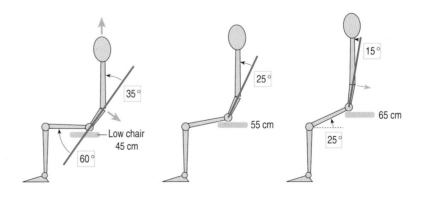

Figure 10.6   The low table increases the flexion of the lumbar region. (From *Human Factors* 1982; 24: 257–269, with permission of The Human Factors Society Inc.)

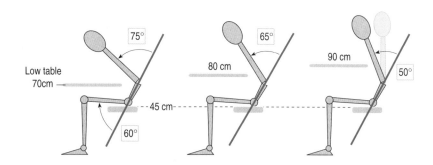

Arm rests

Supporting the arms on arm rests or a desk in front reduces both spinal muscular activity and intradiscal pressure, particularly when writing, but also when typing (Andersson et al, 1975).

LIFTING

The UK Health and Safety Commission (1991) reports that more than 25% of workplace accidents involve handling goods, while Hayne (1981) states that 30% of all industrial injuries are due to manual transport of loads. Those most likely to sustain back injuries are the unprepared, the unskilled, young people and those in the first year or so of a new job (Blow and Jackson, 1971; Magora, 1974). There is an increased risk of back pain in workers who lift a 25 kg load more than 15 times a day (Hoogendoorn et al, 2000).

LOAD ON THE SPINE IN LIFTING

Leverage

When the trunk moves in the sagittal plane, the intervertebral discs act as a series of fulcra of movement, the lumbosacral disc usually being referred to as the main fulcrum in the spine. The force exerted on it is the product of the weight to be lifted (which includes the weight of the trunk above the disc) and its distance from the fulcrum. The lever, which has to balance and lift the weight, is shorter, being provided by the back muscles. Therefore, the greater the distance of the weight from the body, in effect the heavier the weight becomes and the stronger the force required in lifting it. As the weight is progressively brought closer to the body, the lever exerted by the lift weight becomes shorter. In the initial stages of a lift, if the weight is a substantial distance from the body, the force required to lift it can be considerable. This distance is significantly more important than the actual method of lifting in determining the load on the spine.

Muscle activity

Prior to lifting a weight from the floor, the lumbar spine is lowered into flexion, erector spinae contracting eccentrically until a critical point is reached (see p. 138), when the muscles become electrically silent. As flexion continues, the muscles sustain tension together with the thoracolumbar fascia and posterior ligaments. If the weight to be lifted is very heavy (over 68.4 kg), the lumbar spine is initially flexed further, when inertia has to be overcome and ground reaction forces are greatest (Fig. 10.7) (Frievalds et al, 1984). The lift is then continued by the powerful hip and knee extensors, the activity of erector spinae being nil in the early stages. It is thought that the back muscles alone, even with maximal contraction, are unable to provide the power to raise the trunk at this stage, and a combination of three 'back support mechanisms' comes into play to enable the lift to be completed without injury to the spine.

Later in the lift, when the back muscles do contract to extend the spine, they also have a compressive effect on the vertebral column, which raises intradiscal pressure. The further away from the body the weight is, the greater the amount of erector spinae activity required in lifting it, and there is a proportionate increase in intradiscal pressure.

If a load is carried high on the back, the trunk automatically tends to lean forward slightly to prevent imbalance, causing increased activity in the lower back muscles. If, however, the load is placed lower on the back, the activity of the back muscles is reduced (Carlsöö, 1964).

A loaded spine does not have the same ability as an unloaded one to compensate for even a minor sudden extra strain (Hirsch, 1955). When not under pressure from carrying a weight, the intervertebral discs usually absorb strains, such as a fall, relatively easily, since the demands on the elasticity of the disc are less in an individual bearing only his or her own body weight. If, on the other hand, the spine is under pressure (as in carrying a heavy weight), the disc is compressed closer to its elastic limit. A sudden extra strain (e.g. losing a grip on a bulky object which is difficult to hold) will cause additional compression, which may at its maximum amplitude exceed the elastic limit of the collagen system somewhere in the annulus, or the end plate, or the attachment of the collagen to bone with the result that rupture may occur.

Many manual handling injuries occur when the spine is subjected to unexpected events such as a fall or slip (Bridger, 2003, pp. 89–120). Spinal loads are significantly greater (up to 70%) when the spine is

Figure 10.7 Features of typical lift of heavy weight from floor to standing position, beginning with the knees flexed. (Adapted from Troup JDG 1979 Biomechanics of the vertebral column. *Physiotherapy* 65: 241.)

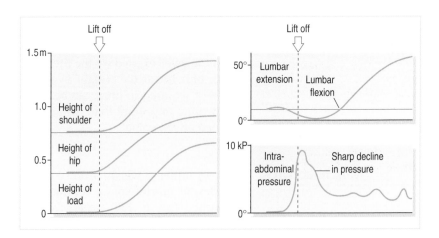

exposed to unexpected loading (Marras et al, 1987) probably because the spine is unprepared for the sudden loading and the back muscles over-compensate with increased activity, resulting in additional forces acting on the spine.

BACK SUPPORT MECHANISMS

A combination of the following mechanisms is considered to assist the back muscles in the initial phase of a lift:

1. Intra-abdominal pressure
2. Supportive role of the thoracolumbar fascia
3. Passive support of ligaments

Intra-abdominal pressure

Heavy weight lifting is always associated with a marked increase in intratruncal – that is, intra-abdominal and intrathoracic – pressure. This is usually brought about by a reflex contraction of transversus abdominis primarily (and, to a lesser extent, the oblique abdominal muscles), the muscles of the pelvic floor and the muscles of the larynx, which close the glottis. Electromyographic studies have shown that the recti are inactive in lifting, avoiding additional flexion of the spine. The fluid contents in the abdominal and thoracic cavities are compressed, and this leads to a rise in pressure. The circumferential arrangement of transversus abdominis allows it to have the greatest efficiency in raising intra-abdominal pressure (De Troyer et al, 1990).

Bartelink (1957) first proposed the theory that this raised intra-abdominal pressure (IAP) acted upwards on the diaphragm like a balloon (Fig. 10.8), separating the pelvis from the thoracic cage and serving to lift or support the thorax, especially when the trunk is flexed, thereby

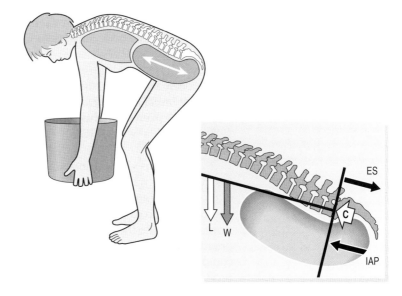

Figure 10.8   The spine, thoracic and abdominal cavities during lifting. The force diagram indicates how the increases in intra-abdominal pressure (IAP) may relieve the intervertebral compression (C) which is equal and opposite to the tensile force in erector spinae (ES) required to raise the load (L) and the upper part of the body (W). (Adapted from Troup JDG 1979 Biomechanics of the vertebral column. *Physiotherapy* 65: 239.)

supplementing the back muscles and providing a trunk extensor moment. This mechanism was considered to have a larger moment arm than the trunk extensor muscles, and hence some of the compressive stress on the lumbar intervertebral discs would be relieved (Bartelink, 1957; Thomson, 1988). It has been calculated that the load on the extensor muscles can be reduced by 12–20% through this mechanism (Thomson, 1988). The intrathoracic pressure acts to stabilize the rib cage during activities of the arms.

Pressure increases are greater when heavier loads are lifted and also when the speed of action is faster (Davis and Troup, 1964). The magnitude of IAP has a linear relationship to the magnitude of the static flexion moments (Morris et al, 1961; Mairiaux et al, 1984). However, studies have failed to find a linear relationship between raised IAP and dynamic loading (Troup et al, 1983; Marras et al, 1985). The IAP is unrelated to training of the abdominal muscles, and increased strength in them has not been shown to result in an increase in their activity when lifting (Hemborg et al, 1983). It should be considered that strengthening regimes for abdominal muscles using solely isometric contractions may be inadequate for training what is essentially a dynamic process of eccentric and concentric contraction.

Another theory for the mechanism through which the IAP provides protection is that it compresses the convex surfaces of the lumbar lordosis, causing the lumbar spine to stiffen (Aspden, 1989).

Greater pressure increases have been demonstrated in patients with back pain than in normal subjects when lifting weights of 5–10 kg, and this was thought to emphasize the supportive role of IAP (Fairbank and O'Brien, 1979).

Generally, pressure increases are active for a very short time only. If there is a need to breathe again when lifting, the contraction of the diaphragm limits the pressure increase to the abdominal cavity and its supporting mechanism to the lumbar spine. However, it is during the initial phases of the lift that the pressures are at their highest, when spinal stress is likely to be at a maximum. As the weight is lifted closer to the body, the lever exerted by it becomes shorter, and it is then within the capacity of the back muscles to lift it.

The supportive role of the thoracolumbar fascia

It has been suggested that increased IAP and tension in the thoracolumbar fascia produce an extension moment of the trunk which could afford some protection during lifting (Grillner et al, 1978; Fairbank et al, 1980; Gracovetsky et al, 1985); recent research has failed to support this theory.

It was proposed that transversus abdominis could produce an extensor moment of the trunk by virtue of the oblique orientation of the fibres of the fascia. Transversus abdominis attaches into the entire lateral raphe and contraction of the muscle increases tension in the middle and posterior layers of the thoracolumbar fascia; it was proposed that the oblique orientation of the fibres of the posterior layer of the thoracolumbar fascia could allow the conversion of lateral tension to longitudinal tension, producing an extensor moment (Gracovetsky et al, 1977, 1985). At any point along the lateral raphe, a fibre of the superficial lamina passes cau-domedially and a fibre of the deep lamina passes caudolaterally towards the spine. These fibres form a series of triangles extending over two lev-els and the force exerted at the basal angle would have a horizontal and vertical vector. It was proposed that when transversus abdominis con-tracts it produces bilateral tension resulting in a vertical and horizontal force at the basal angle of each triangle. The sum of the horizontal vec-tors is zero, while the vertical vectors produce opposite movement approximating the spinous processes and creating trunk extension (Gracovetsky et al, 1977, 1985). Gracovetsky and colleagues calculated that the gain from lateral tension to longitudinal tension was 5:1, con-tributing significantly to trunk extension.

Other mathematical studies have calculated that the contribution from this mechanism is much smaller (McGill and Norman, 1988; Tesh et al, 1987) and when tension was produced in the thoracolumbar fascia of a cadaver no approximation of the spinous processes was produced. At present it seems unlikely that there is a significant contribution from the IAP and thoracolumbar fascia to control the trunk in flexion loading (Richardson et al, 1999).

Transversus abdominis and the thoracolumbar fascia may assist in stabilizing the spine by stiffening intersegmental movement rather than producing movement. Contraction of transversus abdominis increases lateral tension in the thoracolumbar fascia and acts on the transverse and spinous processes of the lumbar vertebrae, limiting translation and rota-tion of the vertebrae (Richardson et al, 1999). It is proposed that when the thoracolumbar fascia is slack, a small amount of vertebral motion is pos-sible in all directions, but when tension increases the available vertebral movement reduces.

Passive support of ligaments

When the lumbar spine is flexed, the posterior ligaments (in particular the supraspinous and interspinous), capsules of the apophyseal joints and thoracolumbar fascia are tense, and are therefore strong enough to sustain large forces. In particular, the density of the thoracolumbar fas-cia suggests that it can act as a major load-bearing structure. In the flexed position, the lumbar spine can be passively used to lift large weights. The power is provided by the hip extensors, which extend the hips and tilt the pelvis backwards; providing the lumbar spine remains flexed, this power is transmitted to the thorax, rotating it posteriorly and executing the early stages of the lift.

Using the ligaments instead of active muscular contraction at this point in the lift reduces the compressive forces on the lumbar interverte-bral discs: the ligaments lie posterior to the back muscles and thus have the mechanical advantage of a longer lever.

As the weight is brought progressively closer to the body, there is a transition from passive support by ligaments to active contraction of the back muscles, which are now able to balance the weight and continue with the lift. As soon as spinal extension begins, the ligaments are relaxed and their supportive role therefore ends.

METHODS OF LIFTING

Although one lifting method alone does not suit every individual or every task, some general rules are widely agreed upon, such as keeping the load close to the body and squat lifting if possible. Rotating or laterally flexing the spine while lifting should be avoided because, when combined with loading, these movements can damage the apophyseal joints and intervertebral discs.

The two methods commonly compared are stoop lifting (with the spine flexed) and squat lifting (with the knees flexed). Although the squat lift is often recommended as good practice, it is often not used in industry because industrial weights are not designed to be lifted from the squatting position (Bridger, 2003). Comparisons of the squat and stoop lift in a crate handling task found that there was no difference in spinal shrinkage between the two techniques (Rabinowitz et al, 1998).

The stoop lift has lower energy expenditure than the squat lift because of the greater body weight displaced vertically (Grieve, 1975; Troup, 1977) and this may explain why it is often used by people who are untrained in lifting techniques.

The squat lift makes it possible for the subject to lift the weight between the legs. This close proximity of the weight to the fulcrum of the lumbosacral disc means that the lever exerted by the weight is short; this is by far the most important factor in reducing both the force required to lift it and the load on the spine. If the hands have to be near to floor level in order to grasp the weight, some degree of lumbar flexion is necessary. One disadvantage of this type of lift is that the compressive forces across the knee joints are high. Squat lifts also require greater coordination and control and place higher demands on the cardiovascular system than other lifting techniques. In most individuals, the spine is flexed to 50% of its maximum in the squatting position (Adams and Dolan, 1995).

Much debate has centred on whether there is an optimum position of the lumbar spine – extension, neutral or flexion – to be used during lifting (Delitto et al, 1987; Hart et al, 1987). Gracovetsky et al (1981) demonstrated that individuals will choose their own unique posture that shares the load between the thoracolumbar fascia, the posterior ligaments and the posterior annulus. This unique posture always reduces the lordosis. Experimental work done on cadaveric intervertebral discs suggests that there might be some benefit in flexing the lumbar spine in heavy lifts as the stress distribution is favourable for sustaining higher compressive loads (Hutton and Adams, 1982). By flexing the lower lumbar spine and extending the thoracic spine, the weight to be lifted can still be kept close to the body.

Clearly there is no single position that suits every individual for every lift, and a flexible approach is necessary when training uninjured workers in lifting techniques, taking into account anthropometric measurements. A 'straight-back' (neutral) position (McGill and Norman, 1986) produces the greatest support; while reducing the compressive forces of an extended spine, it also reduces the ligamentous stress of a flexed spine. Lifting in flexion is difficult to avoid when lifting from the floor, because it is necessary to flex somewhat during this task, in which case the lift should be performed quickly. Where a slower lift is necessary, an extended lumbar spine may be preferable in order to reduce creeping of ligamentous tissue, but pretraining for strength and endurance of the extensor muscles is advisable to make it safe and effective (Scott Sullivan, 1989).

REPETITIVE LOADING OF THE SPINE

Activities such as repetitive heavy lifting and digging subject the spine to fatigue compressive loading. Tyrrell et al (1985) found that, following dynamic lifting, there was a measurable loss of height in the spine, in proportion to the applied load and rate, due to expulsion of fluid from the intervertebral discs. Repetitive lifting led to greater shrinkage than did equivalent static loading, and it was concluded that repeatedly lifting a 50 kg load would induce shrinkage equal to the entire diurnal loss of stature (see p. 80) within 20 minutes (Corlett et al, 1987). Loss of disc height has a clear relevance to structural geometrical changes and changed properties of the spine, such as disc bulging, end plate bulging, the stiffness of the discs, and the load on the apophyseal joints. There could also be a relation to nutritional factors of the disc.

On unloading the spine, either by cessation of lifting or by adopting certain postures, stature is regained relatively quickly (Tyrell et al, 1985). This implies that even if short periods of unloading the spine are allowed in a heavy job, a substantial recovery can take place during these rest periods, and the total shrinkage or disc compression will be diminished.

The recommended maximum weight lifted by an individual in the workplace is dependent on three factors: the biomechanical criterion (e.g. lumbar motion segment compression failure), the psychosocial criterion (e.g. subjective estimates of the maximum weight of lift), and the physiological criterion (e.g. whole-body maximum energy expenditure capability). Ayoub (1992) found that if workers were required to lift loads at a frequency of more than eight lifts per minute, then the metabolic rate at which they expended energy would probably dictate the recommended weight that could be lifted over an 8-hour period. When an individual is required to lift less than three times per minute, biomechanical considerations such as motion segment fatigue will determine the maximum recommended weight to be lifted.

The effect of repetitive heavy loading of the spine has been simulated by testing cadaveric lumbar motion segments to destruction. The outcome depended on the posture used. If the motion segment was compressed and flexed, the lamellae of the annulus sometimes became distorted leading to radial fissures in the discs, which are the precursors to a gradual disc prolapse (Adams and Hutton, 1983). However, not all discs showed these distortions, which indicates that there are individual variations. If the motion segment was compressed and not flexed, the site of the failure was in the vertebral body and end plate (Hardy et al, 1958).

The response of a spine to the stresses of repetitive heavy lifting depends on its pre-existing condition. A spine such as that possessed by an athlete, which has been subjected to repeated strenuous activity, but not to the point of injury, will have responded by developing hypertrophied bone, a thicker vertebral body cortex and a more dense trabecular system, giving the vertebral body and end plate a higher resistance to failure.

LIFTING ABILITY IN MALES/FEMALES

Women are approximately 30% weaker than men of equivalent height, weight and training (Hayne, 1981), and this influences their load tolerance. Guidelines have been laid down recommending maximum weights and workloads which are acceptable to industrial workers (Health and Safety Executive, 1992, 1998).

It has been hypothesized that women may be at a mechanical disadvantage when lifting in a stooped posture: the hip joints in women are located more anteriorly than in men, away from line of gravity. This produces a force couple acting on the lumbosacral joint which means that, in effect, any object handled by a woman would seem approximately 15% heavier than if it were handled by a man of identical stature and strength (Tichauer, 1976).

In the presence of ligamentous laxity, the risk of sacroiliac joint strain when lifting in a stooped posture is increased; this would apply to some women during menstruation or pregnancy.

PUSHING AND PULLING

The capacity of an individual for pushing and pulling depends on body weight, the posture used, the stability of the feet and the ability to transfer energy from the body to the load.

During these activities, there is an increase in intrathoracic and intra-abdominal pressures – more so in pushing than pulling (Davis and Troup, 1964). During pushing, the recti are tense and the load on the lumbosacral disc is less than when pulling. The biomechanical explanation for this is depicted in Figure 10.9. The compressive load on the L5/S1 disc is two to three times larger in pulling than pushing, body weight contributing more to the compressive load in pulling than pushing. Laboratory studies have found pushing a load to be superior to pulling it (Lee et al, 1991).

The pulling force (P_i) is directed anteriorly and increases the bending moment and erector spinae force considerably, because of the short lever arm this muscle has with respect to the axis of rotation. Thus, the load on the disc is also increased. In pushing, however (see Fig. 10.9A), the horizontal pushing force (P_s) is now directed posteriorly. Its bending moment is counterbalanced by the force of the recti. Because these muscles have a larger lever arm compared with erector spinae, their force is relatively less and induces a smaller increase in disc load.

EFFECTS OF LUMBOSACRAL CORSETS

Corsets are sometimes prescribed for patients with back pain, and, in some instances, are of great value in relieving pain when used as

Figure 10.9   Reaction at lumbosacral disc to truncal muscle activity parallel to the spinal axis. A, *Pushing:* effect of weight of upper part of body (W) is countered by activity of erector spinae (ES), the pushing force (P$_s$) by rectus abdominis (RA). The sum of ES and RA is equal and opposite to the force compressing the L5/S1 disc (C). B, *Pulling:* the pulling force P$_i$ is applied and the effect of W is countered by ES which is equal and opposite to C. (Adapted from Troup JDG 1979 Biomechanics of the vertebral column. *Physiotherapy* 65: 239.)

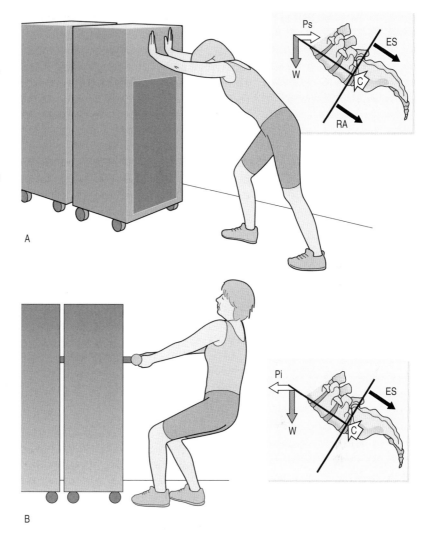

a temporary measure. However, in other instances, patients find corsets uncomfortable to wear, hot, restrictive and ineffective in relieving symptoms.

A large number of lumbosacral supports are available, varying from the light elasticated type to the longer steel-braced type. Both the length of the corset and its construction will influence the effect that it has when worn. Some of the lighter corsets can be surprisingly effective in relieving pain. The reason for this is not really known, and it may be simply that they keep the area warm; alternatively they may act as a placebo or provide psychological support. Industrial workers who wear weightlifter belts and abdominal supports all report an increased sense of security (McGill et al, 1990; Reddell et al, 1992; Magnusson et al, 1996).

MOBILITY

The simple lumbosacral corset does not restrict movement except at the extremes of range (Van Leuven and Troup, 1969). Restricted movement in the lower thoracic and upper lumbar spine can lead to increased movement at the lumbosacral level. Therefore, if the aim is to immobilize an area, it is important to know the precise level of the spinal lesion before prescribing a corset for a patient. Lumbosacral rotation is very slightly restricted when wearing a corset (Lumsden and Morris, 1968).

INTRADISCAL PRESSURE

A tightly fitting corset compresses the abdomen, raising intra-abdominal pressure, and decreases the load on the vertebral column so that intradiscal pressure may be reduced by approximately 30% (Nachemson, 1964).

MUSCLE ACTIVITY

Subjects were found to have decreased activity in the abdominal muscles when wearing an experimentally inflated corset during lifting (Morris and Lucas, 1964). Without a support, these muscles assist during loading in increasing the intra-abdominal pressure. When the longer, non-inflated corsets were worn, they produced increases in intra-abdominal pressure during sitting; the elasticated varieties produced significant increases in intra-abdominal pressure in walking (Grew and Deane, 1982).

McGill et al (1990) measured electromyographic activity and IAP in subjects who were lifting weights while wearing a weightlifter belt. The IAP increased by approximately 20 mmHg, but there was no corresponding decrease in activity of erector spinae. They recorded a small reduction in electromyographic activity in the abdominal muscles during lifting when a belt was worn. When the subjects held their breath while lifting, there was a reduction of electromyographic activity in the back extensors, regardless of whether or not a belt was worn.

Electromyographic activity in erector spinae is not affected during standing and slow walking by wearing a corset, presumably because this muscle inserts much higher in the spine and, therefore, continues to work to keep the spine upright. During fast walking, it was found that wearing a corset increased muscle activity (Waters and Morris, 1970).

There is no evidence that the wearing of corsets for periods varying from 6 months (Walsh and Schwartz, 1990) to 5 years in itself leads to muscle weakness (Nachemson and Lindh, 1969), although there may be a degree of physical dependence (Grew and Deane, 1982).

EFFECTS OF COLLARS

MOBILITY

No splinting device or collar completely immobilizes the neck from the occipito-atlantal junction to C7. There are a variety of collars that provide different degrees of support. These range from very little support provided by the soft cervical collar made from felt or foam rubber, which was found to limit only 5–10% of flexion, extension and lateral flexion and had no effect at all on rotation (Hartman et al, 1975), to more effective support provided by more rigid bracing.

This does not mean that lighter collars are ineffective; in addition to any other effects that they have, they also serve to remind the patient to avoid certain neck movements when wearing one. As with all orthoses, they should only be supplied to the patient if accompanied by instructions as to their purpose.

Orthoses which best immobilize the lower cervical spine allow the upper cervical vertebrae to move in a non-uniform manner (Fisher et al, 1977). It was noted that when subjects attempted flexion of the neck against the orthosis, the upper cervical spine extended and the lower cervical spine flexed. On attempting extension against the orthosis, the upper cervical spine flexed and the lower cervical spine extended. This is particularly important when considering the supply of a collar for a patient with rheumatoid arthritis if there is excessive laxity of the transverse ligament or erosion of the odontoid peg.

Rotation of the upper cervical spine is the movement that is most difficult to restrict because conventional collars end here. The only orthosis that limits rotation to any degree has been found to be the halo orthosis.

MECHANORECEPTORS

Relative immobility of the upper three cervical vertebrae, and a reduction in the normal compressive force of the weight of the head, disturbs the normal pattern of afferent impulses from type I and II mechanoreceptors in ligaments, the apophyseal joints and the uncovertebral joints. These receptors subserve postural control, and their importance in governing the degree of dexterity when performing intricate manual operations has been demonstrated (Wyke, 1965).

ADHESION FORMATION

Following trauma to the neck, e.g. a whiplash injury, excessive immobilization in a collar leads to adhesion formation due to organization of extravasated blood and tissue fluid, shortening of contracted muscles, thickening of periarticular tissues and muscle atrophy (Mealy et al, 1986).

References

Adams MA, Dolan P (1995) Recent advances in lumbar spinal mechanics and their clinical significance. *Clinical Biomechanics* 10: 3–19.

Adams MA, Hutton WC (1980) The effect of posture on the role of the apophyseal joints in resisting intervertebral compressive forces. *Journal of Bone and Joint Surgery (Br.)* 62: 358.

Adams MA, Hutton WC (1983) The effect of fatigue on the lumbar intervertebral disc. *Journal of Bone and Joint Surgery (Br.)* 65: 199.

Alexander FM (1932) *The Use of Self.* Methuen, London.

Andersson BJG, Ortengren R, Nachemson A, et al (1975) The sitting posture: an electromyographic and discometric study. *Orthopedic Clinics of North America* 6: 1, 105.

Andersson BGJ, Murphy RW, Ortengren R, et al (1979) The influence of backrest inclination and lumbar support on lumbar lordosis. *Spine* 4: 52.

Aspden RM (1989) The spine as an arch. A new mathematical model. *Spine* 14: 266–274.

Ayoub MM (1992) Problems and solutions in manual materials handling: The state of the art. *Ergonomics* 35: 713–728.

Bartelink JV (1957) The role of abdominal pressure in relieving the pressure on the lumbar intervertebral discs. *Journal of Bone and Joint Surgery (Br.)* 39: 718.

Bjorksten M, Jonsson B (1977) Endurance limit of force of long-term intermittent static contractions. *Scandinavian Journal of Environmental Health* 3: 23.

Blow RJ, Jackson JM (1971) An analysis of back injuries in registered dock workers. *Proceedings of the Royal Society of Medicine* 64: 735.

Bridger RS (2003) *Introduction to Ergonomics*, 2nd edn. Taylor and Francis, London.

Bridger RS, Orkin D, Henneberg M (1992) A quantitative investigation of lumbar and pelvic postures in standing and sitting: interrelationships with body position and hip muscle length. *International Journal of Industrial Ergonomics* 9: 235–244.

Brunswic M (1984) Ergonomics of seat design. *Physiotherapy* 70: 40.

Burdorf A, Naaktgeboren B, deGroot HCWM (1993) Occupational risk factors for low back pain among sedentary workers. *Journal of Occupational Medicine* 35: 1213–1220.

Carlsöö S (1964) Influence of frontal and dorsal loads on muscle activity and on weight distribution in the feet. *Acta Orthopaedica Scandinavica* 34: 299.

Corlett EN, Eklund JAE, Reilly T, et al (1987) Assessment of workload from measurements of stature. *Applied Ergonomics* 18: 65.

Davis PR, Troup JDG (1964) Pressure in the trunk cavities when pulping, pushing and lifting. *Ergonomics* 7: 465.

Delitto RS, Rose SJ, Apts DW (1987) Electromyographic analysis of two techniques for squat lifting. *Physical Therapy* 67. 1329.

DeTroyer A, Estenne M, Ninane V, et al (1990) Transversus abdominis muscle function in humans. *Journal of Applied Physiology* 68, 1010–1016.

Dolan P, Adams MA, Hutton WC (1988) Commonly adopted postures and their affect on the lumbar spine. *Spine* 13: 197.

Dunlop RB, Adams MA, Hutton WC (1984) Disc space narrowing and the lumbar facet joints. *Journal of Bone and Joint Surgery (Br.)* 66: 706.

Eklund JAE, Corlett EN (1987) Evaluation of spinal loads and chair design in seated work tasks. *Clinical Biomechanics* 2: 27.

Fairbank JCT, O'Brien JP (1979) Intra-abdominal pressure and low back pain. Paper read at Annual Meeting of International Society for the Study of the Lumbar Spine, Gothenburg, June 1979.

Fairbank JCT, O'Brien JP, Davis PR (1980) Intra-abdominal pressure rise during weight lifting as an objective measure of low-back pain. *Spine* 5: 179–184.

Fisher SV, Bowar JF, Awad EA, et al (1977) Cervical orthosis – effect on cervical spine motion: roentgenographic and goniometric method of study. *Archives of Physical Medicine and Rehabilitation* 58: 109.

Floyd WF, Silver PHS (1951) Function of the erectores spinae in flexion of the trunk. *Lancet* I: 133.

Floyd WF, Silver PHS (1955) The function of the erectores spinae muscles in certain movements and postures in man. *Journal of Physiology* 129: 184.

Frievalds A, Chaffin DB, Garg A, et al (1984) A dynamic biomechanical evaluation of lifting maximum acceptable loads. *Journal of Biomechanics* 17: 251.

Gracovetsky S, Farfan H, Lamy C (1977) A mathematical model of the lumbar spine using an optimised system to control muscles and ligaments. *Orthopedic Clinics of North America* 8: 135–153.

Gracovetsky S, Farfan HF, Lamy C (1981) The mechanism of the lumbar spine. *Spine* 6: 249.

Gracovetsky S, Farfan H, Helleur C (1985) The abdominal mechanism. *Spine* 10: 317–324.

Grew ND, Deane G (1982) The physical effects of lumbar spine supports. *Prosthetics and Orthotics International* 6: 79.

Grieco A (1986) Sitting posture: an old problem and a new one. *Ergonomics* 29: 345.

Grieve DW (1975) Dynamic characteristics of man during crouch- and stoop-lifting. In: Nelson RC (ed.) *Biomechanics IV*. University Park Press, Baltimore, pp. 19–29.

Grieve D, Pheasant S (1982) Biomechanics. In: Singleton WL (ed.) *The Body at Work*. Cambridge University Press, Cambridge.

Grillner S, Nilsson J, Thorstensson A (1978) Intraabdominal pressure changes during natural movements in man. *Acta Physiologica Scandinavica* 103: 275–283.

Hardy WG, Lissner HR, Webster JE, et al (1958) Repeated loading tests of the lumbar spine: a preliminary report. *Surgical Forum* IX: 690.

Hart DL, Stobbe TJ, Jaraiedi M (1987) Effects of lumbar posture on lifting. *Spine* 12: 138.

Hartman JT, Palumbo F, Jay Hill B (1975) Cineradiography of the braced normal cervical spine. *Clinical Orthopaedics and Related Research* 109: 97.

Hartvigsen J, Lebeuf-Y de C, Lings S, et al (2000) Is sitting-while-at-work bad for your low back? A systematic, critical literature review. *Scandinavian Journal of Public Health* 28: 230–239.

Hayne C (1981) Manual transport of loads by women. *Physiotherapy* 67: 226.

Health and Safety Commission (1991) *Manual Handling of Loads, Proposals for Regulation and Guidance*. Health and Safety Executive, 1 Chepstow Place, Westbourne Grove, London W2 4TF.

Health and Safety Executive (1992) *The Manual Handling Operations Regulations*. HMSO, London.

Health and Safety Executive (1998) *Manual Handling: Guidance on Regulations*. HMSO, London.

Hellems HK, Keates TE (1971) Measurement of the normal lumbosacral angle. *American Journal of Roentgenology* 113: 642.

Hemborg B, Moritz U, Hamberg J, et al (1983) Intra-abdominal pressure and trunk muscle activity during lifting – effect of abdominal muscle training in healthy subjects. *Scandinavian Journal of Rehabilitation Medicine* 15: 183.

Hirsch C (1955) The reaction of intervertebral discs to compression forces. *Journal of Bone and Joint Surgery (Am.)* 37: 586.

Hoogendoorn W, Bongers PM, de Vet HCW, et al (2000) Flexion and rotation of the trunk and lifting at work are risk factors for low back pain. *Spine* 25: 3087–3092.

Hutton WC, Adams MA (1982) Can the lumbar spine be crushed in heavy lifting? *Spine* 7: 586.

Hutton WC, Stott JRR, Cyron BM (1977) Is spondylolysis a fatigue fracture? *Spine* 2: 202.

Irvin RE (1997) Suboptimal posture: origin of the majority of idiopathic pain of the musculoskeletal system. In: Vleeming A, Mooney V, Dorman T, Snijders C, Stoeckart R (eds) *Movement, Stability and Low Back Pain*. Churchill Livingstone, Edinburgh, Ch. 9, pp. 133–155.

Kappler RE (1982) Postural balance and motion patterns. *Journal of the American Orthopedic Association* 81: 598–606.

Karhu O, Kansi P, Kuorinka I (1977) Correcting working postures in industry: A practical method for analysis. *Applied Ergonomics* 8: 199–201.

Keagy RD, Brumlik J, Bergan JL (1966) Direct electromyography of the psoas major muscle in man. *Journal of Bone and Joint Surgery (Am.)* 48: 1591.

Kendall FP, McCreary E, Provance P (1993) *Muscle Testing and Function*, 4th edn. Williams and Wilkins, Baltimore, p. 71.

Lander C, Korbon GA, DeGood DE, Rowlinson JC (1987) The Balans chair and its semi-kneeling position: an ergonomic comparison with conventional sitting position. *Spine* 12: 269–272.

Lee KS, Chaffin DB, Herrin GD, Walker AM (1991) Effect of handle height and lower-back loading in cart pushing and pulling. *Applied Ergonomics* 22: 117–123.

Link CS, Nicholson GG, Shaddeau SA, Birch RB, Gossman MR (1990) Lumbar curvature in standing and sitting in two types of chairs: relationship of hamstring and hip flexor muscle length. *Physical Therapy* 70: 611–618.

Lord MJ, Small JM, Dinsay JM, Watkins RG (1997) Lumbar lordosis: effects of standing and sitting. *Spine* 22: 2571–2574.

Lumsden RM, Morris JM (1968) An in-vivo study of axial rotation and immobilisation at the lumbo-sacral joint. *Journal of Bone and Joint Surgery (Am.)* 50: 1591.

Lundervold AJS (1951) *Electromyographic Investigations of Position and Manner of Working in Typewriting*. W. Brøggers Boktrykkeri A/S, Oslo.

Magnusson M, Pope MH, Hansson T (1996) Does a back support have a positive biomechanical effect? *Applied Ergonomics* 27: 201–205.

Magora A (1972) Investigation of the relation between low back pain and occupation, 3. Physical requirements: sitting, standing and weight lifting. *Industrial Medicine and Surgery* 41: 5–9.

Magora A (1974) Investigation of the relation between low back pain and occupation, 6. Medical history and symptoms. *Scandinavian Journal of Rehabilitation Medicine* 6: 81.

Mairiaux P, Davis PR, Subbs DA, Baty D (1984) Relation between intra-abdominal pressure and lumbar movements when lifting weights in the erect posture. *Ergonomics* 27: 883–894.

Mandal AC (1984) The correct height of school furniture. *Physiotherapy* 40: 48.

Marras W, Joynt RL, King AI (1985) The force velocity relation and intra-abdominal pressure during lifting activities. *Ergonomics* 28: 603–613.

Marras WS, Rangarajulu SL, Lavender SA (1987) Trunk loading and expectation. *Ergonomics* 30: 551–562.

McGill SM, Norman RW (1986) Partitioning of the L4-5 dynamic moment into disc, ligamentous and muscular components during lifting. *Spine* 11: 666.

McGill SM, Norman RW (1988) Potential of the lumbodorsal fascial forces to generate back extension moments in squat lifts. *Journal of Biomedical Engineering* 10: 312–318.

McGill S, Norman RW, Sharratt MT (1990) The effect of an abdominal belt on trunk muscle activity and intra-abdominal pressure during squat lifts. *Ergonomics* 33: 146–160.

Mealy K, Brennan H, Fenelin GCC (1986) Early mobilization of acute whiplash injuries. *British Medical Journal* 292: 656.

Morris JM, Lucas DB (1964) Biomechanics of spinal bracing. *Arizona Medicine* 21: 170.

Morris JM, Lucas DM, Bresler B (1961) Role of the trunk in stability of the spine. *Journal of Bone and Joint Surgery (Am.)* 43: 327–351.

Nachemson A (1964) *In vivo* measurement of intra-discal pressure. *Journal of Bone and Joint Surgery (Am.)* 46: 1077.

Nachemson A, Lindh M (1969) Measurement of abdominal and back muscle strength with and without low back pain. *Scandinavian Journal of Rehabilitation Medicine* 1: 60.

Rabinowitz D, Bridger RS, Lambert MI (1998) Lifting technique and abdominal belt usage. *Safety Science* 28: 155–164.

Reddell CR, Congleton JJ, Hichingson RD, Montgomery JF (1992) An evaluation of a weight-lifting belt and back injury prevention training class for airline baggage handlers. *Applied Ergonomics* 23: 319–329.

Richardson C, Jull G, Hodges P, Hides J (1999) *Therapeutic Exercise for Spinal Segmental Stabilization in Low Back Pain*. Churchill Livingstone, Edinburgh.

Rohlmann A, Claes LE, Bergmann G, Graichen F, Neef P, Wilke H-J (2001) Comparison of intradiscal pressures and spinal fixator loads for different body positions and exercises. *Ergonomics* 44: 781–794.

Schoberth H (1962) *Sitzhaltung, Sitzschaden, Sitzmöbel*. Springer Verlag, Berlin.

Schuldt K, Ekholm J. Harms-Ringdahl K, et al (1986) Effects of changes in sitting posture on static neck and shoulder muscle activity. *Ergonomics* 29: 1525.

Scott Sullivan M (1989) Back support mechanisms during manual lifting. *Physical Therapy* 69: 1, 52.

Soames R, Atha J (1981) The role of the antigravity musculature during quiet standing in man. *European Journal of Applied Physiology and Occupational Physiology* 47: 159–167.

Tesh KM, ShawDunn J, Evans JH (1987) The abdominal muscles and vertebral stability. *Spine* 12: 501–508.

Thomson KD (1988) On the bending moment capability of the pressurized abdominal cavity during human lifting activity. *Ergonomics* 31: 817–828.

Tichauer ER (1976) Biomechanics sustains occupational safety and health. *Industrial Engineering* 8: 46.

Troup JDG (1977) Dynamic factors in the analysis of stoop and crouch lifting methods: a methodological approach to the development of safe materials handling standards. *Orthopedic Clinics of North America* 8: 201.

Troup JD, Leskiner TP, Stalhammar HR, Kuorinka IA (1983) A Comparison of intraabdominal pressure increases, hip torque, and lumbar vertebral compression in different lifting techniques. *Human Factors* 25 (5): 517–525.

Tyrell AR, Reilly T, Troup JDG (1985) Circadian variation in stature and the effects of spinal loading. *Spine* 10: 161.

Van Leuven RM, Troup J (1969) The instant lumbar corset. *Physiotherapy* 55: 499.

Walsh NE, Schwartz MS (1990) The influence of prophylactic orthosis on abdominal strength and low back injury in the workplace. *American Journal of Physical Medicine and Rehabilitation* 69: 245–250.

Waters RL, Morris JM (1970) Effect of spinal supports on the electrical activity of the muscles of the trunk. *Journal of Bone and Joint Surgery (Am.)* 52: 51.

Wyke M (1965) Comparative analysis of proprioception in left and right arms. *Quarterly Journal of Experimental Psychology* 17: 149.

Index